Renal Cell Carcinoma:
Research and Treatments

Renal Cell Carcinoma: Research and Treatments

Edited by **Barbara Mayer**

FOSTER
ACADEMICS

New Jersey

Published by Foster Academics,
61 Van Reypen Street,
Jersey City, NJ 07306, USA
www.fosteracademics.com

Renal Cell Carcinoma: Research and Treatments
Edited by Barbara Mayer

International Standard Book Number: 978-1-63242-356-6 (Hardback)

Printed in the United States of America.

Contents

Preface

This book has been a concerted effort by a group of academicians, researchers and scientists, who have contributed their research works for the realization of the book. This book has materialized in the wake of emerging advancements and innovations in this field. Therefore, the need of the hour was to compile all the required researches and disseminate the knowledge to a broad spectrum of people comprising of students, researchers and specialists of the field.

Renal cell cancer has experienced tremendous resurgence. This book provides a synopsis of latest research and innovative ideas for the future in this rapidly changing field, which encompasses medicine, surgery, radiation oncology, basic science, pathology, radiology, and supportive care. This book targets clinicians, scientists and professionals who have interest in renal cell cancer. The book comprises of surgery mechanisms, radiation therapy, personal data and existing and emerging therapies of the disease. The objective was to present a detailed account that would act as a credible source for scientists and clinicians; and interpret the domain for trainees in surgery, medicine, radiation oncology and pathology.

At the end of the preface, I would like to thank the authors for their brilliant chapters and the publisher for guiding us all-through the making of the book till its final stage. Also, I would like to thank my family for providing the support and encouragement throughout my academic career and research projects.

Editor

Translational

Molecular Pathogenesis of Renal Cell Carcinoma: A Review

Israel Gomy and Wilson Araújo Silva Jr.
University of São Paulo, Medical School of Ribeirão Preto,
Genetics Department, Ribeirão Preto,
Brazil

1. Introduction

Renal cell carcinomas (RCC) represent almost 90% of all kidney cancers and in about 2% of cases there is a family history of RCC (McLaughlin et al, 1984). Despite their rare incidences, Mendelian hereditary syndromes with RCC have provided important insights into the molecular pathogenesis of this tumor. The cloning of susceptibility genes that are involved in familial predisposition has offered entry points into the signaling pathways that are deregulated in sporadic RCC. Sporadic RCC are extremely heterogeneous and are classified into many histolological subtypes. The most frequent form is clear cell or conventional RCC, accounting for approximately 75% of all cases, whereas the most common non-clear cell tumor is papillary RCC (12% of cases), which is subdivided into types 1 and 2. Other subtypes include chromophobe and oncocytomas, each of them occurring in 4% of patients, collecting-duct (<1%) and rare forms or yet to be classified (< 2%). The correlation between histopathological features and genetic alterations in RCC has been introduced in 1997 with the Heidelberg classification (Kovacs et al, 1997). More recently, expression profiles through microarrays have been done for many of the kidney tumor subtypes and provide the evidence that their expression patterns reflect their histological classifications and demonstrate that various renal tumor subtypes are genetically distinct entities (Higgins et al, 2003).

Generally, there is a good correlation between the genetic causes of familial RCC and their histopathological features as exemplified by the commonest form of hereditary RCC, von Hippel-Lindau (VHL) disease, which invariably presents a clear cell type. Moreover, germline mutations in the *MET* proto-oncogene cause type 1 papillary RCC, whereas type 2 is correlated with germline mutations in the fumarate hidratase gene, which cause hereditary leiomyomatosis. Birt-Hogg-Dubè syndrome is also characterized by susceptibility to RCC but with a mixed chromophobe-oncocytoma histopathology, and is associated with germline mutations in the *BHD* tumor suppressor gene.

All the genes identified so far, which are involved in the molecular pathogenesis of hereditary and sporadic RCC comprise a diverse set of complex biochemical and cell metabolism pathways, such as iron, energy, nutrient and oxygen-sensing (Linehan et al., 2010a). A plenty of biochemical and molecular studies of the numerous signalling pathways disrupted in RCC have already provided reasonable translational approaches and clinical applications of target therapy RCC with promising results (Iliopoulos, 2006). The histopathological and molecular features of RCC are summarized in table 1.

Tumor type	Locus	Gene	Pathway	Syndrome
Clear cell	3p25	VHL	VEGF	von Hippel-Lindau
	3p14	FHIT	TGF-β	Familial clear cell
	3p21	RASSF1A		RCC
	17p11	BHD	AMPK-mTOR	
				Birt-Hogg-Dube
Papillary type 1 type 2	7q31	MET	MET-HGF	Hereditary papillary RCC
	1q42	FH	VEGF	
			TGF-β	Hereditary leiomatosis
	7q31.1	FRA7G		
	9q34	TSC1	mTOR	
	16p13	TSC2	mTOR	
	1q25	HRPT2		Tuberous sclerosis complex
				Tuberous sclerosis complex
				Hyperparathyroidism -jaw tumor
Chromophobe	17p11	BHD	AMPK-mTOR	Birt-Hogg-Dube
Oncocytoma	17p11	BHD	AMPK-mTOR	Birt-Hogg-Dube
	9q34	TSC1	mTOR	Tuberous complex
	16p13	TSC2	mTOR	Tuberous complex
			mTOR	
Collecting duct carcinoma	-1q32,-6p,-8p, -9p,-13q,- 19q32,-21q	unknown	unknown	none
Renal carcinoma associated with Xp11.2 translocation	1p34	PSF-TFE3		
	1q21	PRCC-TFE3		
	17q23	CTLC-TFE3	none	none
	17q25	ASPL-TFE3		
	3q23	?		
	Xq12	NonO-TFE3		
Mucinous tubular and spindle cell carcinoma	-8p,-9p,- 11q,+12q,+16 q+17,+20q	unknown	unknown	none

Table 1. Histopathological and genetic characteristics of RCC

2. The oxygen-sensing pathway: HIF-VHL interaction and clear-cell RCC pathogenesis

Hypoxia-inducible factors (HIF) are oxygen-sensitive basic helix–loop–helix transcription factors, which regulate biological processes that facilitate both oxygen delivery and cellular adaptation to oxygen deprivation. HIF is a heterodimer consisting of unstable a-subunits and stable constitutively expressed b-subunits. HIF-α, together with HIF-β bind to hypoxia-response elements in gene promoters to regulate the expression of genes that are involved in energy metabolism, angiogenesis, erythropoiesis, iron metabolism, cell proliferation, apoptosis and other biological processes. HIF1-α and HIF2-α mediate transcription of a number of downstream genes thought to be important in cancer, including transforming growth factor alpha (*TGF-α*), platelet-derived growth factor (*PDGF*), and vascular endothelial growth factor (*VEGF*) (Linehan et al., 2010a).

In clear-cell renal-cell carcinoma, HIF-α accumulates, resulting in the overexpression of proteins that are normally inducible with hypoxia, acting on neighboring vascular cells and promoting tumor angiogenesis. The augmented tumor vasculature provides additional nutrients and oxygen to promote the growth of tumor cells (Cohen & McGovern, 2005).

Germline mutations in the VHL gene are found in almost all families with VHL disease, an autosomal dominant condition characterized by a plenty of benign and malignant tumors (Figure 1). The most common cancer is clear cell RCC, which affects 25-30% of patients and is a major concern in disease morbity and mortality (Maher et al., 1990). Remarkably, up to

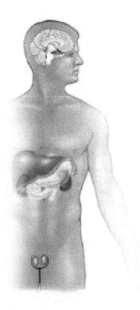

Fig. 1. von Hippel-Lindau disease predisposes to several tumors in brain, spinal cord, eyes, liver, pancreas, kidneys, testes.

91% of patients with sporadic clear cell RCC harbor biallelic VHL inactivation (Gnarra et al, 1994). Somatic mutations are found in approximately 50% of these tumors, whereas inactivation due to promoter hypermethylation has been identified in 10-20% of sporadic clear-cell RCC (Kim & Kaelin, 2004). Therefore, defects in the VHL gene are the major responsible for all cases of RCC.

The product of the VHL gene, VHL protein (pVHL), is part of an intracellular multiprotein complex that contains elongin C and B, Cul2 and Rbx1 and functions as the substrate recognition component of an E3-ubiquitin ligase. This complex selects specific substrates for ubiquitination and targets them for destruction through the proteasome, mainly HIF-α. In normoxia, the a-subunits are the target for prolyl hydroxylation that generates a binding site for pVHL. The interaction between the two proteins causes the polyubiquitynation and subsequent proteosomal degradation of HIF-α. When the cell is hypoxic or iron levels are low, the VHL complex cannot target and degrade HIF and HIF overaccumulates, driving the transcription of a number of genes important in cancer, such as *VEGF*, *PDGF*, and *GLUT1*(Figure 2a). In cells with normal VHL function, the α subunits of HIF are rapidly degraded by the proteasome, whereas in VHL-defective cells HIF-α subunits are constitutively stabilized (Maxwell et al, 1999). When the *VHL* gene is mutated, as in clear cell RCC, the complex cannot target and degrade the α subunits of HIF leading to upregulation of their targets genes (Figure 2b). Therefore, the absence of pVHL mimics hypoxia and results in a constitutive up-regulation of HIF that produces a transcriptional activation of several target genes, such as VEGF, PDGF-B, erythropoietin, TGF-α, and glucose-transporter-1 (GLUT-1).

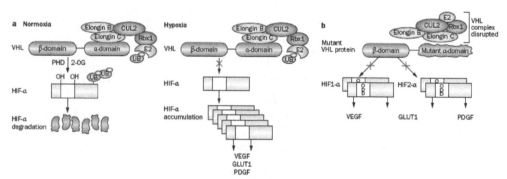

Fig. 2. The HIF-VHL-VEGF pathway. a. HIF- α degradation in normoxic cells and stabilization in hypoxic cells. b. HIF1- α and HIF2- α are not degraded and upregulate the expression of their target genes (VEGF, PDGF, GLUT1)(with permission).

It has been shown that VEGF protein expression in VHL-defective renal cancer cells is mainly induced by HIF-2α activity. The expression of other HIF targets, such as GLUT-1, urokinase-type plasminogen activator receptor (uPAR), and plasminogen activator inhibitor-1 (PAI-1), was also regulated by HIF-2a in these cells. Thus, HIF-2α seems to play a critical role in tumorigenesis of clear-cell RCC mediated by loss of VHL (Kondo et al, 2002). Clear cell kidney cancers (with or without *VHL* mutation) that express both HIF1-α and HIF2-α exhibit enhanced signaling via the mitogen-activated protein kinase (MAPK) and mTOR pathways. Constitutive activation of the Raf/MEK/Erk pathway has been demonstrated in approximately 50% of RCC samples (ref.14. EJC). Conversely, clear cell tumors that express only HIF2-α have elevated activity of the oncogene c-myc (Gordan et al, 2008).

VHL substrates other than HIF have been reported, and although their exact role in kidney carcinogenesis has not been proved to be the same as HIF's, it is possible that they may contribute directly or indirectly to VHL-deficient RCC and/or other solid tumors. VHL has been shown to interact with the RNA polymerase II subunits Rpb1, Rbp6, and Rpb7 at domains that present sequence and structural similarity to the HIF binding domain. Binding of these subunits to pVHL was shown to promote their ubiquitination and decrease transcriptional activity of Pol II (Kuznetsova et al, 2003).

Moreover, pVHL has been shown to influence the content of the extracellular matrix. Fibronectin coimmunoprecipitates with wild type but not mutant pVHL, and pVHL-deficient RCC cell lines fail to assemble extracellular fibronectin, most likely because of a defect in fibronectin maturation (Ohh et al, 1998).

Finally, it was recently shown that VHL is linked to the DNA damage response pathway. pVHL binds directly to p53, inhibits its mdm2-mediated ubiquitination, suppresses p53 nuclear export, and promotes its acetylation by p300 and overall p53 transcriptional activity. Reintroduction of pVHL in VHL-deficient RCC lines enhances p53-mediated G1 arrest and promotes their apoptotic response to genotoxic stress (Roe et al, 2006).

2.1 Therapeutic perspectives

The better understanding of VHL signaling pathway has provided the foundation for the development of therapeutic approaches that target this pathway in patients with advanced clear cell kidney cancer.

Most therapeutic agents currently approved to treat clear cell kidney cancer target either the downstream targets of HiF activity (such as the VEGF receptor) or inhibit mtorC1, which provides translational control of HiF1-α (Thomas et al., 2006). The responses to these agents observed in patients with advanced clear cell kidney cancer is proof of principle that targeting the VHL–HIF pathway can induce tumor regression in humans. However, these agents target only a small proportion of the downstream genes regulated by HIFs. An approach to target HIF transcriptional activity or translation of HIFs themselves — that is, to affect all the genes regulated by HIFs — could potentially provide more-effective therapy. Targeting the HIF2-α pathway is likely to be more successful than solely targeting the HIF1-α pathway. Efforts are currently underway to identify agents that down regulate HIF2-α-induced gene expression (Linehan et al., 2010a). Tyrosine kinase receptors trigger activation of signal transduction pathways involved in cell proliferation and survival of RCCs (Patel et al, 2006). Growth factors, such as VEGF and TGF-a, might bind to the respective tyrosine kinase receptors (EGFR and VEGFR-1) that are expressed in renal cancer cells. Thus, these receptors could potentially be targets of small molecules inhibitors. Nevertheless, many chemotherapeutic and targeted tyrosine kinase approaches are limited by their toxic effects on non-tumor cells. An alternative therapy, might be done by targeting autophagy, a central component of the cell response to nutrient and energy deprivation (Turcotte et al, 2008). By this approach, only those cells with no VHL product would be affected, whereas cells with a wild-type copy of the VHL gene would not. Therefore, this would provide a less-toxic and more-effective form of therapy for patients with advanced renal cancer.

3. The MET-HGF pathway and type-1 papillary renal cancer

Papillary renal-cell carcinoma occurs in several familial syndromes. Hereditary papillary renal carcinoma (HPRC) is an autosomal dominant disorder associated with multifocal papillary renal-cell carcinoma with type 1 histological features and is caused by germline activating mutations in the MET proto-oncogene (Schmidt et al, 1997) (Figure 3).

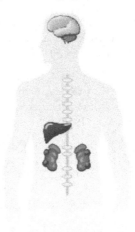

Fig. 3. Hereditary Papillary Renal Carcinoma leads to multiple (even thousands) of papillary tumors. (with permission)

The MET proto-oncogene encodes a receptor tyrosine kinase that is physiologically activated by hepatocyte growth factor (HGF). Binding of HGF to the extracellular portion of the MET receptor triggers autophosphorylation of critical tyrosines in the intracellular tyrosine kinase domain, thus activating a downstream signaling cascade. Activation of the MET/HGF signaling pathway has been shown to be involved in a number of biological activities including cell proliferation, cell motility, branching morphogenesis and epithelial-mesenchymal transition (Boccaccio & Comoglio, 2006).

Mutations of the MET proto-oncogene were detected in germline of all HPRC patients but only in a small subset of cases with sporadic type 1- papillary RCC (Schmidt et al, 1999). Thus, the pathogenesis of hereditary papillary renal carcinoma is usually different from that of sporadic papillary RCC. Tumorigenesis of most sporadic papillary RCCs are not be induced only by MET mutations, but mostly by MET and chromosome 7-related genes dosage. Since the frequency of MET mutations in sporadic papillary RCCs is low, it is possible that other genes might be involved in this form of renal cancer. In this respect, mutations of the KIT proto-oncogene have been described in 68% of papillary RCC patients (Lin et al, 2004). However, the role of KIT in the pathogenesis of this disease needs to be confirmed by functional studies. Furthermore, nutrient-stimulated HGF–MET signaling induces phosphorylation of serine–threonine protein kinase 11 (STK11or LKB1) through the RAS–ERK pathway, implicating *MET* in the LKB1–AMPK–mTOR nutrient and energy sensing pathway (Figure 4).

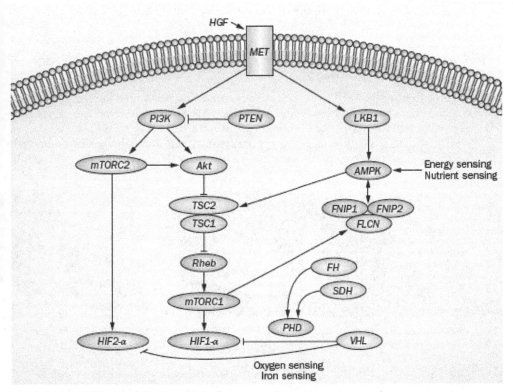

Fig. 4. HGF-MET pathway. Crosslinks between other energy, iron and oxygen-sensing pathways. (with permission)

Of particular interest for renal carcinogenesis is the observation that MET and VHL signaling pathways intersect via pVHL-mediated regulation of HIF function. HIF stabilization through hypoxia or loss of VHL function results in transcriptional upregulation, and therefore promotion of the transforming potential of the *c-MET* receptor (Pennacchietti et al, 2003). This crosstalk between VHL and c-MET pathways may explain why clear-cell and papillary histologies often coexist in the same tumor (Iliopoulos et al, 2006).

3.1 Therapeutic perspectives

The therapeutic implications of inhibiting *c-MET* signaling are promising, as activating mutations or copy number–overexpression of *c-MET* underlies a significant subset of type 1 papillary RCC.

A clinical trial is currently underway to determine the effect of foretinib, a kinase inhibitor of both *MET* and *VEGF* receptors, in patients with either hereditary or sporadic papillary kidney cancer. Early evidence shows the efficacy of this agent in patients with germline mutations in the tyrosine kinase domain of *MET* (Srinivasan et al, 2009). Response to such an agent with activity against *MET* might be seen in tumors that are characterized by a mutation in the tyrosine kinase domain of *MET*; this drug might also have some activity in tumors that have *MET* amplification (Linehan et al., 2010b).

4. The mitochondrial metabolic pathway: The FH gene and type-2 papillary renal cancer and the SDH gene

Germline mutations of the *FH* gene, which encodes mitochondrial fumarate hydratase, have been detected in most individuals with hereditary leiomyomatosis renal cell carcinoma (HLRCC), who are susceptible to develop cutaneous and uterine leiomyomas, uterine leiomyosarcoma and, most often solitary and unilateral renal tumors, which may present different histological patterns, particularly type-2 papillary RCC (Tomlinson et al, 2002) (Figure 5).

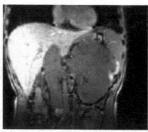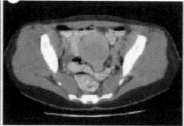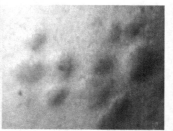

Fig. 5. Hereditary Leiomyomatosis Renal Cell Carcinoma predisposes to type-2 papillary RCC (left), uterine (middle) and cutaneous (right) leiomyomas (with permission).

FH is an enzyme component of the mitochondrial tricarboxylic acid or Krebs cycle, which has an important role in energy metabolism. In patients with FH deficient cells, it has been proposed that the inactivation of this enzyme might lead to a hypoxic environment that can favour renal carcinogenesis. FH inactivating mutations increase fumarate levels, and consequently the concentration of the fumarate precursor succinate. The high levels of succinate in the cytoplasm lead to stabilization of HIF-1α subunits and transcriptional upregulation of hypoxia-inducible genes, such as *VEGF* and *GLUT1* (which encodes the glucose transporter type 1) (Figure 6). Thus, these factors are critically important to increase vasculature and glucose transport in RCC cells, thereby contributing to the highly aggressive nature of HLRCC-associated renal tumors (Iliopoulos et al, 2006).

The inhibition of HIF-1α by the increased levels of fumarate provides a VHL-independent mechanism for dysregulation of HIF degradation in FH-deficient HLRCC-associated kidney cancers. FH-deficient kidney cancer cell lines are glucose-dependent and have significantly impaired oxidative phosphorylation. The glucose-mediated generation of cellular reactive oxygen species in an FH-deficient kidney cancer cell line results in stabilization of HIF1-α (Sudarshan et al, 2009). The impaired oxidative phosphorylation in FH-deficient kidney cancer results in a nearly total dependence on glycolysis for energy production.

Succinate dehydrogenase *(SDH)* is another Krebs cycle enzyme gene that has been associated with the development of familial tumors. Familial paraganglioma/ pheochromocytoma kindreds have been found to have germline mutations in the mitochondrial complex II genes *SDHB*, *SDHC*, and *SDHD*. Renal carcinoma, along with pheochromocytoma/paraganglioma, has been found to be a component of the familial pheochromocytoma/paraganglioma complex associated with germline *SDHB* mutations (Neumann et al, 2004), and a recent report described germline *SDHB* mutations in a family with renal cancer with no history of pheochromocytoma (Ricketts et al, 2008). The inactivation of SDH increases levels of succinate, which has been shown to affect HIF stability (Isaacs et al, 2005). It would be expected to severely impair oxidative phosphorylation and lead to glucose dependence of SDH-deficient kidney tumors, which are likely to be as sensitive to glucose as FH-deficient tumors (Linehan et al., 2010a) (Figure 6).

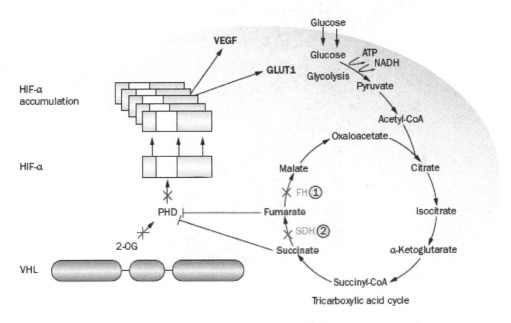

Fig. 6. FH and SDH genes and the metabolic mitochondrial pathway crosslinking with the HIF-VHL pathway (with permission).

4.1 Therapeutic perspectives

Both enhanced tumor angiogenesis and glucose transport could be the best targets for the treatment of either FH-deficient or SDH-deficient renal tumors, because they are extremely dependent on glucose transport for energy production. Whereas targeting the vasculature in patients with advanced VHL-deficient clear cell kidney cancer has only resulted in modest success, targeting the vasculature in both FH and SDH-deficient tumors could provide a powerful and effective approach to disrupt the fundamental metabolic machinery of these aggressive cancers (Linehan et al., 2010a).

5. The *FLCN* gene and chromophobe renal cell carcinomas-oncocytomas

The *FLCN* gene is impaired in Birt-Hogg-Dubè syndrome, a rare autosomal dominant disorder characterized by hair-follicle hamartomas (fibrofolliculomas) of the face and neck, spontaneous pneumotorax, lung cysts and RCCs, particularly chromophobe RCC (33%), hybrid oncocytic renal cell carcinoma (50%), clear-cell RCC (9%) and oncocytomas (5%) (De Luca et al, 2008) (Figure 7).

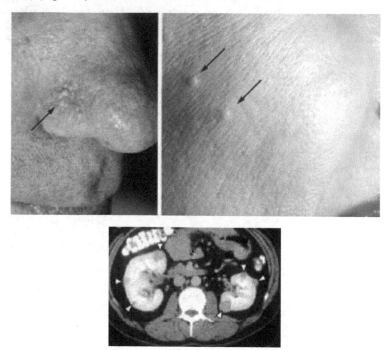

Fig. 7. Birt-Hogg-Dubè syndrome. Fibrofolliculomas on the face and bilateral RCC (with permission).

The *FLCN* gene encodes a protein called folliculin, which has no significant homology to any known human protein, although it is highly conserved across species (Nickerson et al, 2002). All described germline *FLCN* mutations are insertions, deletions, nonsense and splice-site mutations that predict truncation of the protein (Schmidt et al, 2005). In addition, somatic mutations in the second copy of BHD or loss of heterozygosity at the FLCN locus were observed in 70% of patients with germline mutations, thus suggesting *FLCN* to play a role as a tumor suppressor gene (Vocke et al, 2005).

In sporadic cases, somatic mutations are rare, but promoter methylation has been observed, indicating the involvement of *FLCN* in sporadic RCC tumorigenesis (Khoo et al, 2003).The function of folliculin has not been completely elucidated yet, but recent findings have showed that folliculin interacts with FNIP1, which binds to the 5' AMP-activated protein kinase (AMPK), an energy sensor that negatively regulates mammalian target of rapamycin (mTOR) (Baba et al, 2006). When folliculin functions normally, the FLCN–FNIP1–FNIP2 complex binds to AMPK so *FLCN* is phosphorylated by a rapamycin-sensitive kinase (mTORC1). Conversely, when folliculin is deficient, AKT, mTORC1 and mTORC2 are activated, thus stimulating tumorigenesis (Figure 8). These findings suggest a potential role of folliculin in regulating the activation of this cell survival pathway.

The research in murine models of Birt–Hogg–Dube syndrome would suggest that rapamycin analogs such as sirolimus might be potential therapeutic agents against renal tumors (Linehan et al, 2010a).

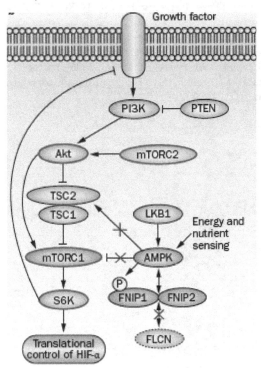

Fig. 8. FLCN interacts with AMPK-mTOR pathway. FLCN deficiency allows activation of proto-oncogenes (red circles) (with permission).

6. The AMPK-mTOR nutrient and energy sensing pathway and Tuberous Sclerosis Complex

Germline mutations in either TSC1 or TSC2 genes lead to the Tuberous Sclerosis Complex, an autosomal dominant genodermatosis characterized by multiple hamartomatous lesions that affect the skin, retina, brain, lungs and kidneys (Figure 9).

Eighty percent of children with TSC have renal lesions including benign angiomyolipomas (70%), cysts (20%), and oncocytoma (<1%) (Ewalt et al, 1998). Renal angiomyolipomas are most often multiple and bilateral, but rarely transform to a malignant tumor (<1%). The cumulative renal cancer incidence is 2.2%–4.4% (4,5) and the average age at diagnosis is 28 years, with occasional early childhood cases (Washecka et al, 1991). The renal abnormalities in TSC are unusual in patients that develop epithelial lesions, such as cysts, oncocytomas and clear cell, papillary, or chromophobe carcinomas as well as mesenchymal lesions (angiomyolipomas), suggesting that TSC genes regulate early differentiation and proliferation of renal precursor cells (Henske, 2004).

The TSC1 gene encodes hamartin and TSC2 encodes tuberin. Both proteins form a heterodimer, which interacts with many cellular pathways, including the AMPK-mTOR nutrient and energy sensing pathway. TSC1-TSC2 acts as a GTPase-activating protein toward rheb, a ras-family GTPase that activates mMTORC1. GTPase activity of the TSC1–TSC2 complex on rheb results in inhibition of mTOR activity. *TSC1*-deficient and *TSC2*-deficient tumors exhibit increased phosphorylation of p70s6 kinase, s6 ribosomal protein and 4e-BP1, downstream effectors of mtorC1 activation, and readouts for initiation of mRNA translation and protein synthesis (Crino et al, 2006). Lack of TSC1–TSC2 inhibition of mTOR would presumably also result in HIF accumulation through increased *HIF* mRNA translation by activated mTORC1 (Figure 10).

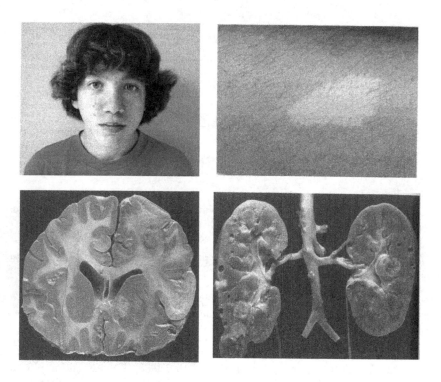

Fig. 9. Tuberous Sclerosis Complex. Hamartomatous lesions on skin (top left), hypomelanotic macules (top right), cortical tubers (bottom left) and angiomyolipomas (bottom right).

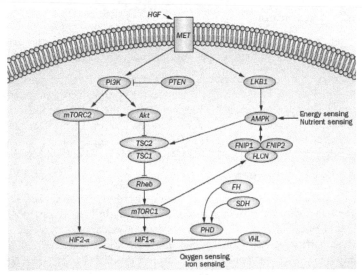

Fig. 10. TSC1-TSC2 tumor suppressor complex interacts with AMPK-mTOR nutrient and energy sensing pathway (with permission).

6.1 Therapeutic perspectives

Currently, there are a number of trials that evaluate the role of sirolimus in patients with Tuberous Sclerosis Complex. This agent has been demonstrated to cause the regression of angiomyolipomas, through the inhibition of the mTOR signaling pathway. Nevertheless, after the treatment was stopped, most renal tumors tended to growth again. In spite of that, this study provided the grounds for a molecular approach to the treatment of renal tumors associated with the *TSC1–TSC2* pathway (Linehan et al., 2010b).

7. Collecting-duct carcinomas

Collecting duct carcinomas (CDC) are uncommon and aggressive tumors thought to arise from cells of the distal nephron.

Their genetic defects have not been completely elucidated; however, they have shown cytogenetic and molecular alterations different from other renal tumors (Kennedy et al, 1990).

Nonetheless, some molecular findings suggest that these cancers are heterogeneous and can exhibit features similar to more common types of RCC as well as to urothelial carcinoma.

Genetic studies have shown monosomy of chromosomes 1, 6, 14, 15 and 22 and frequent allelic loss of 1q, 6p, 8p, 13q and 21q. Monosomy of 8p has been associated with high stage and aggressive behavior and might be responsible for the poor prognosis of CDC (Fuzesi et al, 1992). Loss of heterozygosity (LOH) of 3p is rarely detectable in these tumors, although *VHL* allelic loss has been occasionally reported. Moreover, some studies have found 9p LOH in half of CDC cases, whereas other studies have not. Mutations of the *RB* gene and LOH of 13q have also been observed in some CDC but its role in the pathogenesis of CDC needs to be clarified (Fogt et al, 1998).

8. Tubulocystic carcinomas

The molecular pathogenesis of tubulocystic carcinoma, a rare renal tumor composed of tubular and cystic structures, remains poorly understood.

The genomic defects of tubulocystic carcinoma are similar to those of papillary RCC, as it often exhibits trisomy of chromosome 17. It has been hypothesized that it may represent a lowgrade collecting duct carcinoma of the kidney despite the lack of enough citogenetic and molecular evidence, such as trisomy of 7, monosomy of 1, 6, 14, 15, and 22, allelic loss on 1q, 6p, 8p, 13q, and 21q, which are often found in CDC (Yang et al, 2008).

9. Renal medullary carcinomas

Renal medullary carcinoma is considered as an aggressive variant of collecting duct carcinoma, a rare and rapidly growing tumor of the medulla of kidneys. This tumor is frequently seen in young male with African ancestry and carriers of sickle cell trait. In a study of nine tumors through comparative genomic hybridization (CGH), eight depicted no changes and only one presented monosomy of chromosome 22 (Swartz et al, 2002).

10. TFE translocation carcinomas family

Accordingly with the WHO classification of renal tumors (Eble et al, 2004), an entity recently defined by chromosomal translocations involving the Xp11.2 region is responsible for about one third of renal carcinomas in children and young adults. These cancers resemble clear cell RCC and seems to have a benign evolution, even with metastasis, while others may behave aggressively. They are also known as the TFE translocation carcinoma family (MTTCF) (Tomlinson et al, 1991).

All translocations result in the production of quimeric proteins containing the *TFE3* product , such as those from *PRCC, ASPL, PSF,* and *NonO (p54nrb)* genes. For instance, translocation of Xp to chromosome 1 forms an in-frame fusion of the *TFE3* gene on Xp11.2 to a novel gene *PRCC* on chromosome 1(Camparo et al, 2008).

Because the normal TFE3 protein has a DNA-binding domain, fusion proteins composed of this gene product and the ubiquitously expressed PRCC and ASPL proteins result in the overexpression of an abnormal transcription factor that causes aberrant expression of cellular genes. Another subset of renal tumors are associated with a translocation t(6;11)(p21;q12) involving the transcription factor TFEB(Camparo et al, 2008).

Some gene expression profiling studies indicated a distinct subgroup of tumors. For example, TRIM 63 glutathione S-transferase A1 and alanyl aminopeptidase are the main differentially expressed genes for MTTCF (Camparo et al, 2008).

Therefore, the correct classification of these tumors may pose important prognostic and therapeutical implications. For instance, tumors with the ASPL-TFE3 translocation particularly present at an advanced stage associated with lymph node metastases. In addition, some tumors with *PRCC-TFE3* fusion have been shown to lack a normal mitotic checkpoint control, which may turn them more sensitive to chemotherapeutic agents that target microtubules, such as vincristine and paclitaxel (Lopez-Beltran et al, 2010).

11. Mucinous tubular and spindle renal cell carcinomas

These are rare and morphologically distinctive tumors, although they share some features of type I papillary RCC.

The main molecular differences between them have been studied through CGH expression microarrays. Two studies found multiple genetic abnormalities in all cases, such as losses of chromosomes 1, 4, 6, 8, 9,13, 14, 15, 18 and 22. The major differential diagnosis is papillary RCC with solid growth, whose gains of chromosomes 7 and 17 and losses of chromosome Y are typical, but lack in mucinous tubular and spindle RCC (Rakozy et al, 2002).

12. Renal cell carcinomas with sarcomatoid transformation

Sarcomatoid transformation has been seen in all of the common types of RCC: clear cell, papillary, chromophobe and collecting duct, but its specific molecular mechanisms remain poorly understood.

It is hypothesized that the sarcomatoid components of RCCs represent areas of dedifferentiation, and it seems that the genomic changes associated with a specific type of RCC should be conserved within the dedifferentiated sarcomatoid RCC component. In a recent study, the allelic loss profile between clear cell and sarcomatoid components of RCCs was compared and showed the same pattern of nonrandom X-chromosome inactivation in most cases. The results suggested that both clear cell and sarcomatoid components of RCCs are derived from the same progenitor cell. Some other studies suggest a link between mutation of the TP53 tumor suppressor gene and sarcomatoid morphology. Major differential diagnosis is poorly differentiated urothelial carcinoma of the renal pelvis, which presents peculiar genetic profiles, specifically, gains of chromosome 3, 7, 17 and losses of 9p21 (Lopez-Beltran et al, 2010).

13. Acquired cystic disease-associated renal tumors

Interestingly, in kidneys that have developed acquired cystic disease and, consequently, resulting in end-stage renal disease, two distinctive types of renal neoplasm have been found to occur: 'acquired cystic disease-associated RCC' and 'clear cell papillary RCC' (Cossu-Rocca et al, 2010).

Acquired cystic disease-associated RCCs are morphologically heterogeneous with abundant eosinophilic cytoplasm and variably solid , cribriform, tubulocystic with papillary architecture. Chromosomal aberrations have been found in these tumors in few studies, such as gains of chromosomes 1, 2, 6, 7, 10 and 17 (Cossu-Rocca et al, 2010).

Clear cell papillary RCC presents with papillary structures proliferating within cystic spaces, both lined by cells with clear cytoplasm. Through interphase FISH analysis, a study found all tumors to lack the gains of chromosome 7 and loss of Y, which are peculiar for papillary RCC and, in addition, there was no 3p deletion, which is typical of clear cell RCC.

The other major differential diagnoses are: tubulocystic carcinoma (trisomic for 17 but not for 7), chromophobe RCC (multiple chromosomal losses) and oncocytoma (loss of chromosome 1) (Lopez-Beltran et al, 2010).

14. Thyroid-like follicular renal cell carcinoma

Recently, there have been reports of an uncommon renal tumor, which had not been classified under a known subtype of RCC (Lopez-Beltran et al, 2010). It shows similar histology to thyroid follicular carcinoma and seems to affect more often women without previous lesions in the thyroid.

Chromosomal gains of 7q36, 8q24, 12, 16, 17p11-q11, 17q24, 19q, 20q13, 21q22.3, and Xp and losses of 1p36, 3, and 9q21-33 were identified through CGH. However, a recent report did not found any chromosomal alterations on CGH analysis. It is speculated that thyroid-like follicular RCC may represent a unique histological subtype of RCC of low malignant potential (Lopez-Beltran et al, 2010).

15. Conclusion

Currently, there is sufficient evidence that kidney cancer is essentially a disease of dysregulated cellular metabolism (Linehan et al, 2010a).

Germline mutations in each of the seven genes involved in inherited kidney cancer syndromes lead to the dysregulation of at least one metabolic pathway that is mediated by oxygen, iron, energy or nutrient sensing (Figure 11).

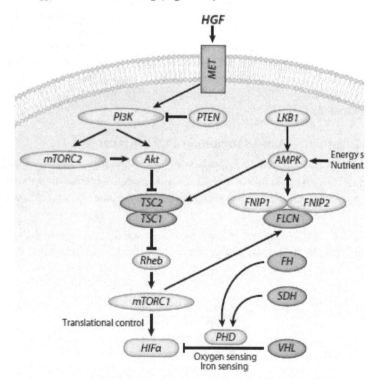

Fig. 11. The metabolic pathways mediated by the seven tumor suppressor genes mutated in hereditary cancer syndromes (with permission)

The shared consequence of *VHL, FH* and *SDH* mutations is the stabilization of HIFs through inactivation of the prolyl-hydroxilase domain, which leads to the transcriptional activation of genes that stimulate tumor growth, neovascularization, invasion and metastasis. HIF overexpression is also triggered by the upregulation of the mTOR pathway, either through inactivating mutations in the tumor suppressor genes *TSC1,TSC2* and *FLCN*, or activating oncogenic "signalling pathways".

By targeting HIF and its downstream genes, a first-line therapeutic approach to VHL-deficient renal tumors may be feasible and can also be applied to FH-deficient and SDH-deficient tumors. To date, novel agents focusing on the VHL pathway have been approved for the treatment of patients with advanced kidney cancer (Table 2) (Linehan et al, 2010b). Unfortunately, however, most of them occasionally present progression and rarely promote long-term complete responses.

In conclusion, the pursuit of a thorough understanding of the molecular pathogenesis and the intricate metabolic pathways of advanced renal cell carcinoma may provide the foundation for the development of novel approaches that might possibly increase the response and survival rates of patients with this extremely heterogeneous disease.

Histology	Gene	Drug
Clear cell	VHL	Sunitinib, sorafenib, bevacizumab, temsirolimus, everolimus, axitinib
Type 1 papillary	MET	Foretinib
Type 2 papillary	FH	Targeting VEGF
Chromophobe Oncocytoma Hibrid oncocytic	FLCN or BHD	Rapamycin
Angiomyolipoma	TSC1, TSC2	Sirolimus

Table 2. Targeted therapies for the most common renal cell carcinomas

16. References

Baba, M.; Hong, S.; Sharma, N. (2006). Folliculin Encoded by the BHD Gene Interacts with a Binding Protein, FNIP1, and AMPK, and is Involved in AMPK and mTOR Signaling. *Proc Natl Acad Sci U S A*, Vol.103, pp. 15552–15557.

Boccaccio, C. & Comoglio, P. (2006). Invasive Growth: a MET-driven Genetic Programme for Cancer and Stem Cells. *Nat Rev Cancer*, Vol.6, pp. 637–645.

Camparo, P.; Vasiliu, V.; Molinie, V. (2008). Renal Translocation Carcinomas: Clinicopathologic, Immunohistochemical, and Gene Expression Profiling Analysis of 31 Cases with a Review of the Literature. *Am. J.Surg. Pathol.*, Vol.32, pp. 656–670.

Cohen, H. & McGovern, F. (2005). Renal-Cell Carcinoma. *N Engl J Med*, Vol.353, pp. 2477-2490.

Cossu-Rocca, P.; Eble, J.; Zhang, S.; Martignoni, G.; Brunelli, M. & Cheng, L. (2010). Acquired Cystic Disease-associated Renal Tumors: an Immunohistochemical and Fluorescence in situ Hybridization Study. *Mod. Pathol.*, Vol.19, pp.780-787.

Crino, P. B.; Nathanson, K. L. & Henske, E. P.(2006). The Tuberous Sclerosis Complex. *N. Engl. J.Med.* Vol.355, pp. 1345-1356.

De Luca, A.; Carotenuto, P.; D'Alessio, A.; Normanno, N. (2008). Molecular Biology of Renal-Cell Carcinoma. *European Journal of Cancer,* Vol.6, pp. 30-34.

Eble, J.; Sauter, G.; Epstein, J. & Sesterhenn, I. (2004). *Pathology and Genetics. Tumors of the Urinary System and Male Genital Organs.* IARC Press, Lyon, France.

Ewalt, D.; Sheffield, E.; Sparagana, S.; Delgado, M. & Roach, E. (1998). Renal Lesion Growth in Children with Tuberous Sclerosis Complex. *J Urol.*, Vol.160, No.1, pp. 141-145.

Fogt, F.; Zhuang, Z.; Linehan, W. & Merino, M. (1998). Collecting Duct Carcinomas of the Kidney: a Comparative Loss of Heterozygosity Study with Clear Cell Renal Cell Carcinoma. *Oncol. Rep.*, Vol.5, pp. 923-926.

Fuzesi, L.; Cober, M. & Mittermayer, C. (1992). Collecting Duct Carcinoma: Cytogenetic Characterization. *Histopathology* vol.21, pp. 155-160.

Gnarra, J.; Tory, K.; Weng, Y. (1994). Mutations of theVHL Tumor Suppressor Gene in Renal Carcinoma. *Nat. Genet,* Vol.7, pp. 85-90.

Gordan, J. D. *et al.* (2008). HIF-alpha Effects on c-Myc Distinguish Two Subtypes of Sporadic VHL-deficient Clear Cell Renal Carcinoma. *Cancer Cell,* Vol.14, pp. 435-446.

Henske, E. (2004). The genetic basis of kidney cancer: why is tuberous sclerosis complex often overlooked? *Curr Mol Med.* Vol. 4, No.8, pp. 825-831.

Higgins, J.; Shinghal, R.; Gill, H. (2003). Gene Expression Patterns in Renal Cell Carcinoma Assessed by Complementary DNA Microarray. *Am J Pathol*, Vol.162, pp. 925-932.

Iliopoulos O. (2006). Molecular Biology of Renal Cell Cancer and the Identification of Therapeutic Targets. *J Clin Oncol.*, Vol.24, pp. 5593-5600.

Isaacs, J.; Jung, Y.; Mole, D. (2005). HIF Overexpression Correlates with Biallelic Loss of Fumarate Hydratase in Renal Cancer: Novel Role of Fumarate in Regulation of HIF Stability. *Cancer Cell,* Vol. 8, pp. 143-153.

Kennedy, S.; Merino, M.; Linehan, W.; Roberts, J.; Robertson, C. & Neumann, R.(1990). Collecting Duct Carcinoma of the Kidney. *Hum. Pathol.*, Vol.21, pp. 449-456.

Khoo, S.; Kahnoski, K.; Sugimura, J. (2003). Inactivation of BHD in Sporadic Renal Tumors. *Cancer Res*, Vol.63, pp. 4583-4587.

Kim, W. & Kaelin, W. (2004). Role of VHL Gene Mutation in Human Cancer. *J Clin Oncol,* Vol.22, pp. 4991-5004.

Kondo, K., Klco, J., Nakamura, E., Lechpammer, M. & Kaelin, W. G. Jr. (2002). Inhibition of HIF is Necessary for Tumor Suppression by the von Hippel-Lindau Protein. *Cancer Cell,* Vol.1, pp. 237-246.

Kovacs G.; Akhtar, M.; Beckwith, B. (1997). The Heidelberg Classification of Renal Cell Tumours. *J Pathol* Vol.183, pp.131-133.

Kuznetsova, A.; Meller, J.; Schnell, P. (2003). Von Hippel-Lindau Protein Binds Hyperphosphorylated Large Subunit of RNA Polymerase II Through a Proline Hydroxylation Motif and Targets it for Ubiquitination. *Proc Natl Acad Sci USA* Vol.100, pp. 2706-2711.

Lin, Z.; Han, E.; Lee, E. (2004). A Distinct Expression Pattern and Point Mutation of c-kit in Papillary Renal Cell Carcinomas. *Mod Pathol,* Vol.17, pp. 611-616.

Linehan, W.; Srinivasan, R. & Schmidt, L. (2010a). The Genetic Basis of Kidney Cancer: a Metabolic Disease. *Nature Reviews Urology*, Vol.7, (May 2010), pp. 277-285.

Linehan, W.; Bratslavsky, G. ; Pinto, P. ; Schmidt, L. ; Neckers, L. ; Bottaro, D. & Srinivasan, R. (2010b). Molecular Diagnosis and Therapy of Kidney Cancer. *Annual Review of Medicine*, Vol.61, pp. 329-343.

Lopez-Beltran, A.; Montironi, R. ; Egevad, L. ; Caballero-Vargas, M. ; Scarpelli, M. ; Kirkali, Z. & Cheng, L. (2010). Genetic Profiles in Renal Tumors. *Internation Journal of Urology*, Vol.17, pp. 6-19.

Maher, E.; Yates, J.; Harries, R. (1990). Clinical Features and Natural History of von Hippel-Lindau Disease. *Q.J.Med*, Vol.77, pp. 1151-1163.

Maxwell, P.; Wiesener, M.; Chang, G. (1999). The Tumour Suppressor Protein VHL Targets Hypoxia-inducible Factors for Oxygen-dependent Proteolysis. *Nature*, Vol.399, pp. 271-275.

McLaughlin, J.; Mandel, J.; Blot, W.; Schuman, L.; Mehl, E. & Fraumeni, J. (1984). A Population-based Case-control Study of Renal Cell Carcinoma. *J Natl Cancer Inst*, Vol.72, pp. 275-284.

Neumann, H.; Pawlu, C.; Peczkowska, M. (2004). Distinct Clinical Features of Paraganglioma Syndromes Associated with SDHB and SDHD Gene Mutations. *JAMA* Vol.292, pp. 943-951.

Nickerson, M.; Warren, M.; Toro, J. (2002). Mutations in a Novel Gene Lead to Kidney Tumors, Lung Wall Defects, and Benign Tumors of the Hair Follicle in Patients with the Birt-Hogg-Dube Syndrome. *Cancer Cell*, Vol.2, pp. 157-164.

Ohh, M.; Yauch, R.; Lonergan, K. (1998). The von Hippel-Lindau Tumor Suppressor Protein is Required for Proper Assembly of an Extracellular Fibronectin Matrix. *Mol Cell*, Vol.1, pp. 959-968.

Patel, P.; Chadalavada, R.; Chaganti, R. (2006). Targeting von Hippel-Lindau Pathway in Renal Cell Carcinoma. *Clin Cancer Res*, Vol.12, pp. 7215-7220.

Pennacchietti, S.; Michieli, P.; Galluzzo M. (2003). Hypoxia Promotes Invasive Growth by Transcriptional Activation of the MET Protooncogene. *Cancer Cell*, Vol.3, pp. 347-361.

Rakozy, C.; Schmahl, G.; Bogner, S. & Storkel, S. (2002). Low-grade Tubular-mucinous Renal Neoplasms: Morphologic, Immunohistochemical, and genetic features. *Mod. Pathol.*, Vol.15, pp. 1162-1171.

Ricketts, C.; Woodward, E.; Killick, P. (2008). Germline SDHB Mutations and Familial Renal Cell Carcinoma. *J. Natl. Cancer Inst.*, Vol.100, pp. 1260-12662.

Roe, J.; Kim, H.; Lee, S. (2006). p53 Stabilization and Transactivation by a von Hippel-Lindau Protein. *Mol Cell*, Vol.22, pp. 395-405.

Schmidt, L.; Duh, F.; Chen, F. (1997). Germline and Somatic Mutations in the Tyrosine Kinase Domain of the MET Protooncogene in Papillary Renal Carcinomas. *Nat Genet*, Vol.16, pp. 68-73.

Schmidt, L.; Junker, K.; Nakaigawa, N. (1999). Novel Mutations of the MET Proto-oncogene in Papillary Renal Carcinomas. *Oncogene*, Vol.18, pp. 2343-2350.

Schmidt, L.; Nickerson, M.; Warren, M. (2005). Germline BHD Mutation Spectrum and Phenotype Analysis of a Large Cohort of Families with Birt-Hogg-Dube Syndrome. *Am J Hum Genet*, Vol.76, pp. 1023-1033.

Srinivasan, R.; Choueiri, T.; Vaishampayan, U. (2008). A Phase II Study of the Dual MET/VEGFR2 Inhibitor XL880 in Patients with Papillary Renal Carcinoma. *J. Clin. Oncol.* Vol.27 (Suppl), pp.15s.

Sudarshan, S.; Sourbier, C.; Kong, H. (2009). Fumarate Hydratase Deficiency in Renal Cancer Induces Glycolytic Addiction and HIF-1α Stabilization by Glucose-dependent Generation of Reactive Oxygen Species. *Mol. Cell Biol.* Vol.15, pp. 4080–4090.

Swartz, M.; Karth, J.; Schneider, D.; Rodriguez, R.; Beckwith, J. & Perlman, E. (2002). Renal Medullary Carcinoma: Clinical, Pathologic, Immunohistochemical, and Genetic Analysis with Pathogenetic Implications. *Urology,* Vol.60, pp. 1083–1089.

Thomas, G.; Tran, C.; Mellinghoff, I. (2006). Hypoxia-inducible Factor Determines Sensitivity to Inhibitors of mTOR in Kidney Cancer. *Nat. Med.,* Vol.12, pp. 122–127.

Tomlinson, G.; Nisen, P.; Timmons, C. & Schneider, N. (1991). Cytogenetics of a Renal Cell Carcinoma in a 17-month-old Child. Evidence for Xp11.2 as a Recurring Breakpoint. *Cancer Genet. Cytogenet.,* Vol.57, pp. 11–17.

Tomlinson, I.; Alam, N.; Rowan, A. (2002). Germline Mutations in FH Predispose to Dominantly Inherited Uterine Fibroids, Skin Leiomyomata and Papillary Renal Cell Cancer. *Nat. Genet.* Vol.30, pp. 406–410.

Turcotte, S. *et al.* (2008). A Molecule Targeting VHL-deficient Renal Cell Carcinoma that Induces Autophagy. *Cancer Cell* Vol.14, pp. 90–102.

Vocke, C.; Yang, Y.; Pavlovich, C. (2005). High Frequency of Somatic Frameshift BHD Gene Mutations in Birt–Hogg–Dube Associated Renal Tumors. *J Natl Cancer Inst,* Vol.97, pp. 931–935.

Washecka, R. & Hanna, M. (1991). Malignant Renal Tumors in Tuberous Sclerosis. *Urology,* Vol.37, No.4, pp. 340–343.

Yang, X.; Zhou, M.; Hes, O. (2008). Tubulocystic Carcinoma of the Kidney: Clinicopathologic and Molecular Characterization. *Am. J. Surg. Pathol.,* Vol.32, pp. 177–187.

2

Molecular Portrait of Clear Cell Renal Cell Carcinoma: An Integrative Analysis of Gene Expression and Genomic Copy Number Profiling

Cristina Battaglia et al.[*]

Dept. of Biomedical Sciences and Technologies, University of Milano, Milano,
Doctoral School of Molecular Medicine, University of Milano, Milano,
Italy

1. Introduction

Renal cell carcinoma (RCC) incidence accounts for about 3 to 10 cases per 100,000 individuals with a predilection for adult males over 60 year old (1.6:1 male/female ratio) (Chow, 2010; Nese, 2009). In Europe, about 60,000 individuals are affected by RCC every year, with a mortality rate of about 18,000 subjects and an incidence rate for all stages steadily rising over the last three decades. Although inherited forms occur in a number of familial cancer syndromes, as the well-known von Hippel-Lindau (VHL) syndrome, RCC is commonly sporadic (Cohen & McGovern, 2005; Kaelin, 2007) and, as recently highlighted by the National Cancer Institute (NCI), influenced by the interplay between exposure to environmental risk factors and genetic susceptibility of exposed individuals (Chow et al., 2010). Being poorly symptomatic in early phases, many cases become clinically detectable only when already advanced and, as such, therapy-resistant (Motzer, 2011). Based on histology, RCC can be classified into several subtypes, i.e., clear cell (80% of cases), papillary (10%), chromophobe (5%) and oncocytoma (5%), each one characterized by specific histo-pathological features, malignant potential and clinical outcome (Cohen & McGovern, 2005). Patient stratification is normally achieved using prognostic algorithms and nomograms based on multiple clinico-pathological factors such as TNM stage, Fuhrman nuclear grade, tumor size, performance status, necrosis and other hematological indices (Flanigan et al., 2011), although the most efficient predictors of survival and recurrence are based on nuclear grade alone (Nese et al., 2009). As recently reviewed by Brannon et al. (Brannon & Rathmell, 2010), a finer RCC subtype classification could be obtained exploiting the vast amount of

[*] Eleonora Mangano[3], Silvio Bicciato[4], Fabio Frascati[3], Simona Nuzzo[4], Valentina Tinaglia[1,2], Cristina Bianchi[5], Roberto A. Perego[5] and Ingrid Cifola[3]
[1]*Dept. of Biomedical Sciences and Technologies, University of Milano, Milano, Italy;*
[2]*Doctoral School of Molecular Medicine, University of Milano, Milano, Italy*
[3]*Institute for Biomedical Technologies, National Research Council, Segrate, Italy*
[4]*Center for Genome Research, University of Modena and Reggio Emilia, Modena, Italy;*
[5]*Dept. of Experimental Medicine, University of Milano-Bicocca, Milano, Italy*

genomic and transcriptional data that have been presented in numerous studies. For instance, several authors proposed a molecular classification of RCC based on differential gene expression profiles, with any subtype characterized by the activation of distinct gene sets (Brannon, 2010; Furge, 2004; Skubitz, 2006; Sültmann, 2005; Zhang, 2008), while others identified RCC-specific biomarkers (e.g. CA9, ki67, VEGF proteins, phosphorylated AKT, PTEN, HIF-1α). Lately, it has been reported that microRNAs, a small class of non coding RNA molecules, could contribute to RCC development at different levels and may represent a new group of potential tumor biomarkers (Redova et al., 2011). Despite the numerous efforts in dissecting the molecular features of RCC through functional genomics, not a single transcriptional signature or biomarker has gained approval for clinical application yet (Arsanious, 2009; Eichelberg, 2009; Lam, 2007; Yin-Goen, 2006), so that the identification of novel molecular markers to improve early diagnosis and prognostic prediction and of candidate targets to develop new therapeutic approaches remains of primary importance for this pathology.

Among the RCC histotypes, clear cell renal carcinoma (ccRCC) is the most frequent and aggressive subtype and is characterized by a specific pattern of chromosomal alterations (Yoshimoto et al., 2007) that represents a molecular fingerprint potentially useful for diagnostic and prognostic applications (Klatte et al., 2007). Nowadays, the standard clinical treatment comprises surgical resection followed by IFN- and/or IL2-based immunotherapy, although therapy toxicity still represents a major problem (Molina & Motzer, 2011). The development of approaches targeting specific biological pathways, typically deregulated in this tumor, is opening the way to new opportunities for therapeutic intervention (Pal et al., 2010). One of the most investigated processes is the hypoxia pathway (Cohen & McGovern2005; Kaelin, 2007; Wouters & Koritzinsky, 2008) that is genetically linked to ccRCC through one of its key players, i.e., the VHL (von Hippel-Lindau) gene, completely inactivated in all inherited forms and in 80% of sporadic cases. Cloned in 1993, the VHL gene (located at the 3p25.3 locus) is currently known as the main tumor suppressor gene involved in the very early steps of RCC pathogenesis (Banks et al., 2006). Normally, the VHL function is to ubiquinate the two hypoxia-inducible factors HIF-1α and HIF-2α, addressing them to proteasome degradation (Kaelin, 2008). In ccRCC, the bi-allelic VHL inactivation, by combination of deletion and mutation/methylation (Banks et al., 2006), prevents the degradation of HIF-1α and HIF-2α that, in turn, can activate the transcription of a series of hypoxia-inducible genes, such as VEGF, VEGFR, EGFR, PDGF, IGF, GLUT-1, CXCR4, TGF-α, CA9 and EPO, involved in processes like angiogenesis, survival, cell motility, pH-regulation and glucose metabolism (Baldewijns et al., 2010). The complete loss of VHL function results in the up-regulation of a panel of genes that contributes to the ccRCC phenotype and represents a list of potential prognostic markers (Klatte et al., 2007) and/or therapeutic targets (Gong et al., 2010). Additionally, the transcription factor HIF-1α is commonly activated in cancer (Semenza, 2008) and is linked to oncogenic/tumor suppressor molecules implicated in cross-communication, such as the tubular sclerosis complex (TSC) and the mammalian target of rapamycin (mTOR) (Maxwell, 2005). As such, ccRCC represents an ideal model for developing novel targeted therapies directed against the hypoxia pathway and many molecules are already used in clinical trials targeting either HIF-1α, or the upstream pathways regulating HIF (as the Akt-mTOR signal transduction pathway), or the downstream genes induced by HIF (e.g., VEGF and VEGFR) (Baldewijns et al., 2010). Intriguingly, recent evidences indicate that also 20% of RCC sporadic cases with

Molecular Portrait of Clear Cell Renal Cell Carcinoma: An Integrative Analysis of Gene Expression and
Genomic Copy Number Profiling

25

wild-type VHL (and active VHL function) present a peculiar pattern of altered genes, suggesting the involvement of other, still partially unknown, alternative regulatory mechanisms (Gordan et al., 2008).

At DNA level, studies based on traditional cytogenetic and comparative genomic hybridization (CGH) techniques identified a panel of chromosomal aberrations typical of ccRCC (Höglund, 2004; Klatte, 2009). Moreover, high-density single nucleotide polymorphism (SNP) array technology, interrogating thousands of SNP markers distributed throughout the whole human genome, has significantly improved the detection of chromosomal aberrations and offered the opportunity to detect regions with loss of heterozygosity (LOH), an important information for the identification of novel tumor suppressor genes. SNP-arrays have been widely applied to characterize tumor genomic instability (Brenner & Rosenberg, 2010; Lisovich, 2011) and recently to perform the genome-wide DNA profiling of ccRCC tissue samples (Beroukhim, 2009; Chen, 2009; Cifola, 2008). Overall, ccRCC is characterized by recurrent genetic anomalies at characteristic chromosomes, such as deletions with LOH on chromosomes 3p (involving also the VHL locus), 6q, 8p, 9p, and 14q, and duplications of chromosomes 5q and 7. Many evidences suggest that this peculiar pattern of genomic instability represents a tumor-specific molecular fingerprint that has a role in cancer pathogenesis and may be useful in diagnostic and prognostic applications (Gunawan, 2001; Klatte, 2009; Perego, 2008). Furthermore, a comprehensive study showed that cytogenetic alterations could be associated to ccRCC tumorigenesis and malignant progression (Zhang et al., 2010b).

Advances in high-throughput genome-wide profiling technologies allowed an unprecedented comprehensive view of the cancer genome landscape. In particular, high-density microarrays and sequencing-based strategies have been widely used to identify genetic (gene dosage, allelic status, and mutations in gene sequence) and epigenetic (DNA methylation, histone modification, and microRNA) aberrations in cancer (Majewski & Bernards, 2011). The integrative approach of analyzing parallel dimensions has enabled the identification of genes that are often disrupted by multiple mechanisms but at low frequencies by any one mechanism and of pathways that are often disrupted at multiple components but at low frequencies at individual components (Chari et al., 2010). In these last years, there is an increasing tendency to combine genome-wide DNA copy number (CN) analysis with transcriptional profiles to investigate how alterations in DNA content (aneuploidy) can influence global expression patterns. In cancer research, this combined approach helps filtering the large amount of array-based data and, by narrowing down the hundreds of differentially expressed genes to those whose altered expression is attributable to underlying chromosomal alterations, allows highlighting candidate genes that are actively involved in the causation or maintenance of the malignant phenotype. This approach was applied in a wide range of tumor types, including breast (Hyman, 2002; Pollack, 2002), bladder (Harding et al., 2002), prostate (Saramäki et al., 2006), pancreas (Heidenblad et al., 2005), rectal (Grade et al., 2006) and melanoma (Akavia et al., 2010), demonstrating a strong genome-wide correlation between aneuploidy-associated genomic imbalances and global gene expression levels. Most studies focused on amplified and over-expressed genes and calculated that a fraction ranging from 44% to 62% of amplified genes showed concomitant up-regulated expression levels (Hyman et al., 2002). This suggests the presence of an aneuploidy-induced deregulation of the cancer transcriptome that occurs in addition to the transcriptional and mutational deregulation of oncogenes and tumor suppressor genes. This combined approach is exemplified in the study by Garraway et al., in which the analysis of CN data obtained by SNP arrays drives the investigation of pre-existing gene expression profiles (Garraway et al., 2005). Specifically, CN data were used to organize cancer samples into subgroups characterized by specific chromosomal aberrations associated to contiguous SNP chromosomal clusters. This genomic-based sub-grouping constituted the new phenotypic labeling of the samples in the gene expression analysis, i.e. samples from the NCI-60 cancer cell lines panel were re-grouped into two new classes based on the presence or absence of amplification at 3p14-p13 before performing the supervised analysis. The differential expression profiles, inside the SNP cluster characterizing the amplification at 3p14-p13, identified MITF gene as a novel melanoma-specific oncogene. This study clearly demonstrated the usefulness of an integrative approach to investigate candidate regions and genes specifically involved in tumor etiology and potentially useful as novel specific cancer biomarkers.

Clearly, to allow the rapid development of these innovative analytical procedures, it is necessary to implement novel and even more sophisticated mathematical and statistical algorithms. For instance, an important issue is to understand how combining and comparing microarray expression data of single genes with DNA copy number data of whole chromosomal regions. Thus, there is an increasing interest for developing computational tools able to link single differentially expressed genes to their chromosomal location, in order to calculate differentially expressed chromosomal regions and thus assemble regional transcriptional activity maps (Akavia, 2010; Schäfer, 2009). To address the integrative analysis of gene expression and copy number data in tumor samples, we recently developed a computational tool named Position RElated Data Analysis (*preda*, Ferrari et al., 2011). *preda* is particularly suited for the identification of chromosomal regions with concomitant and coordinated copy number and transcriptional imbalances (SODEGIRs, Bicciato et al., 2009), thus providing an opportunity for upgrading the information content of genomic data and for discovering novel cancer biomarkers.

In this chapter, we describe a general framework for depicting the molecular portrait of ccRCC through the integrative analysis of gene expression and copy number profiles obtained from publicly available datasets. The chapter is structured in Methods, Results and Discussion and addresses three major issues: i) the analysis and the functional characterization of a large compendium of gene expression data; ii) the identification of chromosomal alterations in ccRCC samples from SNP copy number data; iii) the integrative analysis of gene expression and copy number data.

2. Methods

2.1 Gene expression analysis of ccRCC

To characterize the transcriptional portrait of ccRCC, we retrieved 12 datasets containing microarray gene expression data of clear cell renal carcinoma and normal samples annotated with clinical information. All data were measured on several releases of the Affymetrix Human Genome HG-U133 arrays (i.e., HG-U133A; HG-U133 Plus 2.0, HG-U133A 2.0 and HT-HG-U133A) and have been downloaded from the public microarray data repositories Gene Expression Omnibus (GEO, http://www.ncbi.nlm.nih.gov/geo/; 11 datasets) and

Molecular Portrait of Clear Cell Renal Cell Carcinoma: An Integrative Analysis of Gene Expression and
Genomic Copy Number Profiling

27

ArrayExpress (http://www.ebi.ac.uk/arrayexpress/; 1 dataset). Prior to analysis, we re-organized all datasets by manually annotating and tagging all samples, and re-named any original dataset after the first author's name of the corresponding publication. This re-organization resulted in a compendium of 426 samples comprising 320 ccRCCs and 106 normal renal tissues (Table 1). ccRCC samples have been further annotated according to nuclear grade and divided into a low-grade (n=197) and a high-grade (n=123) class, with the low-grade class comprising 29 G1 and 168 G2 samples and the high-grade class including 97 G3 and 26 G4 samples.

| Microarray repository code | Dataset name | Samples | | References |
		ccRCC	normal	
GSE781[a]	Lenburg	9	8	Lenburg et al., 2003
GSE15641[a]	Jones	---	23	Jones et al., 2005
GSE6344[a]	Gumz	---	10	Gumz et al., 2007
GSE7023[b]	Furge	---	13	Furge et al., 2007
GSE14762[b]	Wang	---	12	Wang et al., 2009
GSE2109[b]	Bittner	188	---	International Genomics Consortium
GSE11151[b]	Yusenko	---	3	Yusenko et al., 2009
E-TAM-282[b]	Cifola	16	11	Cifola et al., 2008
GSE17895[b]	Dalgliesh	83	13	Dalgliesh et al., 2010
GSE12606[b]	Stickel	3	3	Stickel et al., 2009
GSE11904[c]	Gordan	21	---	Gordan et al., 2008
GSE14994[d]	Beroukhim	26[e]	11	Beroukhim et al., 2009

Table 1. Independent datasets included in the ccRCC compendium. The Affymetrix platforms used to obtain the original data are: [a]HG-U133A, [b]HG-U133 Plus 2.0, [c]HG-U133A 2.0, and [d]HT-HG-U133A. Samples from Beroukhim dataset ([e]) were used only in the integrative analysis of gene expression and copy number, since no grading annotation was available.

The integration and normalization of gene expression signals, obtained using different types of microarray in different experiments, is the most critical step for the meta-analysis of public available data since their direct integration may result in misleading results, due to dissimilar experimental conditions, laboratory-dependent bias, etc. Although Robust Multiarray Analysis (RMA; Irizarry et al., 2003) is the most effective signal quantification method, it cannot be applied to data obtained from different platforms (e.g., the HG-U133A and the HG-U133 Plus 2.0 arrays), due to differences in number, type and physical position of probes. As such, we implemented a procedure, called the Virtual Chip, to create a custom and virtual microarray grid that integrates the geometry and probe content of two or more types of Affymetrix arrays (Fallarino et al., 2010). Once defined the virtual grid, all raw data (represented by the so called CEL files) are re-organized to match a single platform, i.e. the virtual chip. At this point, raw data, originally from different types of microarrays, become homogeneous in terms of platform and can be preprocessed and normalized adopting standard approaches, as RMA. The Virtual Chip method allows combining data directly at the level of probe fluorescence intensity and presents the advantage that gene expression signals are generated with a single step of background correction, normalization and summarization. The construction of the virtual grid is inspired by the generation of custom Chip Definition Files (CDFs), i.e., of ad-hoc probe designs and array topologies. In custom CDFs, probes matching the same transcript, but belonging to different probe sets, are aggregated into putative custom-probe sets, each one including only those probes with a unique and exclusive correspondence with a single transcript. Similarly, probes matching the same transcript but located at different coordinates on different types of arrays may be merged in custom-probe sets and arranged in a virtual platform grid, whose geometry can be arbitrarily set. As for any other microarray geometry, this virtual grid may be used as a reference to create a virtual CDF file containing the probes of the Virtual Chip and their coordinates on the virtual platform. The probes included in the virtual CDF are those shared among the platforms of interest, with the additional condition of generating custom probe set of at least 4 probes. The virtual CDF can be derived from any custom CDF, e.g., those developed by Dai and publicly accessible at the Molecular and Behavioral Neuroscience Institute Microarray Lab (Dai et al., 2005). Finally, the virtual CDF can be used as the geometry file in RMA as far as the original CEL files are properly re-mapped to match the topology described in the virtual CDF. Re-mapped CEL files, called virtual CEL files, are homogeneous in terms of platform and gene expression data can be generated with a single step of background correction, normalization and summarization directly from the fluorescence signals of all microarrays composing the meta-dataset. In this particular case, expression values of the meta-dataset were generated from intensity signals using the combined HG-U133A/HG-U133 Plus 2.0/HG-U133A 2.0/HT-HG-U133A virtual-CDF file, the custom definition files for Affymetrix human arrays based on Entrez (version 12.1.0; http://brainarray.mbni.med.umich.edu/Brainarray/Database/CustomCDF/12.1.0/entrezg .asp), and the transformed virtual-CEL files. Intensity values of meta-probe sets have been background adjusted, normalized using quantile normalization, and gene expression levels calculated using median polish summarization (RMA algorithm; Irizarry et al., 2003). The final meta-dataset comprised gene expression values for a total of 11809 Entrez gene IDs and 426 samples.

The meta-dataset was analyzed using the Analysis of Variance (ANOVA) package of Partek Genomics Suite software (Version 6.5, http://www.partek.com/; Partek Inc., St Louis, MO, USA) to identify a list of differentially expressed genes (DEGs) between ccRCC samples and normal renal tissues. Specifically, genes have been defined as differentially expressed if the average expression values in the two groups differed of at least 2-folds and the False Discovery Rate (FDR; Benjamini-Hochberg method) of the statistical comparison was less than 0.05. Differentially expressed genes have been functionally characterized in term of Gene Ontology (GO) biological process (BP) using DAVID tool (http://david.abcc. ncifcrf.gov/; (Huang, 2009a, 2009b) with an FDR≤0.001. Ingenuity Pathways Analysis (IPA, version 9.0) has been applied to assess functional connections that are statistically overrepresented among the differentially expressed genes. Briefly, in IPA, a p-value, calculated by a right tailed Fisher's Exact Test, quantifies the probability of observing the fraction of the focus genes in the canonical pathway as compared to the fraction expected by chance in the reference set, with the assumption that each gene is equally likely to be picked by chance. Finally, we investigated whether expression levels in ccRCCs and normal tissues were associated with elevated expression of biologically relevant gene sets using Gene Set Enrichment Analysis (GSEA, http://www.broadinstitute.org/gsea/index.jsp; Subramanian et al., 2005) on the meta-dataset. In particular, 217 BioCarta and 186 KEGG gene sets were

Molecular Portrait of Clear Cell Renal Cell Carcinoma: An Integrative Analysis of Gene Expression and
Genomic Copy Number Profiling

29

taken from the Molecular Signatures Database (http://www.broadinstitute.org/gsea/msigdb/index.jsp; version 3.0) and a list of 145 genes associated to HIF and VHL genes was downloaded from the NCBI Pathway Interaction Database (http://pid.nci.nih.gov). Gene sets have been considered significantly enriched at FDR≤0.25 when using Signal2Noise as metric and 1,000 permutations of phenotype labels.

2.2 Genomic copy number analysis of ccRCC

To assess copy number alterations in ccRCC, we used two datasets composed of 27 sporadic ccRCC samples profiled by Affymetrix Human Mapping 100K SNP arrays and downloaded from AE (E-TAM-283, E-TAM-284; Cifola et al., 2008) and 26 sporadic ccRCC samples profiled by Affymetrix Human Mapping 250K Sty SNP array and downloaded from GEO (GSE14994; Beroukhim et al., 2009). The genomic copy number values were quantified using Partek Genomics Suite and the presence of copy number alterations, i.e., chromosomal segments affected by amplification or deletion, was calculated using Partek Genomic Segmentation (GS) algorithm. Partek baseline generated from 90 Mapping 100K Hind/Xba HapMap trio samples (available at Affymetrix website; http://www.affymetrix.com/support/technical/sample_data/hapmap_trio_data.affx) and 270 Mapping 250K Sty HapMap samples (available at GEO, GSE5173) were used as diploid reference. In the Genomic Segmentation analysis, the cut-off values to identify gains and losses were set to 2.3 and 1.7, respectively, each segment was computed using a minimum of 10 consecutive filtered probe sets, and the threshold p-value and the signal to noise ratio were set to 0.001 and 0.5, respectively.

2.3 Integrative analysis of gene expression and genomic copy number in ccRCC

To address the integrative analysis of gene expression and copy number data we applied *preda* (Position RElated Data Analysis) tool, an R package for detecting regional variations of genomic features from high-throughput data (Ferrari et al., 2011). *preda* is particularly suited for the identification of chromosomal regions with coordinated copy number and transcriptional imbalances (SODEGIRs, Bicciato et al., 2009). In *preda*, custom-designed data structures allow to efficiently manage different types of genomics signals and annotations, different choices of smoothing functions and statistics empower a variety of flexible and robust workflows, and tabular and graphical representations facilitate downstream biological interpretation of results. The computational framework directly integrates copy number and gene expression profiles at genome-wide level, by statistically assessing the gene dosage and transcription statuses on common genomic positions. We applied *preda* to both Cifola and Beroukhim datasets (Table 1). Briefly, Cifola dataset comprises a subset of 11 ccRCC cases profiled by both Affymetrix Human Mapping 100K and HG-U133 Plus 2.0 arrays (Cifola et al., 2008), while Beroukhim dataset includes 26 ccRCC and 11 normal samples analyzed using both Affymetrix Human Mapping 250K and HT-HG-U133A arrays (Beroukhim et al., 2009). Copy number log-ratios were calculated using CNAG software (version 3.3.0.1, http://www.genome.umin.jp/; Nannya, 2005; Yamamoto, 2007), while gene expression levels were estimated using RMA algorithm. Both types of data were used as input to *preda* to identify regions harboring both down-regulated genes and CN loss or both up-regulated genes and CN gain (SODEGIR deleted and SODEGIR amplified signatures, respectively). To further validate the presence of areas of deletion and amplification in a larger panel of samples, we intersected the list of genes associated to the SODEGIR signatures with the list of differentially expressed genes obtained from the ANOVA comparison of the 320 ccRCCs with the 106 normal samples of the meta-dataset (Table 1). Differentially expressed genes and genes comprised in the SODEGIR signatures were annotated using GeneDistiller 2 tool (http://www.genedistiller.org; Seelow et al., 2008). Literature mining was performed using PubMatrix tool (http://pubmatrix.grc.nia.nih.gov/; Becker et al., 2003) and applying specific keywords such as *cancer, renal cell carcinoma, amplification, methylation, oncogene, tumor suppressor and biomarker.*

3. Result

3.1 Differential gene expression profiling of ccRCC

The aim of this analysis was to functionally characterize the transcriptional profiles that differentiate cancer specimens from normal tissues. We based our initial analysis on the weight of gene expression data, taking advantage of bioinformatics techniques that allow direct interrogation of differentially expressed genes for activation of specific signaling pathways. The cohort of 426 samples composing the meta-dataset was analyzed by ANOVA to identify a list of differentially expressed genes between ccRCC and normal renal tissues. This comparison resulted in 1036 genes specifically modulated more than 2 folds in ccRCC cancers and that showed 95% of statistical confidence for differential expression. The fold change distribution ranged from -210 to 41, although the majority of DEGs showed an expression modulation varying from 2 to 4 folds. As depicted in the clustering map of Figure 1, the 534 up-regulated and 502 down-regulated genes grouped the meta-dataset samples into two clearly defined differential patterns of transcriptional activation in tumor samples as compared to normal tissues.

The functional and biological characterization of the 1036 differentially expressed genes using Gene Ontology (GO) annotation highlighted that the most significant processes and pathways altered in ccRCC are consistent with the important role of aerobic metabolism typically associated to epithelial cancers (Figure 2). In particular, we observed a down regulation of genes associated to metabolism and transport counteracted by the up regulation of genes associated to signal transduction and cell communication. The GO functional characterization indicated that ccRCC decrements the expression of genes related to oxido-reductase activity, amine catabolism, amine and exose biosynthesis, fatty acid metabolism, excretion and secretion, response to hormone, ion transport (Figure 2, panel A) while induces the transcription of genes related to the immune response, response to wounding, defense response, angiogenesis, response to oxygen level, cell proliferation, chemotaxis, cell adhesion and motility, and T-cell activation (Figure 2, panel B).

A further functional characterization of the differentially expressed genes using the knowledge database of Ingenuity Pathway Analysis (IPA) pointed out *cancer* and *genetic disorder* as the most significant enriched categories (p-value≤0.0001 and more than 200 genes). Specifically, IPA analysis associated the modulated genes to the categories of *renal cancer* (ACAT1, BTG2, C7orf68, CA9, CD70, CDH6, CLCNKB, CP, CSF1R, DEFB1, EDNRA, EGF, EPCAM, FGFR3, GPC3, IGF2BP3, IGFBP2, INHBB, KDR, KNG1, MME, MMP9, MUC1, MYC, NR3C1, PDGFRA, RRM2, SFRP1, SLC6A3, TIMP1, TOP2A, TUBA1A, TUBB2A, VEGFA), *cancer progression* (AHR, BCL6, CCND1, CDKN1B, CXCL12, IFI16, KIF2A, MYC, NR4A1, PLAGL1, TGFB1), *angiogenesis* (ANGPTL3, ANGPTL4, ANXA3, APOH, AQP1, ARHGAP24, BTG1, COL4A2, COL4A3, CXCR4, EGF, ITGA5, KDR, MTDH, SERPINE1, SPARC, VASH1, VEGF), *cell cycle* (AHR, CCND1, DEGS1, NEFL, CDKN1B, MMP9), *cell*

Molecular Portrait of Clear Cell Renal Cell Carcinoma: An Integrative Analysis of Gene Expression and
Genomic Copy Number Profiling

31

binding (ABCA1, CAV1, CD2, COL4A3, CXCL12, CXCR4, FGF1, GPC3, IGFBP3, ITGA5, ITGAM, ITGB2, KNG1, SCARB1, SDC1, SERPINE1, SLC6A3, SPARC, ST6GAL1, TGFB1, TLR2, UMOD, VCAM1, VEGFA, VWF), *cell adhesion* (ADAM10, ADAM9, ANGPT2, C3, CCL5, CD93, CDH13, CR2, CXCL12, CYFIP2, FXYD5, INHBB, ITGA4, ITGA5, ITGAM, ITGB2, KDR, KLK6, MARCKS, PECAM1, PLAU, PLXND1, POSTN, ROCK1, SERPINE1, SLIT2, TGFB1, TIMP1, VCAM1, VEGFA, ZEB2), *chemotaxis* (ADAM10, CCL20, CCL5, CD36, CDH13, CXCL11, CXCL12, CXCR4, EGF, HMGB2, KDR, PDGFRA, PLAU, RARRES2, SERPINE1, SLIT2, TGFB1, TLR2, VEGFA), and *fragmentation of DNA* (ABCB1, AIFM1, BNIP3, CLU, DNASE1L3, EGF, FAS, NOX4, SFRP1, SOD2). Moreover, the IPA network analysis resulted in 20 networks including, each one, more than 13 focus molecules and confirmed the previous GO findings of functional activities in mechanisms related to *cell death, cell to cell signaling and interaction, cellular movement,* and *cancer*. Table 2 enlists the top four networks that are mainly enriched in up regulated genes.

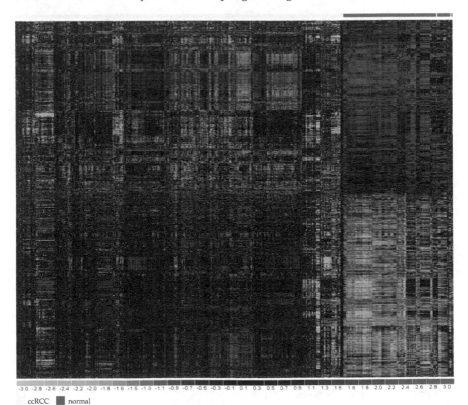

Fig. 1. Clustering map of ccRCC and normal samples based on the list of 1036 differentially expressed genes identified by ANOVA in the comparison between cancer and normal specimens. Each row represents a single gene and each column an experimental sample. Samples are separated into two main groups enriched for ccRCC (upper yellow bar) and normal tissues (upper blue bar). The map has been obtained using the hierarchical clustering of dChip (Li & Wong, 2001) with Pearson correlation and centroid as distance metric and linkage, respectively.

A.

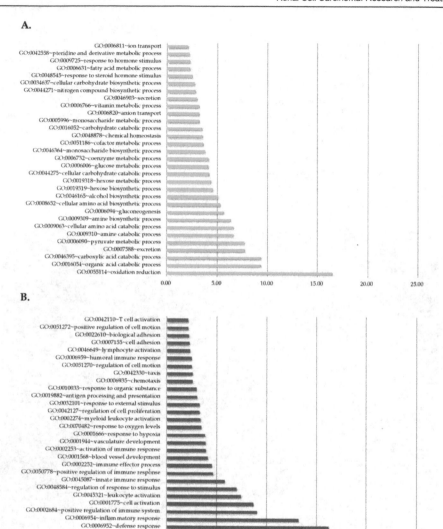

B.

Fig. 2. Functional characterization in terms of GO Biological Process of the 502 down-regulated genes (panel A) and of the 534 up-regulated genes (panel B). On the X-axis the log(FDR) of DAVID enrichment test is reported.

To gain further insight into the biological pathways engaged in ccRCC phenotype, we used bioinformatics classifiers, or gene signatures, that register a modulated activity (either activation or inactivation) of specific signaling pathways in tumor samples. In particular, Gene Set Enrichment Analysis (GSEA) allowed identifying 25 inactivated and 50 activated pathways in cancer samples. The inactivated signaling modules relate to aminoacid metabolism, glucose and lipid metabolism, molecule transport, drug metabolism, glycolysis and gluconeogenesis, oxidative metabolism and immune signaling (Table 3).

Molecules in Network	Score[a]	Focus Molecules[b]	Top Functions
ACTN1, ANGPTL4, ARPC1B, BARD1, BTG1, CASP1, CASP4, CD2, CD70, CLU, CORO1C, CSTA, DNASE1L3, EDN1, GLIPR1, GLUL, GPR65, IFIH1, IL7, IL7R, KDM3A, LGALS1, MAL, NOL3, NR3C1, PLAGL1, PLP2, SCARB1, SERPINB1, SERPINE1, STAT5a/b, TMSB10/TMSB4X, TNFAIP6, TNFAIP8, TNFRSF1B	34	34	Cell Death, Inflammatory Response, Cellular Growth and Proliferation
APOH, BCR, CCL5, CD14, COL4A1, COL4A2, DDX58, Fibrinogen, HLA-F, IFN Beta, IL12 (complex), ISG15, ITGAM, ITGB2, KNG1, LY96, MMP9, NFkB (complex), P38 MAPK, PLAT, PLAU, POSTN, PYCARD, ROCK1, TAP1, TGFB1, TIMP1, TLR1, TLR2, TLR3, TLR7, TNIP1, TRAF3IP2, TRIB3, VCAM1	26	30	Cell-To-Cell Signaling and Interaction, Inflammatory Response, Hematological System Development and Function
ADAM10, AHR, Akt, ANXA1, BAZ1A, C3, C3AR1, CASR, CDH13, CR2, CXCL12, CXCR4, EGF, EIF4EBP1, ERBB4, ERK1/2, GJB1, IGFBP2, IGFBP3, IL1RL1, ITGA5, KDR, KL, LDL, MYOF, PI3K (complex), PLG, PRKCZ, PTPRC, Ras homolog, RCAN1, SLC6A3, TCF4, VDR, VEGFA	26	30	Cellular Movement, Inflammatory Disease, Cellular Growth and Proliferation
ACTG2, AGTR1, ANK2, AUH, BDKRB2, CCNDBP1, CLMN, COL5A1, COL5A2, COL5A3, CSDA, CTH, FBL, GNL2, ID2, IL7, MYH10, NAP1L1, NCL, NTRK2, PLK2, PMP22, PTPN3, RB1, RRAD, S100A2, SPTBN1, TNFRSF1B, TOP2A, TP53, TP73, TP53I3, TSPAN1, TUBA1A, UBE2D1	16	23	Cancer, Neurological Disease, Cellular Development

Table 2. Top four significant networks identified by the IPA network analysis on the list of differentially expressed genes (red, up-regulated DEG; green, down-regulated DEG; black, not regulated). [a] The score column indicates the -log(p-value), while [b] the focus molecules column quantifies the number of modulated genes in the network.

Among the most activated pathways (Table 4), we found association to cancer (renal cell carcinoma and chronic myeloid leukemia) and oncogenic signatures characterized by the presence of several well-known cancer genes (CCND1, MYC, RB1, TP53, RUNX1, AKT2, KRAS, CRKL, CSK, MDM2, NRAS, MET, RAP1A, APC, SHC1, PTEN, ATR, ATM, VAV1, LYN, ROCK1). Some of these signatures are inter-connected through key genes, as the tumor suppressor gene TP53 and the oncogene MYC. As expected, given the fundamental role of hypoxia in renal cell carcinoma, the *HIF and VHL* gene set resulted activated in ccRCC, as illustrated by the high ES score and by the clear-cut pattern of expression of HIF- and VHL- regulated genes in ccRCCs and normal tissues (Table 4 and Figure 3). Among the most active players of this signature, there are genes associated to *angiogenesis* (EDN1, VEGFA), *cell survival* (ATM, MYC), *glucose influx* (SLC2A1), *pH control* (CA9), *oxidative and iron metabolism* (PGK1, HK2, CP, HMOX1) and *HIF processing* (EGLN3, EGLN1). Additional gene sets were related to *cell fate and survival*, *cell to cell signaling* and *kinase signaling*. Furthermore, several pathways activated in ccRCC are associated to *immune signaling*,

Biological context	GSEA gene set	ES	FDR
Amino acid metabolism	Valine leucine and isoleucine degradation	-0.807	0.141
	Propanoate metabolism	-0.804	0.168
	Beta alanine metabolism	-0.769	0.138
	Glycine serine and threonine metabolism	-0.723	0.133
	Arginine and proline metabolism	-0.695	0.153
	Tryptophan metabolism	-0.655	0.152
	Histidine metabolism	-0.654	0.157
	Alanine aspartate glutamate metabolism	-0.604	0.144
	Lysine degradation	-0.580	0.140
	Selenoamino acid metabolism	-0.572	0.145
	Cysteine and methionine metabolism	-0.492	0.174
Differentiation	Taste transduction	-0.601	0.227
	Cardiac muscle contraction	-0.462	0.198
Drug metabolism	Drug metabolism cytochrome P450	-0.662	0.137
	Metabolism of xenobiotics by cytochrome P450	-0.638	0.139
Glyco-metabolism	Pyruvate metabolism	-0.624	0.141
	Glycolysis and gluconeogenesis	-0.504	0.227
Immuno signaling	Vibrio cholerae infection	-0.465	0.185
Lipid metabolism	Glycerolipid metabolism	-0.517	0.152
	Fatty acid metabolism	-0.691	0.150
Mitochondrial metabolism	Citrate cycle TCA cycle	-0.718	0.196
Molecule transport	Aldosterone regulated sodium reabsorption	-0.612	0.213
	Peroxisome	-0.588	0.143
Oxidative metabolism	Butanoate metabolism	-0.763	0.171
	Retinol metabolism	-0.641	0.168

Table 3. List of pathways identified as inactivated in the cancer phenotype by GSEA. All pathways belong to gene sets derived from the KEGG pathway database. The ES and FDR columns indicate the enrichment score (i.e., the degree to which a gene set is overrepresented at the top or bottom of a ranked list of genes) and the statistical significance (i.e., the estimated probability that a gene set with a given ES represents a false positive finding).

Molecular Portrait of Clear Cell Renal Cell Carcinoma: An Integrative Analysis of Gene Expression and
Genomic Copy Number Profiling

35

including for instance NFKB, TOLL like receptor, T cell receptor, and NK cell, in which also many cytokines (i.e. IL18, CCL5, IL8, CCL4, IL7) and their receptors (i.e. IL7R, IL2RG) are involved. Finally, the enrichment analysis evidenced a role for genes involved in *DNA repair and replication* (e.g. MSH2, POLD2, RFC2, RFC4, RFC5, PCNA, SSBP1, LIG1).

Biological context	GSEA gene set	ES	FDR
Angiogenesis	VEGF pathway	0.478	0.222
Cancer	Chronic myeloid leukemia	0.410	0.216
	Renal cell carcinoma	0.441	0.206
Cell differentiation	Notch signaling pathway	0.388	0.245
	Calcineurin pathway	0.539	0.235
	Dorso ventral axis formation	0.586	0.232
Cell fate and survival	Apoptosis	0.372	0.232
	Raccycd pathway	0.479	0.243
	PTEN pathway	0.550	0.220
	Chemical pathway	0.555	0.246
	PML pathway	0.601	0.192
Cell to cell signaling	Systemic lupus erythematosus	0.510	0.233
	Viral myocarditis	0.544	0.155
	Leishmania infection	0.621	0.196
	Graft versus host disease	0.682	0.148
	Asthma	0.687	0.166
	Allograft rejection	0.711	0.180
DNA repair	Nucleotide excision repair	0.513	0.152
	DNA replication	0.682	0.205
	Mismatch repair	0.687	0.242
Glyco-metabolism	Type I diabetes mellitus	0.636	0.173
	Glycosaminoglycan biosynthesis chondroitin sulfate	0.666	0.157
Hypoxia	HIF and VHL	0.518	0.197
Immuno signaling	T cell receptor signaling pathway	0.413	0.227
	NFKB pathway	0.449	0.232
	Natural killer cell mediated cytoxicity	0.457	0.211
	HIVNEF pathway	0.460	0.240
	TOLL like receptor signaling pathway	0.486	0.224
	HCMV pathway	0.503	0.241
	NOD like receptor signaling pathway	0.510	0.235
	Cytosolic DNA sensing pathway	0.540	0.230
	IL7 pathway	0.565	0.239
	CSK pathway	0.577	0.248
	Autoimmune Thyroid disease	0.596	0.237
	Intestinal immune network for IGA production	0.609	0.207
	NKT pathway	0.618	0.227
	NKCELLS pathway	0.645	0.219
	NO2IL12 pathway	0.684	0.237
	TH1TH2 pathway	0.733	0.221

Kinase signaling	PAR1 pathway	0.419	0.241
	P38MAPK pathway	0.459	0.219
Molecule transport	Snare interactions in vesicular transport	0.455	0.232
Oncogenic signaling	MTOR signaling pathway	0.431	0.226
	FCER1 pathway	0.443	0.239
	WNT pathway	0.458	0.230
	GCR pathway	0.471	0.245
	P53 signaling pathway	0.559	0.166
	GSK3 pathway	0.566	0.236
	ARF pathway	0.572	0.231
	ATRBRCA pathway	0.627	0.185
Transcription	RNA degradation	0.482	0.231

Table 4. List of pathways identified as activated in the cancer phenotype by GSEA. All pathways belong to gene sets derived from BioCarta and KEGG pathway databases, with the exception of the HIF and VHL list that has been derived from NCBI Pathway Interaction Database. The ES and FDR columns indicate the enrichment score (i.e., the degree to which a gene set is overrepresented at the top or bottom of a ranked list of genes) and the statistical significance (i.e., the estimated probability that a gene set with a given ES represents a false positive finding).

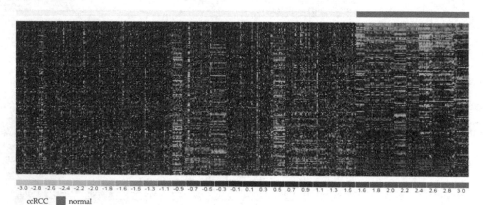

-3.0 -2.8 -2.6 -2.4 -2.2 -2.0 -1.8 -1.6 -1.5 -1.3 -1.1 -0.9 -0.7 -0.5 -0.3 -0.1 0.1 0.3 0.5 0.7 0.9 1.1 1.3 1.5 1.6 1.8 2.0 2.2 2.4 2.6 2.8 3.0

ccRCC   ■ normal

Fig. 3. Standardized gene expression levels of the 145 genes composing the HIF and VHL signaling pathway in ccRCC (upper yellow bar) and normal samples (upper blue bar). Each row represents a single gene and each column an experimental sample. Genes are ordered according to GSEA enrichment score. The map has been obtained using the hierarchical clustering of dChip (Li & Wong, 2001).

We finally investigated whether exists a grade-dependent specific transcriptional signature and compared the two groups of ccRCC cases previously classified as high (G3 and G4) and low grade (G1 and G2) classes. ANOVA differential analysis identified 44 differentially expressed genes (10 up-regulated and 34 down-regulated genes in high grade) that have been grouped according to their cellular localization to highlight putative grade-dependent clinical biomarkers (Table 5). Among the modulated genes, we found *transporters* (COPG, SLC27A2, FABP4, SLCO2A1, SLC17A4, SLC47A1, SLC17A3, SLC6A3), *enzymes* (SOD2,

Molecular Portrait of Clear Cell Renal Cell Carcinoma: An Integrative Analysis of Gene Expression and
Genomic Copy Number Profiling

37

BHMT, HAO2, ADH1B, MGAM, FMO2, ALDOB, GBA3, BBOX1, ABP1, DNASE1L3), *G-protein coupled receptors* (EDNRB, AGTR1, RGS5), *growth factors* (IGFBP1, PDGFD), *transmembrane receptors* (TMEM204, OSMR) and five *transcription regulators* (TFPI2, PPP1R1A, EMX2, NAT8, RCAN2).

Cellular location	Up-regulated	Down-regulated
Cytoplasm	PPP1R1A, COPG, KRT19, SOD2	PCK1, FABP4, BBOX1, GBA3, C13orf15, C5orf23, ALDOB, SCGN, ADH1B, HAO2, BHMT, APOLD1
Endoplasmic Reticulum Membrane		FMO2, SLC27A2, SLC17A3
Extracellular Space	SPOCK1, IGFBP1, TFPI2, MT1X	EMCN, ABP1, PDGFD, UMOD
Nucleus		DNASE1L3, EMX2, XIST, AUTS2, RCAN2
Plasma Membrane	RARRES, OSMR	SLC6A3, AGTR1, RGS5, SLC47A1, SLC17A4, EDNRB, SLCO2A1, TMEM204, MGAM, NAT8

Table 5. Cellular location of the 44 differentially expressed genes identified between high and low grade samples.

Despite the intrinsic heterogeneity of the meta-dataset (due to the combination of different experimental sets), when applied to cluster the 320 ccRCC samples, the grade-dependent specific transcriptional signature was able to segregate the high-grade phenotypes in an homogenous group characterized by a general down regulation of gene expression (Figure 4).

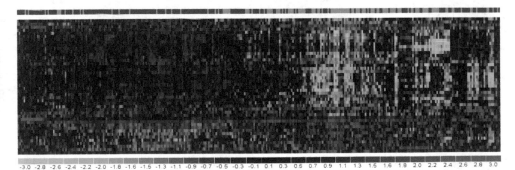

-3.0 -2.8 -2.6 -2.4 -2.2 -2.0 -1.8 -1.6 -1.5 -1.3 -1.1 -0.9 -0.7 -0.5 -0.3 -0.1 0.1 0.3 0.5 0.7 0.9 1.1 1.3 1.5 1.6 1.8 2.0 2.2 2.4 2.6 2.8 3.0

▪ low grade   ▪ high grade

Fig. 4. Clustering map of high and low grade ccRCC samples based on the list of 44 differentially expressed genes identified by ANOVA in the comparison between high and low grade samples. Each row represents a single gene and each column an experimental sample. Samples are separated into two main groups enriched for low (upper blue bars) and high grade (upper orange bars). The map has been obtained using the hierarchical clustering of dChip (Li and Wong2001) with Pearson correlation and centroid as distance metric and linkage, respectively.

3.2 Copy number profiling of ccRCC

Genetic studies on ccRCC clinical samples characterized some recurrent alterations in precise chromosomal regions (i.e. deletions of chromosomes 3p, 6q, 8p, 9p, 14q, and amplifications of chromosomes 5q and 7). To confirm the copy number signature of ccRCC, we analyzed the CN profile of two independent datasets by SNP array technology with different resolution level. As showed in Figure 5, the genome-wide assessment of copy number alterations characterizing 27 and 26 sporadic ccRCC samples profiled by Affymetrix Human Mapping 100K and 250K Sty Array, respectively, revealed that all autosomes were affected by either CN gain or loss or both of them. In Cifola dataset (panel A), the most frequently amplified regions were on chromosomes 4q, 5 (p and q arms), 7 (p and q arms), 11p and 12q, whereas the most recurrent deleted region was identified on chromosome 3p. The longest recurrent amplifications resulted on chromosomes 1 (p and q arms), 2 (p and q arms), 3q, 11q, 16q, 18q and 19p, often spanning two or more consecutive megabases. These DNA alterations presented frequencies ranging from 6 to 12 samples. Similarly, the CN profile of Beroukhim dataset (panel B), obtained with a denser SNP array, showed that the most frequently amplified regions were on chromosomes 5 (p and q arms), 7 (p and q arms), 11p, 12q, 19 and 20, whereas the most recurrent deleted regions were identified on chromosomes 3p, 6, 8q, 9 and 14. Overall, we observed that the CNA profile obtained from the two datasets were globally overlapping, so confirming the typical ccRCC genomic signature. Due to the higher density of SNP array used in their study, Beroukhim et al. were able to better discriminate some CNAs as compared to Cifola dataset (i.e. the loss on chromosomes 8p, 11q, 14q, 15, and the gain on chromosomes 11p, 12, 19, 20).

A.   **B.**

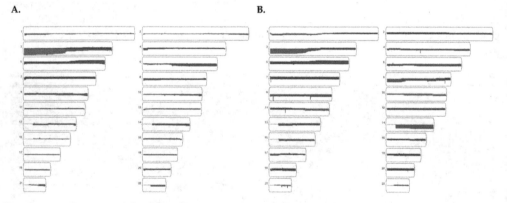

Fig. 5. Visualization of the CNA frequencies occurring in Cifola (panel A) and Beroukhim datasets (panel B). Regions of DNA copy number gain (red bar) and copy number loss (blue bar) are represented along each chromosome (from 1 to 22, ordered horizontally). X chromosome was omitted from this analysis.

3.3 Integrative analysis of gene expression and copy number data

In order to identify chromosomal regions with coordinated copy number and transcriptional imbalances (SODEGIRs), we performed the integrative analysis on the two independent datasets with paired gene expression and copy number data (namely, Cifola and Beroukhim). In Cifola dataset, *preda* analysis revealed segments of amplified

Molecular Portrait of Clear Cell Renal Cell Carcinoma: An Integrative Analysis of Gene Expression and
Genomic Copy Number Profiling

39

SODEGIR located at 5q21.3-q35.3 (from 130 to 180Mb) and a single deleted SODEGIR at 3p14.1-p22.3 (from 35 to 60 Mb) (Figure 6, panel A). Similar imbalanced regions were found for chromosomes 3 and 5 in Beroukhim dataset (Figure 6, panel B), although the lower probe density of the gene expression platform utilized in this study (i.e., the HG-U133A arrays) did not allow a finer resolution of the chromosomal segments as compared to Cifola dataset.

A.   **B.**

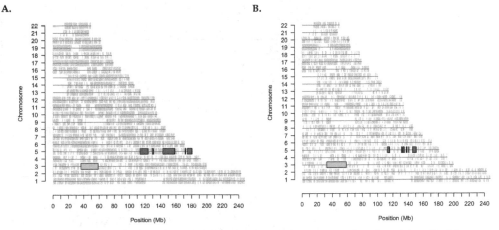

Fig. 6. SODEGIR amplified (red) and deleted (green) chromosomal regions identified by *preda* in the integrative analysis of gene expression and copy number data for Cifola (panel A) and Beroukhim dataset (panel B).

To further study the influence of gene dosage associated to structural position as one of the mechanism of transcriptional regulation, the genes located at SODEGIR signature (199 and 147 genes in deleted and amplified SODEGIRs, respectively) were intersected with the list of differentially expressed genes, identified by ANOVA in the comparison between ccRCC and normal tissues of meta-dataset. Overall, we found that 68% of the genes associated to the deleted signature (136 out of 199 genes) resulted down-regulated in the meta-dataset, while 61% of the genes associated to amplified signature (90 out of 147 genes) were up regulated at a statistically significant level. The most differentially down-regulated genes ranged from -2 to -10 fold changes (PTH1R, ACY1, ACOX2, IL17RB, HYAL1, UQCRC1, ACAA1, DNASE1L3, SEMA3G, ABHD14A, AMT, APEH, ALS2CL, CISH, MYL3, SEMA3B, HIGD1A, PLXNB1, PDHB), while the most up regulated ranged from 2 to 3.5 fold changes (TNFAIP8, LOX, SPARC, CSF1R, TCERG1, LOXL2, SPARCL1, YIPF5, RPS14, ABLIM3, TNIP1, STK10, CLK4). IPA annotation grouped these genes in the biological categories of *transcription and translation regulator, transmembrane receptor, enzyme* and *kinase* (Table 6), while Gene Distiller and PubMatrix highlighted that genes of the deleted SODEGIR are associated to *tumor suppressor function* (DLEC1, TMEM158, PTHR1, SEDT2, LIMD19, FAM107A, BAP1), *epigenetic modification* (STAC, CTDSPL, DLEC1, PRSS50, SEDT2, IP6K1, SEMA3B, TUSC2, PARP3, PRKCD) and *chromosomal deletion* (DLEC1, LIMD1, LTF, RBM6, IRFd2, TUSC2, COL7A1), and genes of the amplified SODEGIR are enriched in *oncogenes* (CSF1R, PDGFRB, LOX, DUSP1, SPARC, ITK, FLT4, GNB2L1, LARS, CD74, F12, MAML1, SQSTM1) and associated to *gene amplification* (CSF1R, PDGFRB, LOX, NSD1).

Biological category	Deleted SODEGIR 3p14.1-p22	Amplified SODEGIR 5q21.3-q35.3
Transcription and translation regulator	RAD54L2, LIMD1, ZNF197, ZNF35, SMARCC1, EIF1B	TCERG1, FEM1C, CNOT8, ZNF354A, NSD1, SQSTM1, MED7, MAML1, SOX30, MXD3, RPS14
Transmembrane receptor	DAG1, NISCH, PLXNB1, IL17RB	CD74, FLT4
Enzyme	HEMK1, ARIH2, TKTL1, GMPPB, PARP3, MLH1, DHX30, SETD2, LARS2, ABHD5, P4HTM, ABHD6, CYB561D2, RPP14, ENTPD3, PLCD1, EXOSC7, ALAS1, PDHB, AMT, ABHD14A, DNASE1L3, ACAA1, UQCRC1, HYAL1, ACOX2	LOX, LOXL2, DDX41, LTC4S, GM2A, THG1L, GNB2L1, DPYSL3, MGAT1, LARS, MGAT4B, HINT1, HNRNPAB, PGGT1B, G3BP1, GFPT2, PPIC, B4GALT7
Kinase	MAP4K2, PRKAR2A, MST1R, OXSR1, ULK4, PRKCD, CAMKV, ACVR2B, NPRL2, MAPKAPK3, NME6, IP6K1	CSF1R, STK10, CLK4, ITK, PDGFRB, CSNK1A1, HK3, CSNK1G3, MAPK9

Table 6. Biological function of the subset of differentially expressed genes located into SODEGIRs.

4. Discussion

In this chapter we illustrated the identification of distinct molecular profiles in ccRCC samples using experimental data available in public repositories and published in peer-reviewed articles (Brannon & Rathmell, 2010). To exemplify how genomic data can be exploited to functionally characterize the molecular characteristics of renal carcinoma, we downloaded more than 500 ccRCC samples from public repositories of genomic data and, after manual selection, we created a compendium (meta-dataset) of gene expression and copy number profiles in 320 ccRCCs, annotated with the nuclear grade information, and 106 normal samples mainly representing adjacent renal tissues from the same surgical specimen. The bioinformatics analysis of gene expression profiles allowed the identification of lists of differentially expressed genes and of gene signatures activated in the cancer phenotype. Additionally, the comprehensive analysis of copy number profiles highlighted characteristic chromosomal aberrations affecting ccRCC cases and the integration of gene expression and copy number data revealed the presence of chromosomal regions with concomitant transcriptional and gene dosage imbalances.

As recently reviewed by Pal et al. (Pal et al., 2010), several gene expression and proteomic studies carried out on fresh and archival ccRCC tissues (Perroud, 2009; Seliger, 2009) evidenced a series of molecular processes and pathways involved in ccRCC tumorigenesis (Banumathy & Cairns, 2010) and indicated that ccRCC progression is strictly associated to the adaptation of cancer cells to low oxygen levels (Baldewijns, 2010; Bristow & Hill, 2008) and to their continuous proliferation even in the presence of compromised DNA repair mechanisms (Semenza, 2008). These results find an additional confirmation from the analysis of genomic data presented in this chapter. Indeed, the application of different bioinformatics tools resulted in a list of genes (e.g., VEGFA, MYC, CA9, SLC2A1, BNIP3, CXCR4, EGLN3 alias PDH3, SERPINA1, KDR, ATM, CP) highly activated in ccRCC and related to hypoxia signaling, known to be targets of the transcription factor HIF-1α or involved in cancer and pathways (as apoptosis and angiogenesis) which have been already targeted for therapeutic intervention in RCC (Pantuck et al., 2003). As expected, among the up-regulated genes, there is the well-known cancer gene MYC (Gordan, 2007, 2008) that several studies indicated as modulated by HIF-1α (Dang, 2008; Gordan, 2007; Podar & Anderson, 2010) and playing a fundamental role in ccRCC proliferation (Tang et al., 2009).

Focusing the investigation to genes and pathways more specifically associated to ccRCC, the analysis of molecular profiles confirmed the presence of the *adipogenic signature* characterized by the up-regulation of genes such as FABP7, NR3C1, ANGPTL4, CAV2, CAV1, and the down-regulation of FABP1 and of the transcription factors TFCP2L1 and GATA3, as previously reported by Tun et al. (Tun et al., 2010). Loss of cell-cell adhesion and cell polarity is commonly observed in epithelial tumors and correlates with their invasion into adjacent tissues and generation of metastases. Many evidences indicate that loss of cell polarity and cell-cell adhesion may also be important in early stages of neoplastic transformation (Coradini et al., 2011). Disruption of intercellular junctions and alterations in cell polarity are specific hallmarks of epithelial cancer cells. In fact, most human tumors arising in epithelial tissues gradually lose their polarized morphology and acquire a mesenchymal phenotype (*epithelial-mesenchymal transition*, EMT) (Thiery, 2003, 2009). Accordingly, and in concordance with Tun et al. (Tun et al., 2010), we observed the up-regulation of several EMT-associated genes (TGFB1, SPARC, VIM, MTHFD2, HSPG2, PROCR, COL3A1, ZEB2), indicating the involvement of this biological process in cancer cell progression and spreading in host tissues, as confirmed very recently by a study on the protein expression of important EMT mediators in ccRCC (Mikami et al., 2011). Among the other up-regulated genes and pathways (Table 4), the up regulation of gene transcription factor 4 (TCF4) confirmed previous evidences of the interplay between Wnt/β-catenin and PI3K/Akt signaling cascades and its involvement in tumor development and progression (Chen et al., 2011). Furthermore, the activation of a series of *immuno pathways*, especially antigen presenting and processing pathways, is quite striking in ccRCC and has been recently demonstrated by the proteomic identification of tumor antigen-derived peptides in RCC (Seliger et al., 2011). In particular, the CD74 up-regulation is suggested to be linked to the PI3K/Akt- and MEK/ERK-dependent intracellular signaling cascades, both associated with NF-kB nuclear translocation and DNA-binding activity (Liu et al., 2008).

Overall, the elucidation of the functional role of the ccRCC activated signaling pathways could be useful for the identification of novel cancer markers or for the development of molecular–targeted therapeutic agents. Taking into account the biological localization and functional roles of genes up regulated in ccRCC, we propose a series of genes that could represent candidate biomarkers for further investigations (Table 7).

Symbol	Description	References
ANXA4	annexin A4	Shi et al., 2004; Jones et al., 2005; Seliger et al., 2009
CA9	carbonic anhydrase IX	Atkins et al., 2004; Pantuck et al., 2005; Zhao et al., 2006; Osunkoya et al., 2009; Zhou et al., 2010
CAV1	caveolin-1	Campbell et al., 2003; Waalkes et al., 2011
CD70	CD70 molecule	Junker et al., 2005; Law et al., 2009
CD74	class II major histocompatibility complex-associated invariant chain	Young et al., 2001; Liu et al., 2008
CDH6	cadherin 6, type 2, K-cadherin (fetal kidney)	Shimazui et al., 2004; Paul et al., 2004
CP	ceruloplasmin (ferroxidase)	Osunkoya et al., 2009;
CXCR4	CXC chemokine receptor-4	Staller et al., 2003; Struckmann et al., 2008
ENGL3	prolyl hydroxylase-3 (PHD3)	Zhao et al., 2006; Sato et al., 2008; Tanaka et al., 2011; Dalgliesh et al., 2010
IGFBP3	insulin-like growth factor binding protein 3	Yao et al., 2005; Takahashi et al., 2005; Chuang et al., 2008
MMP9	matrix metallopeptidase 9 (gelatinase B, 92kDa gelatinase, 92kDa type IV collagenase)	Struckmann et al., 2008; Mikami et al., 2011
NNMT	nicotinamide N-methyltransferase	Yao et al., 2005; Seliger et al., 2009; Kim et al., 2010; Teng et al., 2011
STC2	stanniocalcin 2	Meyer et al., 2009
VEGFA	vascular endothelial growth factor A	Skubitz & Skubitz, 2002; Lam et al., 2005; Liu et al., 2010; Zhou et al., 2010

Table 7. List of candidate biomarker genes up regulated in ccRCC.

In particular, *Annexin A4* (ANXA4) is a member of the annexin family of calcium-dependent phospholipid binding proteins and can exist as a soluble protein as well as a membrane-associated protein. ANXA4 could play an important role in regulating the cellular functions at the level of cell–cell interaction, cell adhesion and motility and, although increased protein expression level of ANXA4 has been confirmed in ccRCC by global proteomic analysis (Seliger et al., 2009), its possible implication in the carcinogenesis of RCC deserves further studies. *Carbonic anhydrase 9* (CA9) is a transmembrane member of the carbonic anhydrase family that catalyses the reversible hydration of carbon dioxide into bicarbonate and a proton, thus enabling tumor cells to maintain a neutral pH despite an acidic microenvironment. CA9 is not expressed in healthy renal tissue but is expressed in most ccRCCs through HIF-1α accumulation driven by hypoxia and inactivation of the VHL gene.

Molecular Portrait of Clear Cell Renal Cell Carcinoma: An Integrative Analysis of Gene Expression and
Genomic Copy Number Profiling

43

CA9 expression can be detected in the tumor by immunohistochemistry (IHC) and in blood and tissue by ELISA assay and RT-PCR (Truong & Shen, 2011). In metastatic disease, high CA9 expression reported by IHC was indicated as a powerful prognostic marker for better survival and sensitivity to IL-2 treatment, although the robustness of this association is still debated (Atkins, 2004; Pantuck, 2005). Almost no data are currently available about the association of CA9 expression and response to targeted drugs. The prognostic value of CA9 in ccRCC could be explained by the frequent VHL gene inactivation driving an early activation of the HIF pathway. The poorer prognosis associated with low CA9 expressing tumors could be attributed to the simultaneous over-expression of EGFR contributing to the activation of Akt-mTOR pathways. Targeting CA9 by inhibitors, radioimmunotherapy, monoclonal antibodies or vaccination is promising and offers new avenues for clinical research (Tostain et al., 2010). Recently, it was reported that serum CA9 levels are significantly higher in ccRCC than in non-ccRCC samples and may help in the differential diagnosis of RCC. Serum CA9 levels also correlate with tumor size in ccRCC patients (Zhou et al., 2010). The role of *caveolin-1* (CAV1) in RCC pathogenesis is still controversial, as it is considered involved in both suppression and promotion of tumor growth and development. However, its increased expression has been used as marker of less favorable outcome in patients with both clinically confined ccRCC (Campbell et al., 2003) and distant metastasis (Waalkes et al., 2011), thus suggesting to be a candidate prognostic marker for RCC aggressiveness. *CD70 protein* (CD70) is a type II transmembrane protein belonging to the tumor necrosis factor family. It represents the ligand for CD27, a glycosylated transmembrane protein of the tumor necrosis factor receptor family. CD70 protein has been found expressed at a high level in ccRCCs by IHC (Junker et al., 2005). The role of this protein in tumorigenesis and its utility as diagnostic marker in serum and urine or as therapeutic tool certainly deserves further studies. *Cadherin-6* (CDH6) is an adhesion molecule that was proved to be marker of poor prognosis and metastases development in ccRCC (Paul, 2004; Shimazui, 2004). *Ceruroplasmin* (CP) is a protein involved in iron metabolism, is regulated by HIF-1α (Martin et al., 2005) and has been associated to metastatic potential and tumor progression. Serum CP protein level has been found elevated in RCC and other malignancies as compared to healthy controls, indicating its potentiality as a cancer biomarker (Osunkoya et al., 2009). *CXC chemokine receptor-4* (CXCR4) is a target of the VHL-HIF pathway and Staller et al. (Staller, 2003; Struckmann, 2008) demonstrated that its high expression is associated to poor survival. *Prolyl hydroxylase-3* (PHD3/ENGL3) is a member of the PHD family, which is involved in the degradation of HIF proteins in cooperation with VHL protein under normoxic conditions. PHD3 was found frequently over-expressed in RCC tissues, with high specificity to cancer samples (Zhao et al., 2006) and its usefulness as a novel tumor antigen for RCC immunotherapy has been recently demonstrated in clinical serum samples from RCC patients (Sato, 2008; Tanaka, 2011). *Insulin-like growth factor binding protein 3* (IGFBP3) is one of the most over-expressed genes in ccRCC (Takahashi, 2005; Yao, 2005) and its increased protein expression has been demonstrated in 74% of ccRCCs by IHC and associated with higher Fuhrman nuclear grade (Chuang et al., 2008). *Matrix metallopeptidase 9* (MMP9) has been reported increased in ccRCC and associated to survival. Statistical analysis indicated that elevated Snail, MMP2 and MMP9 protein expression are significantly correlated to worse disease-free and disease-specific survival of RCC patients (Mikami et al., 2011). MMP9, TIMP1 and CXCR4 have been studied both in vitro and in vivo and the data strongly indicated that VHL coordinately regulates the expression of metastasis-associated genes CXCR4/CXCL12 and

MMP2/MMP9, but the exact regulatory molecular mechanism remains to be determined (Struckmann et al., 2008). Some of the genes here mentioned have been validated at protein level, as *nicotinamide n-methyltransferase* (NNMT) and *enolase 2* (ENO2) proteins whose expression was found increased in RCC by Western blot (Teng et al., 2011). Increased cytoplasmic expression of *stanniocalcin 2* (STC2) was found correlated to other conventional indicators of RCC aggressiveness and to shorter overall survival. STC2 could become an additional tissue biomarker that may be useful in the post-operative risk stratification of RCC patients (Meyer et al., 2009). The increased expression of vascular *endothelial growth factor A* (VEGFA) was predictive of distant metastases development and lymph node involvement and was significantly associated with poor survival (Lam et al., 2005). These studies have paved the way for the development of new therapeutic agents to block VEGF signaling and the cascade of events leading to tumor formation. In a randomized phase II clinical trial on 116 metastatic ccRCC patients, the use at high doses of a neutralizing antibody against VEGFA (bevacizumab) resulted in a significant prolongation of the time to progression of disease (Yang et al., 2003).

According to the canonical classification of ccRCC (Flanigan et al., 2011), the Furhman nuclear grade is one of the most important parameters for RCC prognosis prediction (Nese et al., 2009), together with stage, age, tumor position and size, necrosis and other few molecular biomarkers (e.g., CA9). Noticeably, recent grade-dependent proteomic characterization reported that MYC, HIF-1α and p53 are the major hubs of the network obtained analyzing formalin-fixed paraffin embedded ccRCC tissues (Perroud et al., 2009). Chen et al (Chen et al., 2009) analyzed the correlation between chromosome aberrations and clinical pathological variables, including tumor stage and nuclear grade, and observed a significant association between LOH at chromosomes 9, 14q and 18q and higher nuclear grade. In the present study, we identified SOD2, KRT19 and OSM as potential grade-dependent ccRCC biomarkers. Briefly, *manganese superoxide dismutase* (SOD2) belongs to the antioxidant gene family and has emerged as a key enzyme with a dual role in tumorigenic progression (Hempel et al., 2011). Recently, SOD2 has been indicated as marker for circulating tumor cells in prostate cancer (Giesing et al., 2010) and potentially predictive for lymph node metastasis in tongue squamous cell carcinoma (Liu et al., 2010). *Keratin 19* (KRT19) encodes for one of the cytoskeleton cytokeratins and has been identified as a novel candidate tumor suppressor gene epigenetically inactivated in RCC cell lines and primary tumors (Morris et al., 2008). This gene was found to be functionally related to miR-492 and crucially involved in neoplastic progression of malignant embryonic liver tumors (von Frowein et al., 2011). *Oncostatin M* (OSM) is a member of the IL-6 cytokine family implicated in signal transduction; its receptor (OSMR) was found increased at both gene copy number and expression levels in gastric cancer (Junnila et al., 2010) and cervical squamous cell carcinomas, in association with poor survival (Scotto et al., 2008). However, to our knowledge, no previous studies exist that link OSMR to renal carcinogenesis. The clinical application of these genes as potential ccRCC grade-dependent biomarkers deserves further investigation in well curate and extensive collections of ccRCC cases.

The analysis of copy number levels in a total of 53 ccRCC samples profiled with SNP arrays (Beroukhim, 2009; Cifola, 2008) identified and confirmed the typical genomic signature of ccRCC, as recently showed by higher density SNP arrays (Dalgliesh et al., 2010). The most frequent CN alterations in ccRCC samples are the deletion of 3p and the amplification of 5q.

Similarly, Chen et al. detected gains of chromosome 5q33.1-qter and losses of chromosome 3p21.31-p22.3 in 58% and 80% of the 80 RCC samples analyzed using Illumina 317K SNP arrays (Chen et al., 2009), respectively. Noticeably, these regions have great influence on the expression levels of the resident genes as previously demonstrated by integrative genomic studies (Beroukhim, 2009; Bicciato, 2009; Cifola, 2008; Furge, 2004). In accordance, the comprehensive integrative analysis pinpointed that the two most significant chromosomal regions with coordinated copy number and transcriptional imbalances (SODEGIRs) are localized at the same chromosomal arms (Figure 6). Although the integrative analysis presented here was conducted using a completely different approach from that applied by Beroukhim et al. (Beroukhim et al., 2009), both studies identified 12 over-expressed genes located at the 5q peak region (GNB2L1, MGAT1, RUFY, RNF130, MAPK9, CANX, SQSTM1, LTC4S, TBC1D9B, HNRPH1, FLT4). Among them, the ubiquitin-binding protein *sequestosome 1* (SQSTM1) was found also in the focal amplification region at 5q35.3 by Chen et al. (Chen et al., 2009) and was reported over-expressed in breast and prostate tumors (Kitamura, 2006; Thompson, 2003). Moreover, we confirmed that, as previously evidenced by Cifola and co-workers (Cifola et al., 2008) and recently confirmed at proteomic level (Liu et al., 2010), *lyxyl oxidase* (LOX) is over-expressed in ccRCC. LOX is one of the critical HIF-1α targets mediating tumor progression and catalyzes the cross-linking of collagens and elastin in the extracellular matrix, thereby regulating tissue tensile strength (Erler & Giaccia, 2006). Paradoxically, LOX has been reported to be both up-regulated and down-regulated in cancer cells, especially in colorectal cancer (Baker, 2011; Pez, 2011). Mechanistic investigations revealed that LOX activates the PI3K-Akt signaling pathway, thereby up-regulating HIF-1α protein synthesis in a manner requiring LOX-mediated hydrogen peroxide production. Concordantly with these results, cancer cell proliferation was stimulated by secreted and active LOX in a HIF-1α-dependent fashion (Pez et al., 2011). Our data suggest that the transcriptional modulation of LOX might be also driven by genomic imbalance. Among the significant down-modulated genes located at the deleted SODEGIR on chromosome 3p14.1-p22, it is worthwhile mentioning two potential tumor suppressor genes, i.e. *deleted in lung cancer* (DLEC1), previously reported as candidate tumor suppressor silenced by methylation in RCC cell lines and primary tumors and with growth inhibitory function tested in in vitro experiments (Zhang et al., 2010a), and *SET domain containing 2* (SETD2), encoding for an histone H3 methyltransferase and found affected by inactivating mutations in 12-17% of ccRCCs, together with other components of the chromatin modification machinery (Dalgliesh et al., 2010).

Although some of these genes could represent novel candidate biomarkers, their role in ccRCC etiology requires further investigations and, given the heterogeneity of tumor tissues, the functional analysis of molecular mechanisms associated to ccRCC progression should be likely conducted on primary cultures as in vitro model of ccRCC. Indeed, primary cultures from RCC and normal tissues at early passages retain the phenotypic features (Bianchi,2010; Perego, 2005) and genomic profile (Cifola et al., 2011) of corresponding original tissues, while providing a more homogeneous cytological material. The integrative analysis of molecular profiles of RCC primary cultures may be particularly useful to elucidate the role of some of the many genes and pathways found typically deregulated in this pathology and to highlight key players in RCC biology.

5. Conclusion

As showed in this chapter, the availability of high-density molecular data as gene expression and copy number profiles, and of bioinformatics approaches for their analysis, allows depicting a finer molecular portrait of ccRCC and confirming previous findings about important genes and gene regulatory pathways associated to this renal cancer subtype. The genome-wide integration of DNA copy number data and transcriptional profiles elucidates the interplay between DNA content and global expression patterns and highlights candidate genes that are actively involved in the causation or maintenance of the malignant phenotype. Altogether, these data indicate the presence of candidate *driver* genes important for ccRCC development that undoubtedly deserve further investigation since they may constitute novel specific cancer biomarkers.

6. Acknowledgment

This work was supported by grants from the Italian Ministry of University and Research: FIRB 2003 (n. RBLA03ER38_004); PRIN 2008 (GDB); FIRB 2007 (Rete nazionale per lo studio del proteoma umano, n. RBRN07BMCT); AIRC Special Program Molecular Clinical Oncology "5 per mille".VT is recipient of a fellow of Scuola di dottorato di medicina molecolare,Università degli Studi di Milano. SN is a PhD student of the School of Biosciences and Biotechnology, curriculum Genetics and Molecular Biology of Development, University of Padova.

7. References

Akavia, U. D., Litvin, O., Kim, J., Sanchez-Garcia, F., Kotliar, D., Causton, H. C., Pochanard, P., Mozes, E., Garraway, L. A., & Pe'er, D. (2010). *An integrated approach to uncover drivers of cancer.* Cell, 143(6):1005–1017.

Arsanious, A., Bjarnason, G. A., & Yousef, G. M. (2009). *From bench to bedside: current and future applications of molecular profiling in renal cell carcinoma.* Mol Cancer, 8:20.

Atkins, M., Regan, M., Stanbridge, E., Upton, M., Youmans, A., Febbo, P., Lechpammer, M., & Signoretti S. (2004). *Carbonic anhydrase IX (CAIX) expression predicts for renal cell cancer (RCC) patient response and survival to IL-2 therapy.* In Journal of Clinical Oncology. 22(Supplement 14):4512.

Baker, A. M., Cox, T. R., Bird, D., Lang, G., Murray, G. I., Sun, X. F., Southall, S. M., Wilson, J. R., & Erler, J. T. (2011). *The role of lysyl oxidase in src-dependent proliferation and metastasis of colorectal cancer.* J Natl Cancer Inst, 103(5):407–424.

Baldewijns, M. M., van Vlodrop, I. J. H., Vermeulen, P. B., Soetekouw, P. M., van Engeland, M., & de Bruïne, A. P. (2010). *VHL and HIF signalling in renal cell carcinogenesis.* J Pathol, 221(2):125–138.

Banks, R. E., Tirukonda, P., Taylor, C., Hornigold, N., Astuti, D., Cohen, D., Maher, E. R., Stanley, A. J., Harnden, P., Joyce, A., Knowles, M., & Selby, P. J. (2006). *Genetic and epigenetic analysis of von Hippel-Lindau (VHL) gene alterations and relationship with clinical variables in sporadic renal cancer.* Cancer Res, 66(4):2000–2011.

Banumathy, G. & Cairns, P. (2010). *Signaling pathways in renal cell carcinoma.* Cancer Biol Ther, 10(7):658–664.

Becker, K. G., Hosack, D. A., Dennis, G., Lempicki, R. A., Bright, T. J., Cheadle, C., & Engel, J. (2003). *PubMatrix: a tool for multiplex literature mining.* BMC Bioinformatics, 4:61.

Beroukhim, R., Brunet, J. P., Napoli, A. D., Mertz, K. D., Seeley, A., Pires, M. M., Linhart, D., Worrell, R. A., Moch, H., Rubin, M. A., Sellers, W. R., Meyerson, M., Linehan, W. M., Kaelin, W. G., & Signoretti, S. (2009). *Patterns of gene expression and copy-number alterations in von-Hippel Lindau disease-associated and sporadic clear cell carcinoma of the kidney.* Cancer Res, 69(11):4674–4681.

Bianchi, C., Bombelli, S., Raimondo, F., Torsello, B., Angeloni, V., Ferrero, S., Stefano, V. D., Chinello, C., Cifola, I., Invernizzi, L., Brambilla, P., Magni, F., Pitto, M., Zanetti, G., Mocarelli, P., & Perego, R. A. (2010). *Primary cell cultures from human renal cortex and renal-cell carcinoma evidence a differential expression of two spliced isoforms of annexin A3.* Am J Pathol, 176(4):1660–1670.

Bicciato, S., Spinelli, R., Zampieri, M., Mangano, E., Ferrari, F., Beltrame, L., Cifola, I., Peano, C., Solari, A., & Battaglia, C. (2009). *A computational procedure to identify significant overlap of differentially expressed and genomic imbalanced regions in cancer datasets.* Nucleic Acids Res, 37(15):5057–5070.

Brannon, A. R. & Rathmell, W. K. (2010). *Renal cell carcinoma: where will the state-of-the-art lead us?* Curr Oncol Rep, 12(3):193–201.

Brannon, A. R., Reddy, A., Seiler, M., Arreola, A., Moore, D. T., Pruthi, R. S., Wallen, E. M., Nielsen, M. E., Liu, H., Nathanson, K. L., Ljungberg, B., Zhao, H., Brooks, J. D., Ganesan, S., Bhanot, G., & Rathmell, W. K. (2010). *Molecular stratification of clear cell renal cell carcinoma by consensus clustering reveals distinct subtypes and survival patterns.* Genes Cancer, 1(2):152–163.

Brenner, B. M. & Rosenberg, D. (2010). *High-throughput SNP/CGH approaches for the analysis of genomic instability in colorectal cancer.* Mutat Res, 693(1-2):46–52.

Bristow, R. G. & Hill, R. P. (2008). *Hypoxia and metabolism. hypoxia, DNA repair and genetic instability.* Nat Rev Cancer, 8(3):180–192.

Campbell, L., Gumbleton, M., & Griffiths, D. F. R. (2003). *Caveolin-1 overexpression predicts poor disease-free survival of patients with clinically confined renal cell carcinoma.* Br J Cancer, 89(10):1909–1913.

Chari, R., Thu, K. L., Wilson, I. M., Lockwood, W. W., Lonergan, K. M., Coe, B. P., Malloff, C. A., Gazdar, A. F., Lam, S., Garnis, C., MacAulay, C. E., Alvarez, C. E., & Lam, W. L. (2010). *Integrating the multiple dimensions of genomic and epigenomic landscapes of cancer.* Cancer Metastasis Rev, 29(1):73–93.

Chen, L., Huang, K., Han, L., Shi, Z., Zhang, K., Pu, P., Jiang, C., & Kang, C. (2011). *β-catenin/tcf-4 complex transcriptionally regulates AKT1 in glioma.* Int J Oncol, 39(4):883–890.

Chen, M., Ye, Y., Yang, H., Tamboli, P., Matin, S., Tannir, N. M., Wood, C. G., Gu, J., & Wu, X. (2009). *Genome-wide profiling of chromosomal alterations in renal cell carcinoma using high-density single nucleotide polymorphism arrays.* Int J Cancer, 125(10):2342–2348.

Chow, W. H., Dong, L. M., & Devesa, S. S. (2010). *Epidemiology and risk factors for kidney cancer.* Nat Rev Urol, 7(5):245–257.

Chuang, S. T., Patton, K. T., Schafernak, K. T., Papavero, V., Lin, F., Baxter, R. C., Teh, B. T., & Yang, X. J. (2008). *Over expression of insulin-like growth factor binding protein 3 in clear cell renal cell carcinoma.* J Urol, 179(2):445–449.

Cifola, I., Bianchi, C., Mangano, E., Bombelli, S., Frascati, F., Fasoli, E., Ferrero, S., Stefano, V. D., Zipeto, M. A., Magni, F., Signorini, S., Battaglia, C., & Perego, R. A. (2011). *Renal cell carcinoma primary cultures maintain genomic and phenotypic profile of parental tumor tissues.* BMC Cancer, 11:244.

Cifola, I., Spinelli, R., Beltrame, L., Peano, C., Fasoli, E., Ferrero, S., Bosari, S., Signorini, S., Rocco, F., Perego, R., Proserpio, V., Raimondo, F., Mocarelli, P., & Battaglia, C. (2008). *Genome-wide screening of copy number alterations and LOH events in renal cell carcinomas and integration with gene expression profile.* Mol Cancer, 7:6.

Cohen, H. T. & McGovern, F. J. (2005). *Renal-cell carcinoma.* N Engl J Med, 353(23):2477–2490.

Coradini, D., Casarsa, C., & Oriana, S. (2011). *Epithelial cell polarity and tumorigenesis: new perspectives for cancer detection and treatment.* Acta Pharmacol Sin, 32(5):552–564.

Dai, M., Wang, P., Boyd, A. D., Kostov, G., Athey, B., Jones, E. G., Bunney, W. E., Myers, R. M., Speed, T. P., Akil, H., Watson, S. J., & Meng, F. (2005). *Evolving gene/transcript definitions significantly alter the interpretation of GeneChip data.* Nucleic Acids Res, 33(20):e175.

Dalgliesh, G. L., Furge, K., Greenman, C., Chen, L., Bignell, G., Butler, A., Davies, H., Edkins, S., Hardy, C., Latimer, C., Teague, J., Andrews, J., Barthorpe, S., Beare, D., Buck, G., Campbell, P. J., Forbes, S., Jia, M., Jones, D., Knott, H., Kok, C. Y., Lau, K. W., Leroy, C., Lin, M. L., McBride, D. J., Maddison, M., Maguire, S., McLay, K., Menzies, A., Mironenko, T., Mulderrig, L., Mudie, L., O'Meara, S., Pleasance, E., Rajasingham, A., Shepherd, R., Smith, R., Stebbings, L., Stephens, P., Tang, G., Tarpey, P. S., Turrell, K., Dykema, K. J., Khoo, S. K., Petillo, D., Wondergem, B., Anema, J., Kahnoski, R. J., Teh, B. T., Stratton, M. R., & Futreal, P. A. (2010). *Systematic sequencing of renal carcinoma reveals inactivation of histone modifying genes.* Nature, 463(7279):360–363.

Dang, C. V., Kim, J. W., Gao, P., & Yustein, J. (2008). *The interplay between MYC and HIF in cancer.* Nat Rev Cancer, 8(1):51–56.

Eichelberg, C., Junker, K., Ljungberg, B., & Moch, H. (2009). *Diagnostic and prognostic molecular markers for renal cell carcinoma: a critical appraisal of the current state of research and clinical applicability.* Eur Urol, 55(4):851–863.

Erler, J. T. & Giaccia, A. J. (2006). *Lysyl oxidase mediates hypoxic control of metastasis.* Cancer Res, 66(21):10238–10241.

Fallarino, F., Volpi, C., Fazio, F., Notartomaso, S., Vacca, C., Busceti, C., Bicciato, S., Battaglia, G., Bruno, V., Puccetti, P., Fioretti, M. C., Nicoletti, F., Grohmann, U., & Marco, R. D. (2010). *Metabotropic glutamate receptor-4 modulates adaptive immunity and restrains neuroinflammation.* Nat Med, 16(8):897–902.

Ferrari, F., Solari, A., Battaglia, C., & Bicciato, S. (2011). *Preda: an R-package to identify regional variations in genomic data.* Bioinformatics, 27(17):2446–2447.

Flanigan, R. C., Polcari, A. J., & Hugen, C. M. (2011). *Prognostic variables and nomograms for renal cell carcinoma.* Int J Urol, 18(1):20–31.

Furge, K. A., Chen, J., Koeman, J., Swiatek, P., Dykema, K., Lucin, K., Kahnoski, R., Yang, X. J., & Teh, B. T. (2007). *Detection of DNA copy number changes and oncogenic signaling abnormalities from gene expression data reveals MYC activation in high-grade papillary renal cell carcinoma.* Cancer Res, 67(7):3171–3176.

Molecular Portrait of Clear Cell Renal Cell Carcinoma: An Integrative Analysis of Gene Expression and
Genomic Copy Number Profiling

49

Furge, K. A., Lucas, K. A., Takahashi, M., Sugimura, J., Kort, E. J., Kanayama, H., Kagawa, S., Hoekstra, P., Curry, J., Yang, X. J., & Teh, B. T. (2004). *Robust classification of renal cell carcinoma based on gene expression data and predicted cytogenetic profiles.* Cancer Res, 64(12):4117–4121.

Garraway, L. A., Widlund, H. R., Rubin, M. A., Getz, G., Berger, A. J., Ramaswamy, S., Beroukhim, R., Milner, D. A., Granter, S. R., Du, J., Lee, C., Wagner, S. N., Li, C., Golub, T. R., Rimm, D. L., Meyerson, M. L., Fisher, D. E., & Sellers, W. R. (2005). *Integrative genomic analyses identify MITF as a lineage survival oncogene amplified in malignant melanoma.* Nature, 436(7047):117–122.

Giesing, M., Suchy, B., Driesel, G., & Molitor, D. (2010). *Clinical utility of antioxidant gene expression levels in circulating cancer cell clusters for the detection of prostate cancer in patients with prostate-specific antigen levels of 4-10 ng/ml and disease prognostication after radical prostatectomy.* BJU Int, 105(7):1000–1010.

Gong, K., Zhang, N., Zhang, K., & Na, Y. (2010). *The relationship of erythropoietin overexpression with von hippel-lindau tumour suppressor gene mutations between hypoxia-inducible factor-1⟨ and -2⟨ in sporadic clear cell renal carcinoma.* Int J Mol Med, 26(6):907–912.

Gordan, J. D., Lal, P., Dondeti, V. R., Letrero, R., Parekh, K. N., Oquendo, C. E., Greenberg, R. A., Flaherty, K. T., Rathmell, W. K., Keith, B., Simon, M. C., & Nathanson, K. L. (2008). *HIF-alpha effects on c-MYC distinguish two subtypes of sporadic VHL-deficient clear cell renal carcinoma.* Cancer Cell, 14(6):435–446.

Gordan, J. D., Thompson, C. B., & Simon, M. C. (2007). *HIF and c-MYC: sibling rivals for control of cancer cell metabolism and proliferation.* Cancer Cell, 12(2):108–113.

Grade, M., Ghadimi, B. M., Varma, S., Simon, R., Wangsa, D., Barenboim-Stapleton, L., Liersch, T., Becker, H., Ried, T., & Difilippantonio, M. J. (2006). *Aneuploidy-dependent massive deregulation of the cellular transcriptome and apparent divergence of the Wnt/beta-catenin signaling pathway in human rectal carcinomas.* Cancer Res, 66(1):267–282.

Gumz, M. L., Zou, H., Kreinest, P. A., Childs, A. C., Belmonte, L. S., LeGrand, S. N., Wu, K. J., Luxon, B. A., Sinha, M., Parker, A. S., Sun, L. Z., Ahlquist, D. A., Wood, C. G., & Copland, J. A. (2007). *Secreted frizzled-related protein 1 loss contributes to tumor phenotype of clear cell renal cell carcinoma.* Clin Cancer Res, 13(16):4740–4749.

Gunawan, B., Huber, W., Holtrup, M., von Heydebreck, A., Efferth, T., Poustka, A., Ringert, R. H., Jakse, G., & Füzesi, L. (2001). *Prognostic impacts of cytogenetic findings in clear cell renal cell carcinoma: gain of 5q31-qter predicts a distinct clinical phenotype with favorable prognosis.* Cancer Res, 61(21):7731–7738.

Harding, M. A., Arden, K. C., Gildea, J. W., Gildea, J. J., Perlman, E. J., Viars, C., & Theodorescu, D. (2002). *Functional genomic comparison of lineage-related human bladder cancer cell lines with differing tumorigenic and metastatic potentials by spectral karyotyping, comparative genomic hybridization, and a novel method of positional expression profiling.* Cancer Res, 62(23):6981–6989.

Heidenblad, M., Lindgren, D., Veltman, J. A., Jonson, T., Mahlamäki, E. H., Gorunova, L., van Kessel, A. G., Schoenmakers, E. F., & Höglund, M. (2005). *Microarray analyses reveal strong influence of DNA copy number alterations on the transcriptional patterns in pancreatic cancer: implications for the interpretation of genomic amplifications.* Oncogene, 24(10):1794–1801.

Hempel, N., Carrico, P. M., & Melendez, J. A. (2011). *Manganese superoxide dismutase (SOD2) and redox-control of signaling events that drive metastasis.* Anticancer Agents Med Chem, 11(2):191–201.

Höglund, M., Gisselsson, D., Soller, M., Hansen, G. B., Elfving, P., & Mitelman, F. (2004). *Dissecting karyotypic patterns in renal cell carcinoma: an analysis of the accumulated cytogenetic data.* Cancer Genet Cytogenet, 153(1):1–9.

Huang, D. W., Sherman, B. T., & Lempicki, R. A. (2009). *Bioinformatics enrichment tools: paths toward the comprehensive functional analysis of large gene lists.* Nucleic Acids Res, 37(1):1–13.

Huang, D. W., Sherman, B. T., & Lempicki, R. A. (2009a). *Systematic and integrative analysis of large gene lists using DAVID bioinformatics resources.* Nat Protoc, 4(1):44–57.

Hyman, E., Kauraniemi, P., Hautaniemi, S., Wolf, M., Mousses, S., Rozenblum, E., Ringnér, M., Sauter, G., Monni, O., Elkahloun, A., Kallioniemi, O. P., & Kallioniemi, A. (2002). *Impact of DNA amplification on gene expression patterns in breast cancer.* Cancer Res, 62(21):6240–6245.

Irizarry, R. A., Hobbs, B., Collin, F., Beazer-Barclay, Y. D., Antonellis, K. J., Scherf, U., & Speed, T. P. (2003). *Exploration, normalization, and summaries of high density oligonucleotide array probe level data.* Biostatistics, 4(2):249–264.

Jones, J., Otu, H., Spentzos, D., Kolia, S., Inan, M., Beecken, W. D., Fellbaum, C., Gu, X., Joseph, M., Pantuck, A. J., Jonas, D., & Libermann, T. A. (2005). *Gene signatures of progression and metastasis in renal cell cancer.* Clin Cancer Res, 11(16):5730–5739.

Junker, K., Hindermann, W., von Eggeling, F., Diegmann, J., Haessler, K., & Schubert, J. (2005). *CD70: a new tumor specific biomarker for renal cell carcinoma.* J Urol, 173(6):2150–2153.

Junnila, S., Kokkola, A., Karjalainen-Lindsberg, M. L., Puolakkainen, P., & Monni, O. (2010). *Genome-wide gene copy number and expression analysis of primary gastric tumors and gastric cancer cell lines.* BMC Cancer, 10:73.

Kaelin, W. G. (2007). *The von Hippel-Lindau tumor suppressor protein and clear cell renal carcinoma.* Clin Cancer Res, 13(2 Pt 2):680s–684s.

Kaelin, W. G. (2008). *The von Hippel-Lindau tumour suppressor protein: O2 sensing and cancer.* Nat Rev Cancer, 8(11):865–873.

Kim, D. S., Choi, Y. P., Kang, S., Gao, M. Q., Kim, B., Park, H. R., Choi, Y. D., Lim, J. B., Na, H. J., Kim, H. K., Nam, Y. P., Moon, M. H., Yun, H. R., Lee, D. H., Park, W. M., & Cho, N. H. (2010). *Panel of candidate biomarkers for renal cell carcinoma.* J Proteome Res, 9(7):3710–3719.

Kitamura, H., Torigoe, T., Asanuma, H., Hisasue, S. I., Suzuki, K., Tsukamoto, T., Satoh, M., & Sato, N. (2006). *Cytosolic overexpression of p62 sequestosome 1 in neoplastic prostate tissue.* Histopathology, 48(2):157–161.

Klatte, T., Rao, P. N., de Martino, M., LaRochelle, J., Shuch, B., Zomorodian, N., Said, J., Kabbinavar, F. F., Belldegrun, A. S., & Pantuck, A. J. (2009). *Cytogenetic profile predicts prognosis of patients with clear cell renal cell carcinoma.* J Clin Oncol, 27(5):746–753.

Molecular Portrait of Clear Cell Renal Cell Carcinoma: An Integrative Analysis of Gene Expression and
Genomic Copy Number Profiling

51

Klatte, T., Seligson, D. B., Riggs, S. B., Leppert, J. T., Berkman, M. K., Kleid, M. D., Yu, H.,
Kabbinavar, F. F., Pantuck, A. J., & Belldegrun, A. S. (2007). *Hypoxia-inducible factor
1 alpha in clear cell renal cell carcinoma*. Clin Cancer Res, 13(24):7388–7393.

Lam, J. S., Pantuck, A. J., Belldegrun, A. S., & Figlin, R. A. (2007). *Protein expression profiles in
renal cell carcinoma: staging, prognosis, and patient selection for clinical trials*. Clin
Cancer Res, 13(2 Pt 2):703s–708s.

Lam, J. S., Yu, H., Seligson, D. B., Dong, J., Horvath, S., Pantuck, A. J., Figlin, R. A. &
Belldegrun A. S. (2005). *Expression of the vascular endothelial growth factor family in
tumor dissemination and disease free survival in clear cell renal cell carcinoma*. In Journal
of Clinical Oncology, 23(Supplement 16):4538.

Law, C. L., McEarchern, J. A., & Grewal, I. S. (2009). *Novel antibody-based therapeutic agents
targeting CD70: a potential approach for treating Waldenström's macroglobulinemia*. Clin
Lymphoma Myeloma, 9(1):90–93.

Lenburg, M. E., Liou, L. S., Gerry, N. P., Frampton, G. M., Cohen, H. T., & Christman, M. F.
(2003). *Previously unidentified changes in renal cell carcinoma gene expression identified
by parametric analysis of microarray data*. BMC Cancer, 3:31.

Li, C. & Wong, W. H. (2001). *Model-based analysis of oligonucleotide arrays: model validation,
design issues and standard error application*. Genome Biol, 2(8):RESEARCH0032.

Lisovich, A., Chandran, U. R., Lyons-Weiler, M. A., LaFramboise, W. A., Brown, A. R.,
Jakacki, R. I., Pollack, I. F., & Sobol, R. W. (2011). *A novel SNP analysis method to
detect copy number alterations with an unbiased reference signal directly from tumor
samples*. BMC Med Genomics, 4:14.

Liu, X., Wang, A., Muzio, L. L., Kolokythas, A., Sheng, S., Rubini, C., Ye, H., Shi, F., Yu, T.,
Crowe, D. L., & Zhou, X. (2010). *Deregulation of manganese superoxide dismutase
(SOD2) expression and lymph node metastasis in tongue squamous cell carcinoma*. BMC
Cancer, 10:365.

Liu, Y. H., Lin, C. Y., Lin, W. C., Tang, S. W., Lai, M. K., & Lin, J. Y. (2008). *Up-regulation of
vascular endothelial growth factor-D expression in clear cell renal cell carcinoma by CD74:
a critical role in cancer cell tumorigenesis*. J Immunol, 181(9):6584–6594.

Majewski, I. J. & Bernards, R. (2011). *Taming the dragon: genomic biomarkers to individualize the
treatment of cancer*. Nat Med, 17(3):304–312.

Martin, F., Linden, T., Katschinski, D. M., Oehme, F., Flamme, I., Mukhopadhyay, C. K.,
Eckhardt, K., Tröger, J., Barth, S., Camenisch, G., & Wenger, R. H. (2005). *Copper-
dependent activation of hypoxia-inducible factor (HIF)-1: implications for ceruloplasmin
regulation*. Blood, 105(12):4613–4619.

Maxwell, P. H. (2005). *The HIF pathway in cancer*. Semin Cell Dev Biol, 16(4-5):523–530.

Meyer, H. A., Tölle, A., Jung, M., Fritzsche, F. R., Haendler, B., Kristiansen, I., Gaspert, A.,
Johannsen, M., Jung, K., & Kristiansen, G. (2009). *Identification of stanniocalcin 2 as
prognostic marker in renal cell carcinoma*. Eur Urol, 55(3):669–678.

Mikami, S., Katsube, K. I., Oya, M., Ishida, M., Kosaka, T., Mizuno, R., Mukai, M., & Okada,
Y. (2011). *Expression of snail and slug in renal cell carcinoma: E-cadherin repressor snail is
associated with cancer invasion and prognosis*. Lab Invest .

Molina, A. M., & Motzer, R. J. (2011). *Clinical practice guidelines for the treatment of metastatic
renal cell carcinoma: today and tomorrow*. Oncologist, 16 Suppl 2:45–50.

Morris, M. R., Gentle, D., Abdulrahman, M., Clarke, N., Brown, M., Kishida, T., Yao, M., Teh, B. T., Latif, F., & Maher, E. R. (2008). *Functional epigenomics approach to identify methylated candidate tumour suppressor genes in renal cell carcinoma.* Br J Cancer, 98(2):496–501.

Motzer, R. J. (2011). *New perspectives on the treatment of metastatic renal cell carcinoma: an introduction and historical overview.* Oncologist, 16 Suppl 2:1–3.

Nannya, Y., Sanada, M., Nakazaki, K., Hosoya, N., Wang, L., Hangaishi, A., Kurokawa, M., Chiba, S., Bailey, D. K., Kennedy, G. C., & Ogawa, S. (2005). *A robust algorithm for copy number detection using high-density oligonucleotide single nucleotide polymorphism genotyping arrays.* Cancer Res, 65(14):6071–6079.

Nese, N., Paner, G. P., Mallin, K., Ritchey, J., Stewart, A., & Amin, M. B. (2009). *Renal cell carcinoma: assessment of key pathologic prognostic parameters and patient characteristics in 47,909 cases using the national cancer data base.* Ann Diagn Pathol, 13(1):1–8.

Teng, P. N., Hood, B. L., Sun, M., Dhir, R., & Conrads, T. P. (2011). *Differential proteomic analysis of renal cell carcinoma tissue interstitial fluid.* J Proteome Res, 10(3):1333–1342.

Osunkoya, A. O., Yin-Goen, Q., Phan, J. H., Moffitt, R. A., Stokes, T. H., Wang, M. D., & Young, A. N. (2009). *Diagnostic biomarkers for renal cell carcinoma: selection using novel bioinformatics systems for microarray data analysis.* Hum Pathol, 40(12):1671–1678.

Pal, S. K., Kortylewski, M., Yu, H., & Figlin, R. A. (2010). *Breaking through a plateau in renal cell carcinoma therapeutics: development and incorporation of biomarkers.* Mol Cancer Ther, 9(12):3115–3125.

Pantuck, A. J., Zeng, G., Belldegrun, A. S., & Figlin, R. A. (2003). *Pathobiology, prognosis, and targeted therapy for renal cell carcinoma: exploiting the hypoxia-induced pathway.* Clin Cancer Res, 9(13):4641–4652.

Pantuck, A. J., Fang, Z., Liu, X., Seligson, D. B., Horvath, S., Leppert, J. T., Belldegrun, A. S., & Figlin, R. A. (2005). *Gene expression and tissue microarray analysis of interleukin-2 complete responders in patients with metastatic renal cell carcinoma.* In Journal of Clinical Oncology. *23(Supplement 16):4535.*

Paul, R., Necknig, U., Busch, R., Ewing, C. M., Hartung, R., & Isaacs, W. B. (2004). *Cadherin-6: a new prognostic marker for renal cell carcinoma.* J Urol, 171(1):97–101.

Perego, R. A., Bianchi, C., Corizzato, M., Eroini, B., Torsello, B., Valsecchi, C., Fonzo, A. D., Cordani, N., Favini, P., Ferrero, S., Pitto, M., Sarto, C., Magni, F., Rocco, F., & Mocarelli, P. (2005). *Primary cell cultures arising from normal kidney and renal cell carcinoma retain the proteomic profile of corresponding tissues.* J Proteome Res, 4(5):1503–1510.

Perego, R. A., Corizzato, M., Brambilla, P., Ferrero, S., Bianchi, C., Fasoli, E., Signorini, S., Torsello, B., Invernizzi, L., Bombelli, S., Angeloni, V., Pitto, M., Battaglia, C., Proserpio, V., Magni, F., Galasso, G., & Mocarelli, P. (2008). *Concentration and microsatellite status of plasma DNA for monitoring patients with renal carcinoma.* Eur J Cancer, 44(7):1039–1047.

Perroud, B., Ishimaru, T., Borowsky, A. D., & Weiss, R. H. (2009). *Grade-dependent proteomics characterization of kidney cancer.* Mol Cell Proteomics, 8(5):971–985.

Pez, F., Dayan, F., Durivault, J., Kaniewski, B., Aimond, G., Provost, G. S. L., Deux, B., Clézardin, P., Sommer, P., Pouysségur, J., & Reynaud, C. (2011). *The HIF-1-inducible*

Molecular Portrait of Clear Cell Renal Cell Carcinoma: An Integrative Analysis of Gene Expression and Genomic Copy Number Profiling

53

lysyl oxidase activates HIF-1 via the AKT pathway in a positive regulation loop and synergizes with HIF-1 in promoting tumor cell growth. Cancer Res, 71(5):1647–1657.

Podar, K. & Anderson, K. C. (2010). *A therapeutic role for targeting c-MYC/HIF-1-dependent signaling pathways.* Cell Cycle, 9(9):1722–1728.

Pollack, J. R., Sørlie, T., Perou, C. M., Rees, C. A., Jeffrey, S. S., Lonning, P. E., Tibshirani, R., Botstein, D., Børresen-Dale, A. L., & Brown, P. O. (2002). *Microarray analysis reveals a major direct role of dna copy number alteration in the transcriptional program of human breast tumors.* Proc Natl Acad Sci U S A, 99(20):12963–12968.

Redova, M., Svoboda, M., & Slaby, O. (2011). *MicroRNAs and their target gene networks in renal cell carcinoma.* Biochem Biophys Res Commun, 405(2):153–156.

Saramäki, O. R., Porkka, K. P., Vessella, R. L., & Visakorpi, T. (2006). *Genetic aberrations in prostate cancer by microarray analysis.* Int J Cancer, 119(6):1322–1329.

Sato, E., Torigoe, T., Hirohashi, Y., Kitamura, H., Tanaka, T., Honma, I., Asanuma, H., Harada, K., Takasu, H., Masumori, N., Ito, N., Hasegawa, T., Tsukamoto, T., & Sato, N. (2008). *Identification of an immunogenic ctl epitope of HIFPH3 for immunotherapy of renal cell carcinoma.* Clin Cancer Res, 14(21):6916–6923.

Schäfer, M., Schwender, H., Merk, S., Haferlach, C., Ickstadt, K., & Dugas, M. (2009). *Integrated analysis of copy number alterations and gene expression: a bivariate assessment of equally directed abnormalities.* Bioinformatics, 25(24):3228–3235.

Scotto, L., Narayan, G., Nandula, S. V., Subramaniyam, S., Kaufmann, A. M., Wright, J. D., Pothuri, B., Mansukhani, M., Schneider, A., Arias-Pulido, H., & Murty, V. V. (2008). *Integrative genomics analysis of chromosome 5p gain in cervical cancer reveals target over-expressed genes, including Drosha.* Mol Cancer, 7:58.

Seelow, D., Schwarz, J. M., & Schuelke, M. (2008). *GeneDistiller–distilling candidate genes from linkage intervals.* PLoS One, 3(12):e3874.

Seliger, B., Dressler, S. P., Massa, C., Recktenwald, C. V., Altenberend, F., Bukur, J., Marincola, F. M., Wang, E., Stevanovic, S., & Lichtenfels, R. (2011). *Identification and characterization of human leukocyte antigen class I ligands in renal cell carcinoma cells.* Proteomics, 11(12):2528–2541.

Seliger, B., Dressler, S. P., Wang, E., Kellner, R., Recktenwald, C. V., Lottspeich, F., Marincola, F. M., Baumgärtner, M., Atkins, D., & Lichtenfels, R. (2009). *Combined analysis of transcriptome and proteome data as a tool for the identification of candidate biomarkers in renal cell carcinoma.* Proteomics, 9(6):1567–1581.

Semenza, G. L. (2008). *Hypoxia-inducible factor 1 and cancer pathogenesis.* IUBMB Life, 60(9):591–597.

Shi, T., Dong, F., Liou, L. S., Duan, Z. H., Novick, A. C., & DiDonato, J. A. (2004). *Differential protein profiling in renal-cell carcinoma.* Mol Carcinog, 40(1):47–61.

Shimazui, T., Yoshikawa, K., Uemura, H., Hirao, Y., Saga, S., & Akaza, H. (2004). *The level of cadherin-6 mRNA in peripheral blood is associated with the site of metastasis and with the subsequent occurrence of metastases in renal cell carcinoma.* Cancer, 101(5):963–968.

Skubitz, K. M. & Skubitz, A. P. N. (2002). *Differential gene expression in renal-cell cancer.* J Lab Clin Med, 140(1):52–64.

Skubitz, K. M., Zimmermann, W., Zimmerman, W., Kammerer, R., Pambuccian, S., & Skubitz, A. P. N. (2006). *Differential gene expression identifies subgroups of renal cell carcinoma.* J Lab Clin Med, 147(5):250–267.

Sültmann, H., von Heydebreck, A., Huber, W., Kuner, R., Buness, A., Vogt, M., Gunawan, B., Vingron, M., Füzesí, L., & Poustka, A. (2005). *Gene expression in kidney cancer is associated with cytogenetic abnormalities, metastasis formation, and patient survival.* Clin Cancer Res, 11(2 Pt 1):646–655.

Staller, P., Sulitkova, J., Lisztwan, J., Moch, H., Oakeley, E. J., & Krek, W. (2003). *Chemokine receptor CXCR4 downregulated by von Hippel-Lindau tumour suppressor pVHL.* Nature, 425(6955):307–311.

Stickel, J. S., Weinzierl, A. O., Hillen, N., Drews, O., Schuler, M. M., Hennenlotter, J., Wernet, D., Müller, C. A., Stenzl, A., Rammensee, H.-G., & Stevanović, S. (2009). *HLA ligand profiles of primary renal cell carcinoma maintained in metastases.* Cancer Immunol Immunother, 58(9):1407–1417.

Struckmann, K., Mertz, K., Steu, S., Storz, M., Staller, P., Krek, W., Schraml, P., & Moch, H. (2008). *pVHL co-ordinately regulates CXCR4/CXCL12 and MMP2/MMP9 expression in human clear-cell renal cell carcinoma.* J Pathol, 214(4):464–471.

Subramanian, A., Tamayo, P., Mootha, V. K., Mukherjee, S., Ebert, B. L., Gillette, M. A., Paulovich, A., Pomeroy, S. L., Golub, T. R., Lander, E. S., & Mesirov, J. P. (2005). *Gene set enrichment analysis: a knowledge-based approach for interpreting genome-wide expression profiles.* Proc Natl Acad Sci U S A, 102(43):15545–15550.

Takahashi, M., Papavero, V., Yuhas, J., Kort, E., Kanayama, H. O., Kagawa, S., Baxter, R. C., Yang, X. J., Gray, S. G., & Teh, B. T. (2005). *Altered expression of members of the IGF-axis in clear cell renal cell carcinoma.* Int J Oncol, 26(4):923–931.

Tanaka, T., Kitamura, H., Torigoe, T., Hirohashi, Y., Sato, E., Masumori, N., Sato, N., & Tsukamoto, T. (2011). *Autoantibody against hypoxia-inducible factor prolyl hydroxylase-3 is a potential serological marker for renal cell carcinoma.* J Cancer Res Clin Oncol, 137(5):789–794.

Tang, S. W., Chang, W. H., Su, Y. C., Chen, Y. C., Lai, Y. H., Wu, P. T., Hsu, C. I., Lin, W. C., Lai, M. K., & Lin, J. Y. (2009). *MYC pathway is activated in clear cell renal cell carcinoma and essential for proliferation of clear cell renal cell carcinoma cells.* Cancer Lett, 273(1):35–43.

Thiery, J. P. (2003). *Epithelial-mesenchymal transitions in development and pathologies.* Curr Opin Cell Biol, 15(6):740–746.

Thiery, J. P., Acloque, H., Huang, R. Y. J., & Nieto, M. A. (2009). *Epithelial-mesenchymal transitions in development and disease.* Cell, 139(5):871–890.

Thompson, H. G. R., Harris, J. W., Wold, B. J., Lin, F., & Brody, J. P. (2003). *p62 overexpression in breast tumors and regulation by prostate-derived ETS factor in breast cancer cells.* Oncogene, 22(15):2322–2333.

Tostain, J., Li, G., Gentil-Perret, A., & Gigante, M. (2010). *Carbonic anhydrase 9 in clear cell renal cell carcinoma: a marker for diagnosis, prognosis and treatment.* Eur J Cancer, 46(18):3141–3148.

Truong, L. D. & Shen, S. S. (2011). *Immunohistochemical diagnosis of renal neoplasms.* Arch Pathol Lab Med, 135(1):92–109.

Tun, H. W., Marlow, L. A., von Roemeling, C. A., Cooper, S. J., Kreinest, P., Wu, K., Luxon, B. A., Sinha, M., Anastasiadis, P. Z., & Copland, J. A. (2010). *Pathway signature and cellular differentiation in clear cell renal cell carcinoma.* PLoS One, 5(5):e10696. von Frowein, J., Pagel, P., Kappler, R., von Schweinitz, D., Roscher, A., & Schmid, I.

Molecular Portrait of Clear Cell Renal Cell Carcinoma: An Integrative Analysis of Gene Expression and
Genomic Copy Number Profiling

55

(2011). *MicroRNA-492 is processed from the keratin 19 gene and up-regulated in metastatic hepatoblastoma.* Hepatology, 53(3):833–842.

Waalkes, S., Eggers, H., Blasig, H., Atschekzei, F., Kramer, M. W., Hennenlotter, J., Tränkenschuh, W., Stenzl, A., Serth, J., Schrader, A. J., Kuczyk, M. A., & Merseburger, A. S. (2011). *Caveolin 1 mRNA is overexpressed in malignant renal tissue and might serve as a novel diagnostic marker for renal cancer.* Biomark Med, 5(2):219–225.

Wang, Y., Roche, O., Yan, M. S., Finak, G., Evans, A. J., Metcalf, J. L., Hast, B. E., Hanna, S. C., Wondergem, B., Furge, K. A., Irwin, M. S., Kim, W. Y., Teh, B. T., Grinstein, S., Park, M., Marsden, P. A., & Ohh, M. (2009). *Regulation of endocytosis via the oxygen-sensing pathway.* Nat Med, 15(3):319–324.

Wouters, B. G. & Koritzinsky, M. (2008). *Hypoxia signalling through mTOR and the unfolded protein response in cancer.* Nat Rev Cancer, 8(11):851–864.

Yamamoto, G., Nannya, Y., Kato, M., Sanada, M., Levine, R. L., Kawamata, N., Hangaishi, A., Kurokawa, M., Chiba, S., Gilliland, D. G., Koeffler, H. P., & Ogawa, S. (2007). *Highly sensitive method for genomewide detection of allelic composition in nonpaired, primary tumor specimens by use of Affymetrix single-nucleotide-polymorphism genotyping microarrays.* Am J Hum Genet, 81(1):114–126.

Yang, J. C., Haworth, L., Sherry, R. M., Hwu, P., Schwartzentruber, D. J., Topalian, S. L., Steinberg, S. M., Chen, H. X., & Rosenberg, S. A. (2003). *A randomized trial of bevacizumab, an anti-vascular endothelial growth factor antibody, for metastatic renal cancer.* N Engl J Med, 349(5):427–434.

Yao, M., Tabuchi, H., Nagashima, Y., Baba, M., Nakaigawa, N., Ishiguro, H., Hamada, K., Inayama, Y., Kishida, T., Hattori, K., Yamada-Okabe, H., & Kubota, Y. (2005). *Gene expression analysis of renal carcinoma: adipose differentiation-related protein as a potential diagnostic and prognostic biomarker for clear-cell renal carcinoma.* J Pathol, 205(3):377–387.

Yin-Goen, Q., Dale, J., Yang, W. L., Phan, J., Moffitt, R., Petros, J. A., Datta, M. W., Amin, M. B., Wang, M ., & Young, A. N. (2006). *Advances in molecular classification of renal neoplasms.* Histol Histopathol, 21(3):325–339.

Yoshimoto, T., Matsuura, K., Karnan, S., Tagawa, H., Nakada, C., Tanigawa, M., Tsukamoto, Y., Uchida, T., Kashima, K., Akizuki, S., Takeuchi, I., Sato, F., Mimata, H., Seto, M., & Moriyama, M. (2007). *High-resolution analysis of DNA copy number alterations and gene expression in renal clear cell carcinoma.* J Pathol, 213(4):392–401.

Young, A. N., Amin, M. B., Moreno, C. S., Lim, S. D., Cohen, C., Petros, J. A., Marshall, F. F., & Neish, A. S. (2001). *Expression profiling of renal epithelial neoplasms: a method for tumor classification and discovery of diagnostic molecular markers.* Am J Pathol, 158(5):1639–1651.

Yusenko, M. V., Zubakov, D., & Kovacs, G. (2009). *Gene expression profiling of chromophobe renal cell carcinomas and renal oncocytomas by Affymetrix genechip using pooled and individual tumours.* Int J Biol Sci, 5(6):517–527.

Zhang, Q., Ying, J., Li, J., Fan, Y., Poon, F. F., Ng, K. M., Tao, Q., & Jin, J. (2010). *Aberrant promoter methylation of DLEC1, a critical 3p22 tumor suppressor for renal cell carcinoma, is associated with more advanced tumor stage.* J Urol, 184(2):731–737.

Zhang, Z., Wondergem, B., & Dykema, K. (2010). *A comprehensive study of progressive cytogenetic alterations in clear cell renal cell carcinoma and a new model for ccRCC tumorigenesis and progression.* Adv Bioinformatics, page 428325.

Zhang, Z. F., Matsuda, D., Khoo, S. K., Buzzitta, K., Block, E., Petillo, D., Richard, S., Anema, J., Furge, K. A., & Teh, B. T. (2008). *A comparison study reveals important features of agreement and disagreement between summarized DNA and RNA data obtained from renal cell carcinoma.* Mutat Res, 657(1):77–83.

Zhao, H., Ljungberg, B., Grankvist, K., Rasmuson, T., Tibshirani, R., & Brooks, J. D. (2006). *Gene expression profiling predicts survival in conventional renal cell carcinoma.* PLoS Med, 3(1):e13.

Zhou, G. X., Ireland, J., Rayman, P., Finke, J., & Zhou, M. (2010). *Quantification of carbonic anhydrase IX expression in serum and tissue of renal cell carcinoma patients using enzyme-linked immunosorbent assay: prognostic and diagnostic potentials.* Urology, 75(2):257–261.

3

The Next Challenge in the Treatment of Renal Cell Carcinoma: Overcoming the Resistance Mechanisms to Antiangiogenic Agents

Michele Guida and Giuseppe Colucci
Department of Medical Oncology National Cancer Institute Viale Orazio Flacco Bari
Italy

1. Introduction

In recent years, important advances have been made in the medical therapy of metastatic renal cell carcinoma (mRCC). These advances are due on the one hand to the availability of many new molecules directed at specific biomolecular targets, and on the other hand to the understanding of both the pathogenetic mechanisms which have led to the identification of the key role of some gene mutations and angiogenesis, fundamental mechanisms in the process of tumour proliferation (1,2). In particular, there have been great developments in molecules capable of inhibiting the activity of the pro-angiogenesis receptors of vascular endothelial growth factor (VEGF) and platelet-derived growth factor (PDGF) such as tyrosine-kinase inhibitors (TKI) sunitinib, sorafenib, pazopanib, and monoclonal antibodies bevacizumab. Also inhibitors of specific pathways correlated with tumour growth such as the mTOR inhibitors temsirolinmus and everolimus have become crucial drugs in the management of mRCC (3).

In the last few years, these drugs have radically changed the course of medical therapy of mRCC and other molecules currently in an advanced stage of clinical development will soon further enrich the therapeutic options of mRCC: axitinib (new, powerful anti-tyrosine kinases inhibitor), dovitinib (multi-target inhibitor particularly active against Beta Fibroblast Growth Factor Receptor (FGFR)), volociximab (new chimeric antibody with powerful anti-angiogenic activity directed towards the α5β1integrin), regorafenib, cediranib etc.

As is known, RCC is a highly vascularized neoplasm which is dependent on VEGF-mediated angiogenesis. In fact, mRCC is among neoplasms showing the highest level of circulating VEGF. The importance of VEGF signaling for tumoral growth is also supported by the high frequency of von Hippel-Lindau (VHL) gene mutations found in about 70% of clear cell RCC. The VHL gene product regulates VEGF expression through suppression of the HIF transcription factor. Loss of function mutations in VHL lead to unregulated activation of HIF and overexpression of VEGF and other proangiogenic factors. For these reasons, anti-angiogenic drugs are particularly active in clear cell RCC and these drugs are currently considered the standard of care for first-line treatment. They include the monoclonal antibody bevacizumab which binds to the soluble ligand of VEGF, and the inhibitors of multiple receptor TK for vascular endothelial growth factor receptors (VEGFR-

1, VEGFR-2, and VEGFR-3), PDGFR-α and PDGFR-β, FLT3, the stem cell growth factor receptor KIT, and RET (4).

Despite the efficacy of TKI and bevacizumab therapy, the development of resistance is of major clinical concern; in fact, almost all patients with mRCC develop resistance and the disease inexorably progress.

Conventionally, patients are categorised as "early progressors" when they develop resistance within approximately 6 months of the beginning of first-line therapy, and "late progressors" when they develop resistance later. About 30% of patients present a primary resistance to these drugs with a rapid spreading of disease and a very poor survival (primary refractory). Another 40% of patients, after an initial positive response, exhibit disease progression after about 1 year of treatment (5).

Consequently, the number of patients who receive a second line therapy after anti-angiogenic agents is only about half of the total. In the registrative phase III trial which compared sunitinib to interferon alpha, of 375 patients treated in the sunitinib arm, only 182 patients, corresponding to 56% of the total, received a second line therapy with an anti-mTOR or with a second anti-angiogenic drug (6). Similarly, in the AVOREN study with bevacizumab plus interferon *vs* interferon alone, of 325 patients in the bevacizumab plus interferon arm only 180 patients corresponding to 55% received a second line therapy (7). These data have been confirmed in the similar CALGB 90206 study (8). Notably, outside large controlled studies the percentage of patients receiving a second line treatment after anti-angiogenic agents is much lower. In a recent retrospective analysis of 645 patients from 7 centers and recruited in various studies, only 216 (30%) underwent second line therapy with anti-VEGF/anti-mammalian target of rapamycin (mTOR) drugs (9). Of interest, basal performance status resulted the only significant independent predictor of receiving second-line targeted therapy. Moreover, patients who received a second-line anti-VEGF drug appeared to have a similar overall survival to those who receive a second-line anti-mTOR drug (9).

The adoption of alternative angiogenic signaling pathways to compensate for inhibition of VEGF/VEGFR-mediated signaling seems to be the main, but not the only, common mechanism for the development of cancer resistance to VEGF pathway inhibitors. Nevertheless, to date very few data are available in literature about which alternative pathways are involved in resistant disease. Therefore, understanding the escape mechanisms of resistance to anti-angiogenic agents could improve clinical outcomes and the number of responsive patients.

2. Mechanisms of resistance in MRC

Resistance is generally defined as the capability of tumors to evade the antineoplastic effects of various treatments. About 30% of mRCC have an innate resistance to all available treatments independently from the type of anti-angiogenic agent used. Furthermore, treatment with mTORi as second line therapy results in primary resistance in about 20% of patients.

In this chapter we will attempt to give some partial responses to the numerous questions regarding the significance of resistance in mRCC: what is the definition of resistance? Which mechanisms sustain it? How can we overcome the resistance mechanisms?

2.1 Definition of resistance and its clinical implications

Resistance is divided into primary (also "refractoriness" or "intrinsic responsiveness"), which is characterized by a lack of efficacy to anti-angiogenic agents from the start of therapy, and secondary (also "acquired" or "adaptive" or "evasive" or "angiogenesis escape"), which begins after an initial response to TKI lasting for a period of time of variable length. Notably, early treatment failure involves all anti-angiogenic agents and all type of patients with mRCC.

Nevertheless, primary resistance to TKI in mRCC is heavily influenced by the patient risk score (low-intermediate *vs* poor) and by the type of first line therapy used. Primary refractory patients are about 20% in good-intermediate risk patients treated with different TKI, and it arises over 30% in poor risk patients (6, 8, 10, 11). In addition, the mTORi everolimus generally utilized as second line therapy is characterized by a resistance involving about 20% of patients (12). It is not clear if the patients who present primary resistance are the same as those who also present secondary resistance as data on this topic are not available.

The influence of prior therapies on the risk of primary resistance in patients with mRCC treated with sunitinib as first line has recently been reported in a systemic review and meta-analysis of 10 clinical studies including a total of 4,320 (13). The overall incidence of primary resistance to sunitinib was 22.4%. Moreover, the risk of developing primary resistance was significantly lower in patients with clear-cell cancer compared with non-clear-cell cancer. Notably, patients with prior cytokine therapy exhibited a significantly higher risk of primary progressive disease with sunitinib compared with those who had no prior treatment (RR, 1.18, 95% CI, 1.05-1.34, p=0.007). Although not statistically significant, there was a trend supporting that prior treatment with another mTKI sorafenib increased the risk of resistance to sunitinib in comparison with no prior treatment (RR 1.33, 95% CI: 0.98-1.80, p=0.069).

The conclusions of the Authors are that the risk of primary resistance to sunitinib may vary with tumor histology and prior therapies. In particular, previous exposure to cytokines significantly increased the risk of primary resistance suggesting that an immune mechanism may underlie the resistance to this drug.

A similar meta-analysis was done in patients treated with sorafenib as first line therapy (14). A total of 3,269 patients from 20 studies were included for the analysis. The overall incidence of primary resistance was 22.6% without significant difference between clear cell and non-clear cell nor between prior cytokine therapies and no prior treatment. Notably, patients with prior exposure to sunitinib had a significantly higher incidence of resistance when treated with sorafenib (52.2%). The conclusions of the Authors are that prior exposure to sunitinib but not cytokines significantly increased the risk of resistance with sorafenib in mRCC patients, suggesting that initial therapy with angiogenesis inhibitors may promote the development of resistance to sorafenib.

The conclusive considerations regarding the primary resistance to anti-angiogenic agents in mRCC are that about 30% of mRCC have an innate resistance to all available treatments and the resistance to angiogenic drugs seems to be independent from the type of TKI used.

In second line treatment, resistance to mTORi everolimus occurs in about 20% of patients (12), but when a second TKI was used, the risk of resistance increased to about 50%.

Therefore, considering that only 30%-50% of patients receive second line therapy, the re-challenge with a second TKI is an option available for very few and selected patients.

2.2 The resistance mechanisms

Resistance has yet to be thoroughly understood in kidney cancer. The "angiogenic escape" to anti-VEGF treatment may be dependent both on cancer cell phenomena or endothelial cell phenomena. It is believed that multiple factors affect resistance including factors that decrease angiogenesis and factors that increase angiogenesis. Often these mechanisms are present contemporarily in a single patient. Several of these factors need to be accounted for when developing a comprehensive treatment approach and in understanding why a patient may be resistant to any one approach.

Hypoxia is a known inducer of angiogenic response in a wide variety of tumors. Nevertheless, it is strongly believed that hypoxia is also the key mechanism of angiogenic escape. It involves induction of gene expression via HIF transcription factor of various pro-angiogenic factors including VEGF, FGFs and ephrins. When angiogenesis is inhibited, tumors are in a hypoxic state and develop new alternative pathways to guarantee their further growth (15).

2.3 Primary resistance mechanisms

It is thought that patients with primary resistance to TKI have already activated one or more alternative mechanisms of resistance in response to the selective pressure of their microenvironment. Probably these cases are not, or not only, sustained by angiogenesis mechanisms. Moreover, in patients with primary resistance there is frequently an upregulation of alternative pro-angiogenic pathways mediated by FGFR, interleukin-8 (IL-8), insulin-like GFR, ephrins, and angiopoietins. In particular, FGF/FGFR system has been reported as one of the most important escape pathways of anti-VEGFR therapies.

Other possible mechanisms include the pre-existing inflammatory cell-mediated vascular protection (myeloid cell); an hypovascularity status with consequent indifference toward angiogenesis inhibitors (desmoplastic stroma); the co-option of normal vessels without requisite angiogenesis (4, 16-18).

2.4 Secondary resistance mechanisms

Regarding secondary resistance, many Authors believe that it is precisely the state of **hypoxia** determined by anti-angiogenic drugs which is at the root of the onset of the *escape* mechanisms sustained by new HIF, FGF, IL-8, ephrine etc transcript factors, which lead to the activation of alternative pathways which support a *"new angiogenic wave"* (15). It is notable that during therapy with anti-VEGF the expression of new and ever-increasing pro-angiogenic factors is observed. It is known that the early phase of angiogenesis is generally characterized by a response to anti-VEGF treatment. On the contrary, the late phase of angiogenesis is characterized by the escape to anti-VEGF treatment. This late phase is sustained by FGF, IL-8 and other factors. It has been reported that in the presence of sunitinib the tumor is able to produce until 19 pro-angiogenic factors to rescue endothelia cell proliferation (19,20).

The Next Challenge in the Treatment of Renal Cell Carcinoma: Overcoming the Resistance Mechanisms to
Antiangiogenic Agents

61

Function-blocking antibodies to VEGF receptors R1 and R2 were used to probe their roles in controlling angiogenesis in a mouse model of pancreatic islet carcinogenesis. Inhibition of VEGFR2 but not VEGFR1 markedly disrupted angiogenic switching, persistent angiogenesis, and initial tumor growth. In late-stage tumors, phenotypic resistance to VEGFR2 blockade emerged, as tumors regrew during treatment after an initial period of growth suppression. This resistance to VEGF blockade involves reactivation of tumor angiogenesis, independent of VEGF and associated with hypoxia-mediated induction of other proangiogenic factors, including members of the FGF family. These other proangiogenic signals are functionally implicated in the revascularization and regrowth of tumors in the evasion phase, as FGF blockade impairs progression in the face of VEGF inhibition (15).

Recently, it has been demonstrated that the FGF pathway is important in patients who develop resistance to sunitinib. Welti and collegues (21) reported that FGF2 supports endothelial proliferation and de novo tubule formation in the presence of sunitinib and that FGF2 can suppress sunitinib-induced retraction of tubules. Importantly, these effects of FGF2 were ablated by PD173074, a small molecule inhibitor of FGF receptor signalling. They also showed that FGF2 can stimulate pro-angiogenic signalling pathways in endothelial cells despite the presence of sunitinib. Finally, analysis of clinical renal-cancer samples demonstrated that a large proportion of renal cancers strongly express FGF2. In conclusion, they suggest that therapeutic strategies designed to simultaneously target both VEGF and FGF2 signalling may prove more efficacious than sunitinib in renal cancer patients whose tumours express FGF2.

Interestingly, it has been demonstrated that FGFR is highly expressed in RCC. Tsimafeyeu and collegues analyzed the expression of FGFR1 in 140 patients with mRCC. Expression of FGFR1 was observed in 98% of primary tumors and in 82.5% of lymph node metastases. Moreover, a significant rise in plasma bFGF levels was reported in patients with disease progression but a non-significant fall in patients with response or stable disease. Plasma VEGF-A level increased in patients with response whereas no detectable changes in plasma VEGF-A level was found in patients with progressive disease. The conclusions of the Authors are that plasma levels of bFGF and VEGF-A are altered in MRCC patients receiving sunitinib, and the increases in bFGF levels may represent biomarker of resistance to targeted therapy (22). Recently it has confirmed that the subset of clear cell RCC tumors with increased expression of FGFR1 is associated with a shorter progression free survival (23).

Also the role of IL-8 in resistance mechanisms seems to be determinant. In xenograft models, sunitinib resistance/refractoriness has been reported associated to higher levels of IL-8 (16). Moreover, the resistance to sunitinib was associated with a higher microvessel density, indicating an escape from anti-angiogenesis mechanisms. Finally, the addition of monoclonal antibody anti-IL-8 resensitized the tumor to sunitinib activity. The conclusions of the Authors are that IL-8 mediates resistance to sunitinib and could represent a candidate target to reverse acquired or intrinsic resistance to sunitinib.

Higher levels of IL-8 were associated with shorter progression free survival in mRCC patients treated in phase III trials of pazopanib (24).

Some Authors also demonstrated in pre-clinical models that antiangiogenic drugs could elicit malignant progression of tumors with an increase of local invasion and distant metastasis. In particular, it has been reported that short-term treatment with a potent inhibitor of tumor angiogenesis is able to induce an acceleration of metastasis formation (25). Moreover, other Authors reported that angiogenesis inhibitors targeting the VEGF pathway had antitumor effects in mouse models of pancreatic neuroendocrine carcinoma and glioblastoma, but concomitantly these drugs elicit tumor adaptation and progression to stages of greater malignancy, with heightened invasiveness and in some cases increased lymphatic and distant metastasis (26). Increased invasiveness is also seen by genetic ablation of the VEGF-A gene in both models, substantiating the results of the pharmacological inhibitors. The realization that potent angiogenesis inhibition can alter the natural history of tumors by increasing invasion and metastasis warrants clinical investigation, as the prospect has important implications for the development of enduring antiangiogenic therapies (26).

Other two main mechanisms that could partially explain the ability of the tumor to become resistant to treatment are their capability to epithelial-mesenchimal transformation and the intra-tumoral heterogeneity.

The **epithelial to mesenchymal transition** (EMT) process has been described in different neoplasms and associated with metastatic disease, drug resistance, and develop of angiogenesis (27-30). Treatment-associated tumor hypoxia has been reported to induce an EMT in several tumor models (31). How EMT as a mechanism of acquired resistance occurs in human tumors is unknown and deserves further investigation. In RCC, sarcomatoid phenotype is observed across all histological subtypes, and associated with a poorer prognosis and an increased resistance to VEGF inhibitors. A growing number of interdependent pathways have been linked to the induction of EMT, which, by definition, is a potentially transient/reversible phenotype of epithelial cancers. The reverted histologic phenotype observed in the xenografts also suggests that this escape mechanisms against anti-VEGF therapies may be transient (30, 32, 33).

According to this hypothesis, patients who have initially received clinical benefit from treatment with TKIs and then developed resistant disease may respond again to TKIs following a break from anti-VEGF therapies. The "holiday" period from anti-VEGF therapies may lead to "reset" the tumor microenvironment and reestablish a primarily EGF driven tumor growth. This hypothesis is supported by anecdotic reports of patients who were treated with sunitinib with initial response and subsequent progression who responded again to sunitinib following different targeted therapies such as mTOR inhibitors. The apparent transient/reversible mechanism of resistance to anti-VEGF therapies may also explain why clinical benefit has been reported by sequencing different anti-VEGF therapies despite the fact that these agents target the same VEGF pathway.

Regarding **intratumoral heterogeneity**, it has been demonstrated that mRCC, like other cancer, is characterized by a significant chromosomal instability that creates a selection of multiple clonal tumor subpopulations with an intrinsic multidrug resistance. Multiple intermixed cell subpopulations within one tumour differ by large genomic events as focal amplifications and deletions. For this reason, it is thought that single biopsy is often not representative of mutational landscape of the tumor (34). Recently have been developed methods able to study multiple subpopulations from different anatomic locations of neoplastic tissue (35).

The Next Challenge in the Treatment of Renal Cell Carcinoma: Overcoming the Resistance Mechanisms to
Antiangiogenic Agents

63

Drug/Author	First line	Second line		Predictive factors
	N. Pts	Type of therapy	N. of Pts (%)	
Sunitinib Motzer et al, JCO 2009	375 (sunitinib arm)	Anti-VEGF/ anti-mTOR	182 (56)	-
Beva + IFN Escudier et al, JCO 2010	325 (bevacizumab-IFN arm)	TKI	180 (55)	-
TKI* Vikers et al, Urology 2010	645	Anti-VEGF/ anti-mTOR	216 (30)	Basal PS

* Multi-institutional studies
Abbreviations: PS: Performance status

Table 1. Percentage of patients who access to a second line treatment after TKi in mRCC

Setting	Author	Drug	% of incidence resistance
1a line therapy Good-intermediate prognosis	Motzer, 2007 Ranpura, 2010*	Sunitinib	22.4
	Su, 2010*	Sorafenib	22.6
1a line Poor prognosis	Hudes 2007	Temsirolimus	33
2a line therapy	Motzer, 2008	Everolimus after TKI	20
	Ranpura, 2010*	Sorafenib after Sunitinib	33
	Su, 2010*	Sunitinib after Sorafenib	52.2

*Meta-analysis

Table 2. Percentage of patients with resistance according to the risk score and treatments in mRCC

Due to this genomic instability, it is strongly believed that resistance is a dynamic mechanism changing in different conditions (treatment pressure, hypoxia pressure, etc) and during the tumor growth. This aspect could explain the response obtained in some patients re-challenged with sunitinib. It thought that during treatment interruption, the selective pressure from drugs is removed and drug-sensitive clones re-growth. Recently, Zama and colleagues reported the results of a retrospective study describing 5 partial response (22%) of 23 mRCC patients re-treated with sunitinib (36, 37).

Also a "holiday" period from anti-VEGF therapies it is thought able to determine a reacquired drug-sensitivity by clones become resistant to TKI drugs.

Various genes associated with resistance have been identified which could become a target for future treatments. Recently, Sanjmyatas and colleagues also reported a specific gene expression signature able to characterize the different metastatic potential in ccRCC (38).

It has been demonstrated that some genes are hyperexpressed when there is resistance, for example the gene which encodes sphingosine kinase, calvasculin, chemokine receptor 4 (CXCR4), NNP1, arginase II, hypoxia-inducible protein-2 (HIG2) and VEGF. Other anti-angiogenic genes, however, show reduced expression in resistant tumors, such as the genes which encode cytokines associated with interferon-gamma, in particular IP10 (CXCL10) and Mig (CXCL9) (39). Sphingosine-1-phosphate (S1P), a pleiotropic bioactive lipid derived from sphingosine through sphingosine kinase (SphK) action, is dysregulated in a variety of disease conditions including cancer. S1P is a tumorigenic and angiogenic growth factor produced normally by blood platelets, mast cells and possibly fibroblasts in the tumour microenvironment. It is capable of determining proliferation and migration of endothelial cells, favouring angiogenesis and tumour proliferation. Notably, several tumors up regulate the expression of SPHK1, which may greatly contribute to the putative increased levels of S1P. In experimental models it has been demonstrated that SphK and S1P expression was increased during sunitinib resistance (39).

In xenografts models Bhatt and colleagues provided evidence that resistance to VEGF receptor therapy is due at least in part to resumption of angiogenesis in association with reduction of IFNγ-related angiostatic chemokines, and that this resistance can be delayed by restoration of angiostatic signalling with the concomitant administration of CXCL9 (40).

An emerging area of drug discovery called lipidomic-based therapeutics is in rapid develop. It directly targets pleiotropic bioactive lipids involved in cancer as well as other disorders. It has been postulated that S1P antibodies could represented a potential therapeutic strategies in the treatment of renal cancer (41).

Other mechanisms, not completely known, sustaining secondary resistance in mRCC include: **secondary mutations in tyrosine kinase receptors** (analogous to EGFR TKI); **recruitment of bone marrow-derived pro-angiogenic cells** which can obviate the necessity of VEGF signalling, thereby affecting re-initiaton and continuance of tumour angiogenesis; **increasing of pericyte** coverage of the tumour vasculature, serving to support its integrity and attenuate the necessity for VEGF-mediated survival signalling has been described; activation and enhancement of invasion and metastasis to provide **access to normal tissue vasculature** without obligate neovascularisation (4).

In table 3 are reported the main mechanisms of primary and secondary resistance in mRCC.

3. How can we overcome resistance to anti-angiogenic agents?

Many attempts have been made in the effort to overcome resistance to anti-VEGF treatments, but so far the results are disappointing. They include the use of non cross-resistant drugs, integrating or combining current treatment, optimization of sequential therapies and TKI re-challenge. Finally, several ongoing studies are trying to clarify the optimal sequence of the different drugs and the significance of the rechallenge with TKI in the treatment strategies.

As regards primary resistance, other than new experimental molecules the main route taken up until now has been to the combination of drugs for different biomolecular targets.

The Next Challenge in the Treatment of Renal Cell Carcinoma: Overcoming the Resistance Mechanisms to
Antiangiogenic Agents

65

Primary resistance	- Alternative pro-angiogenic pathways mediated by FGFR, interleukin-8 (IL-8), insulin-like GFR, ephrins, and angiopoietins; - Non angiogenic mechanisms -Pre-existing inflammatory cell-mediated vascular protection (myeloid cell); -Hypovascularity status with consequent indifference toward angiogenesis inhibitors (desmoplastic stroma); -Co-option of normal vessels without requisite angiogenesis -Non clear cell histology
Secondary resistance	- New angiogenic wave induced by hypoxia determined by anti-angiogenic drugs - Epithelial to mesenchymal transition - Intra-tumoral heterogeneity - Gene instability and gene iperexpression - Secondary mutations in tyrosine kinase receptors - Bone marrow-derived pro-angiogenic cells which can obviate the necessity of VEGF signalling; - Increasing of pericyte coverage of the tumour vasculature, serving to support its integrity and attenuate the necessity for VEGF-mediated survival; - Access to normal tissue vasculature without obligate neovascularisation

Note: to bibliographic references see the text

Table 3. Main mechanisms of primary and secondary resistance in mRCC

To overcome secondary resistance, various strategies are being explored: increasing the dose of the current drug, the use of non cross-resistant drugs (for example changing to a mTOR inhibitor such as everolimus after a anti-angiogenic drug), changing to another VEGF inhibitor (for example sunitinib after bevacizumab, or sorafenib after sunitinib, or axitinib after sorafenib), the use of a "drug holiday" (12, 42, 43). However, results obtained so far have been modest, above all because in general the choice of strategy has been empirical rather than determined by a strong biological rationale. It is therefore desirable that new studies are founded on convincing preclinical data.

3.1 Drug combinations

As previously mentioned, several studies using combinations of drugs targeted to different biomolecular targets have been started with the aim of increasing clinical activity. Many attempts have been made to verify if the combination of drugs with different mechanisms of action was able to improve the results of single agent therapy. Unfortunately, so far this strategy has given disappointing or negative results with a heavier profile of toxicity.

Figure 1 shows the possible drug combination strategies in mCRC therapy.

Some combinations have proved to be very toxic and relatively inactive and therefore they were quickly abandoned, as was the case of the combination of TKI and bevacizumab (44, 45).

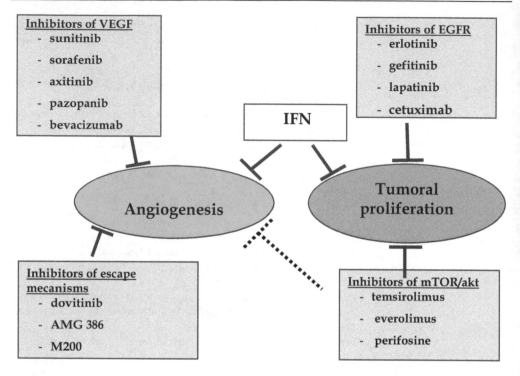

Fig. 1. Possible strategies of drugs association in mRCC

The high expression of EGFR in renal tumours from 50 to 90% (46), has also encouraged the use of anti-EGFR drugs in combination with anti-angiogenic agents. A study has recently been published by Motzer and colleagues at the Memorial Sloan-Kettering Cancer Center in New York in which gefitinib was combined with sunitinib in order to realise a double target. However, the reported results were similar to those obtained with sunitinib alone, but with an increase in toxicity. The Authors therefore discourage further studies on this combination (47).

Another route which seems more promising is the combination of bevacizumab and m-TOR inhibitors. However, after some encouraging early experiences (48-50), more recent studies are re-dimensioning the preliminary results. Of particular note are the results of a randomized phase II trial which compared temsirolimus and bevacizumab *vs* sunitinib *vs* interferon alfa and bevacizumab (TORAVA study). Unfortunately, in view of clearly higher toxicity in the temsirolimus plus bevacizumab arm, superiority of this combination compared to other arms was not reported (51). The conclusions of Authors are that the toxicity of the temsirolimus and bevacizumab combination was much higher than anticipated and limited treatment continuation over time, whereas clinical activity was low compared with the benefit expected from sequential use of each targeted therapy. Thus, this combination cannot be recommended for first-line treatment in patients with mRCC.

The combination of targeted drugs with immunological molecules such as interferon is proving to be more interesting. In particular, encouraging results have been reported on the combination of sorafenib and interferon alpha (52).

The Next Challenge in the Treatment of Renal Cell Carcinoma: Overcoming the Resistance Mechanisms to
Antiangiogenic Agents

67

Generally speaking, even if it is necessary to wait for definitive results of ongoing phase III trials, the results reported so far do not encourage this therapeutic strategy.

Table 4 shows the most significant experiences of the different drug combinations used.

Drugs combinations/ Authors	Setting	N. of pts	PFS (Mo)	OR/SD	Toxicity	Notes
Sorafenib + Interferone Gollob et al, JCO 2007	phase II (1ª e 2ª linc)	40	10	33% PR 29% SD	moderate	50% pts in 2ª line Good activity
Beva + Sunitinib* Garcia et al, ASCO 2008	phase I	31 (varius histology)	-	3/7 mRCC 1/3 melanoma 1 surrene	moderate	Good activity
Beva + Sorafenib Sosman et al, ASCO 2008	phase I-II	48	14	25% PR 18% SD	high (hypertension, stomatite, hand-foot sindrome)	A negative experience
Sunitinib + Gefitinib Motzer et al, AJCO 2010	phase II	42	11	37% OR 34% SD	acceptable (diarrea G3-4 in 14% of pts)	Activity similar to that of sunitinib alone
Beva + Everolimus Whorf et al, ASCO '08 Hainsworth, Whorf, JCO 2010	phase II 1ª e 2ª lines	80	9,1 7,1	30/23% OR 50/64% SD (1ª/2ª linea)	moderate	Good activity
Beva + Temsirolimus Merchan et al, JCO 2009	phae I-II	45	18/5.3	14,5%	acceptable	Long PFS
Beva + Temsirolimus vs Sunitinib vs IFN + Beva	phase II R Beva + Tem		8,2	27,3% OR 47,7% SD	High (41% of pts stop therapy)	Higher toxicity for experimental arm
Escudier et al, ASCO 2010 (TORAVA Trial)	Sunitinib		8,2	23,8% OR 50% SD	As aspected	No confirmed results of phase II studies
	Beva + alpha IFN		16,8	39% OR 34% SD	As aspected	

Abbreviations: PFS: progression free survival.

Table 4. Most significant experiences with drug combinations in mRCC

3.2 New drugs and sequences

Clearly, another approach to overcoming resistance mechanisms is the use of new molecules which have a more powerful anti-angiogenic activity or which are more directly aimed at the targets involved in resistance mechanisms. Axitinib and dovitinib are of particular interest here. In preclinical trials, axitinib has shown much more powerful antiangiogenic activity than other TKIs (53, 54). Furthermore, interesting results have been reported in phase II studies as a second line therapy after sorafenib with an overall response of 23% and a stable disease of 55%; interestingly, the progression free survival was 7.4 months, one of the longest ever reported (42).

Recently, beta FGFR has been identified as a new target for anti-angiogenic therapy. The system FGF/FGF receptor (FGFR) has been frequently reported as one of the most important escape pathways of anti-VEGFR therapies. It is involved in primary and secondary resistance mechanisms. The activation of FGFR3 is associated with cell proliferation and survival in certain cancer cell types. Thus, beta FGFR is proving to be a new interesting target for anti-angiogenic therapy.

Dovitinib, a new small multi-target molecule, is able to strongly binds to FGFR3 and inhibits its phosphorylation, which may result in the inhibition of tumor cell proliferation and the induction of tumor cell death. In addition, this agent may inhibit other members of the TK receptors superfamily, including the VEGFR; FGFR1; PDGFR3; FMS-like tyrosine kinase 3; stem cell factor receptor (c-KIT); and colony-stimulating factor receptor 1; this may result in an additional reduction in cellular proliferation and angiogenesis, and the induction of tumor cell apoptosis. A phase I/II has been recently concluded (55) and a large phase III clinical trial is ongoing to evaluate the efficacy of this drug as third line therapy in mRCC.

Other drugs of great interest are the monoclonal antibody anti-S1P, a molecule directly involved in resistance mechanisms already being developed clinically, and the anti- IL-8 and anti-IL-12 antibodies, which are still being studied in preclinical trials.

Regarding **sequences**, factors that could drive the choice of a more appropriate second line therapy are the response to primary treatment with TKI, the side effects reported in first line therapy, the patient risk score, and the histology of the tumor.

At present, the use of non cross-resistant mTOR inhibitor everolimus is the only registered agent available as second line therapy for mRCC resistant to anti-angiogenic drugs. In fact, the registrative trial showed a significant benefit in terms of PFS of 4.9 months for everolimus *vs* 1.9 months for placebo (12).

A second TKi as second line therapy is another option to consider for patients resistant to antiangiogenetic agents. Nevertheless, it is thought that this treatment must be propose only in carefully selected patients who did not show a rapid progression at the first line TKi. At present, this choice has a weaker recommendation because no definitive data from phase III studies are available yet.

Notably, in the AVOREN study it has been reported a median overall survival of 23.3 months for the sequence alfa interferone/bevacizumab followed by a second antiangiogenetic agent (TKI), with respect to only 21.3 months for the sequence alfa interferone/placebo followed by a TKI (7).

Some Authors believe that better clinical outcomes are correlated with a higher number of lines of treatments used rather than with the sequences utilized. Consequently, they have hypothesize specific sequences with the aim to utilize the maximum of therapeutic options available. Others suppose that the sequence TKI-TKI is to prefer to that with TKI-mTORi on

The Next Challenge in the Treatment of Renal Cell Carcinoma: Overcoming the Resistance Mechanisms to
Antiangiogenic Agents

69

the basis of some preliminary experiences. Also the rechallenge with the same drug has been proposed, especially when a "holiday" period from anti-VEGF therapies is given to the patient. This break could be able to determine a reacquired drug-sensitivity by clones become resistant to TKI. Nevertheless, at present the majority of data are from small and retrospective studies regarding selected patients (36,37,56-61).

Recently, the results of the phase III study with Axitinib as second line therapy have been published (62). Axitinib resulted in significantly longer PFS compared with sorafenib. Nevertheless, in the subgroup of the patients treated previously with the TKI inhibitor the PFS was similar to what has been reported for the mTOR inhibitor everolimus (4.8 vs. 4.9 months).

Of course, further controlled studies are needed to determine the real effect of prior anti-angiogenesis therapy on the development of resistance to further therapies. A series of planned trials are evaluating what are the best sequences and timing.

4. Conclusions

The adoption of alternative angiogenic signaling pathways to compensate for inhibition of VEGF/VEGFR-mediated signaling seems to be the common mechanism for the development of cancer resistance to VEGF pathway inhibitors. Nevertheless, until now very few data are known about which alternative pathways are involved in resistant disease.

Many attempts have been proposed to overcome resistance. These include the use of non cross-resistant drugs, the optimization of sequential therapies, and the use of combined therapies. Unfortunately, all these approaches have given only modest results. Therefore, the overcome resistance mechanisms to antiangiogenic agents remains the next challenge in the treatment of renal cell carcinoma.

5. Acknowledgements

The author would like to thank Caroline Oakley and Silvana Valerio for their assistance with the linguistic revision of this review.

6. References

[1] Rini BI, Small EJ: Biology and clinical development of vascular endothelial growth factor-targeted therapy in renal cell carcinoma. J Clin Oncol 2005; 23:1028-1043.

[2] Motzer RJ, Michaelson MD, Redman BG et al: Activity of SUI 1248, a multitargeted inhibitor of vascular endothelial growth factor receptor and platelet-derived growth factor receptor, in patients with metastatic renal cell carcinoma. J Clin Oncol 2006; 24:1-3.

[3] Schmidinger M, Bellmunt J: Plethora of agents, plethora of targets, plethora of side effects in metastatic renal cell carcinoma. Cancer Treat Rev 2010; 36:416-424.

[4] Bergers G and Hanahan D: Modes of resistance to anti-angiogenic therapy. Nature Reviews 2008; 8(8):592-603.

[5] Rini B, Atkins MB: Resistance to targeted therapy in renal cell carcinoma. Lancet Oncol 2009; 10:992-1000.

[6] Motzer RJ, Hutson TE, Tomczak P, et al: Overall survival and updated results for sunitinib compared with interferon alfa in patients with metastatic renal cell carcinoma. J Clin Oncol. 2009; 27(22):3584-3590.

[7] Escudier B, Bellmunt J, Négrier S et al: Phase III trial of bevacizumab plus interferon alfa-2a in patients with metastatic renai celi carcinoma (AVOREN): final analysis of overall survival. J Clin Oncol 2010; 28:2144-2150.

[8] Rini, BI Halabi S, Rosenberg JE, et al. Phase III trial of bevacizumab plus interferon alfa versus interferon alfa monotherapy in patients with metastatic renal cell carcinoma: final results of CALGB 90206. J Clin Oncol 2010; 28:2137-2143.

[9] Vickers MM, Choueiri TK, Rogers M, et al: Clinical outcome in metastatic renal cell carcinoma patients after failure of initial vascular endothelial growth factor-targeted therapy. Urology 2010; 76(2):430-434.

[10] Hutson, TE, Davis ID, Machiels JP, et al. Efficacy and safety of pazopanib in patients with metastatic renal cell carcinoma.J Clin Oncol 2010 ; 28(3):475-480.

[11] Hudes G, Carducci M, Tomczak P et al: Temsirolimus, interferon alfa, or both for advanced renal-cell carcinoma. N Engl J Med 2007; 356: 2271-2281.

[12] Motzer RJ, Escudier B, Oudard S et al: Efficacy of everolimus in advanced renal cell carcinoma: a double-blind, randomised, placebo-controlled phase III trial. Lancet 2008; 372:449-456.

[13] RanpuraV, Su X, Wu S: Influence of prior therapies on the risk of primary progressive disease in patients with metastatic renal cell carcinoma treated with sunitinib: A meta-analysis. GU ASCO meeting 2010. J Clin Oncol 2011, Abst 347.

[14] Su X, Wu S: Treatment failure secondary to primary progressive disease in patients with metastatic renal cell carcinoma treated with sorafenib: A meta-analysis. GU ASCO 2010, Abst 391.

[15] Casanovas O, Hicklin DJ, Bergers G, Hanahan D: Drug resistance by evasion of antiangiogenic targeting of VEGF signaling in late-stage pancreatic islet tumors. Cancer Cell. 2005; 8(4):299-309.

[16] Sleijfer S, Wiemer E, Seynaeve C, Verweij J: Improved insight into resistance mechanisms to imatinib in gastrointestinal stromal tumors: a basis for novel approaches and individualization of treatment. Oncologist. 2007; 12(6):719-726.

[17] Reichardt P: Novel approaches to imatinib- and sunitinib-resistant GIST. Curr Oncol Rep 2008;10(4):344-349. Review.

[18] Huang D, Ding Y, Zhou M, et al: Interleukin-8 mediates resistance to antiangiogenic agent sunitinib in renal cell carcinoma.. Cancer Res 2010; 70(3):1063-1071.

[19] Folkman J: Principles and practice in Oncology Cancer 2005.

[20] Faivre S, Demetri G, Sargent W, Raymond E: Molecular basis for sunitinib efficacy and future clinical development. Nat Rev Drug Discov. 2007; 6(9):734-745. Review.

[21] Welti JC, Gourlaouen M, Powles T, et al: Fibroblast growth factor 2 regulates endothelial cell sensitivity to sunitinib. Oncogene 2011; 30(10):1183-1193.

[22] Tsimafeyeu I, Demidov L, Ta H, et al: Fibroblast growth factor pathway in renal cell carcinoma. J Clin Oncol 28:15s, 2010 (suppl; abstr 4621).

[23] Ho TH, Wang F, Hoang A, et al: FGFR1) expression and activation in clear cell renal cell carcinoma (ccRCC). ASCO meeting 2011. J Clin Oncol 29: 2011 (suppl; abstr e15015).

[24] Liu Y, Tran HT, Lin Y, et al: Plasma cytokine and angiogenic factors (CAFs) predictive of clinical benefit and prognosis in patients (Pts) with advanced or metastatic renal cell cancer (mRCC) treated in phase III trials of pazopanib (PAZO). ASCO meeting 2011. J Clin Oncol 29: 2011 (suppl 7; abstr 334).

The Next Challenge in the Treatment of Renal Cell Carcinoma: Overcoming the Resistance Mechanisms to
Antiangiogenic Agents

71

[25] Ebos JM, Lee CR, Cruz-Munoz W, et al: Accelerated metastasis after short-term treatment with a potent inhibitor of tumor angiogenesis. Cancer Cell 2009; 15(3):232-239.

[26] Paez-Ribes M, Allen E, Hudock J, et al: Antiangiogenic therapy elicits malignant progression of tumors to increased local invasion and distant metastasis. Cancer Cell 2009; 3;15(3):220-31. Review.

[27] Frederick BA, Helfrich BA, Coldren CD, et al: Epithelial to mesenchymal transition predicts gefitinib resistance in cell lines of head and neck squamous cell carcinoma and non-small cell lung carcinoma. Mol Cancer Ther 2007; 6:1683–1691.

[28] Shah AN, Summy JM, Zhang J, et al: Development and characterization of gemcitabine-resistant pancreatic tumor cells. Ann Surg Oncol 2007; 14:3629–3637.

[29] Kajiyama H, Shibata K, Terauchi M, et al: Chemoresistance to paclitaxel induces epithelial-mesenchymal transition and enhances metastatic potential for epithelial ovarian carcinoma cells. Int J Oncol 2007; 31:277–283.

[30] Ghersi G: Roles of molecules involved in epithelial/mesenchymal transition during angiogenesis. Front Biosci 2008; 13:2335–2355.

[31] Hugo H, Ackland ML, Blick T, et al: Epithelial-mesenchymal and mesenchymal-epithelial transitions in carcinoma progression. J Cell Physiol 2007; 213:374–383.

[32] Hammers HJ, Verheul HM, Salumbides B, et al: Reversible epithelial to mesenchymal transition and acquired resistance to sunitinib in patients with renal cell carcinoma: evidence from a xenograft study. Mol Cancer Ther 2010; 9:1525-1535.

[33] Klymkowsky MW, Savagner P: Epithelial-mesenchymal transition: A cancer researcher's conceptual friend and foe. Am J Pathol 2009; 174:1588–1593.

[34] Lee AJ, Endesfelder D, Rowan AJ, Walther A, et al: Chromosomal instability confers intrinsic multidrug resistance. Cancer Res. 2011; 71(5):1858-70.

[35] Navin N, Kendall J, Troge J, et al: Tumour evolution inferred by single-cell sequencing. Nature 2011; 472(7341):90-94.

[36] Zama IN, Hutson TE, Elson P, et al: Sunitinib rechallenge in metastatic renal cell carcinoma patients. Cancer 2010; 116(23):5400-5406.

[37] Rini BI, Hutson HE, Elson P et al: Clinical activity of sunitinib rechallenge in metastatic renal cell carcinoma. GU ASCO 2010, J Clin Oncol 2010, Abst 396.

[38] Sanjmyatas J, Steiner T, Wunderlich H, et al: A specific gene expression signature characterizes metastatic potential in clear cell renal cell carcinoma. J Urol 2011; 186(1):289-294.

[39] Sabbadini RA: Targeting sphingosine-1 -phosphate for cancer therapy. Br J Cancer 2006; 95:1131-1135.

[40] Bhatt RS, Wang X, Zhang L, et al: Renal cancer resistance to antiangiogenic therapy is delayed by restoration of angiostatic signaling. Mol Cancer Ther. 2010; 9(10):2793-802.

[41] Sabbadini RA. Sphingosine-1-phosphate antibodies as potential agents in the treatment of cancer and age-related macular degeneration. Br J Pharmacol. 2011; 162(6):1225-1238.

[42] Rini BI, Wilding G, Hudes G et al: Phase II study of axitinib in sorafenib-refractory metastatic renal cell carcinoma. J Clin Oncol 2009; 27:4462-4468.

[43] Rini BI, Hutson HE, Elson P et al: Clinical activity of sunitinib rechallenge in metastatic renal cell carcinoma. GU ASCO meeting 2010, J Clin Oncol 2010, Abst 396.

[44] Rini BI, Garcia JA, Cooney MM, et al: Toxicity of sunitinib plus bevacizumab in renal cell carcinoma. J Clin Oncol. 2010; 10;28(17):284-285.

[45] Sosman JA, Flaherty KT, Atkins MB et al: Updated results of phase I trial of sorafenib (S) and bevacizumab (B) in patients with metastatic renal cell cancer (mRCC). ASCO meeting 2008, abst. 5011.

[46] Yoshida K, Hosoya Y, Sumi S, et al: Studies of the expression of epidermal growth factor receptor in human renal cell carcinoma: a comparison of immunohistochemical method versus ligand binding assay. Oncology. 1997; 54(3):220-225.

[47] Motzer RJ, Hudes GR, Ginsberg MS, et al: Phase I/II trial of sunitinib plus gefitinib in patients with metastatic renal cell carcinoma. Am J Clin Oncol 2010; 33(6):614-618.

[48] Whorf RC, Hainsworth JD, Spigel DR, et al: Phase II study of bevacizumab and everolimus (RAD001) in the treatment of advanced renal cell carcinoma (RCC). ASCO meeting 2008, J Clin Oncol 2008, abst 5010.

[49] Hainsworth JD, Spigel DR, Burris HA, et al: Phase II trial of bevacizumab and everolimus in patients with advanced renal cell carcinoma. J Clin Oncol 2010; 28:2131-2136.

[50] Merchan J R, Pitot HC, Qin R, et al: Phase I/II trial of CCI 779 and bevacizumab in advanced renal cell carcinoma (RCC): Safety and activity in RTKI refractory RCC patients. ASCO meeting 2009, J Clin Oncol 2011, Abst 5039.

[51] Négrier S, Gravis G, Pérol D, et al: Temsirolimus and bevacizumab, or sunitinib, or interferon alfa and bevacizumab for patients with advanced renal cell carcinoma (TORAVA): a randomised phase 2 trial. Lancet Oncol. 2011; 12(7):673-680.

[52] Gollob JA, Rathmell WK, Richmond TM., et al: Phase II trial of sorafenib plus interferon alfa-2b as first- or second-line therapy in patients with metastatic renal cell cancer. J Clin Oncol 2007; 25:3288-3295.

[53] Larkin JM, Chowdhury S, Gore ME: Drug insight: advances in renal cell carcinoma and the role of targeted therapies. Nat Clin Pract Oncol. 2007; 4(8):470-479.

[54] Kelly RJ, Rixe O: Axitinib (AG-013736). Recent Results Cancer Res 2010;184:33-44.

[55] Angevin E, Lopez JA, Pande A, et al: TKI258 (dovitinib lactate) in metastatic renal cell carcinoma (mRCC) patients refractory to approved targeted therapies: A phase I/II dose finding and biomarker study. ASCO meeting 2009, J Clin Oncol 2009, Abst 3563.

[56] Dudek AZ, Zolnierek J, Dham A et al: Sequential therapy with sorafenib and sunitinib in renal cell carcinoma. Cancer 2009; 115: 61-67

[57] Di Lorenzo G, Cartenì G, Autorino R et al: Phase II study of sorafenib in patients with sunitinib-refractory metastatic renal cell cancer. J Clin Oncol 2009; 27:4469-4474.

[58] Tamaskar I, Garcia JA, Elson P et al: Antitumor effects of sunitinib or sorafenib in patients with metastatic renal cell carcinoma who received prior antiangiogenic therapy. J Urol 2008; 179:81-86.

[59] Merseburger AS, Simon A, Waalkes S, Kuczyk MA: Sorafenib reveals efficacy in sequential treatment of metastatic renal cell cancer. Expert Rev Anticancer Ther 2009; 9:1429-1434.

[60] Sablin MP, Négrier S, Ravaud A et al: Sequential sorafenib and sunitinib for renal cell carcinoma. J Urol 2009; 182:29-34.

[61] Zimmermann K, Schmittel A, Steiner U et al: Sunitinib treatment for patients with advanced clear-cell renal-cell carcinoma after progression on sorafenib. Oncology 2009; 76:350-354.

[62] Rini BI, Escudier B, Tomczak P, et al: Comparative effectiveness of axitinib versus sorafenib in advanced renal cell carcinoma (AXIS): a randomised phase 3 trial. Lancet. 2011 [Epub ahead of print].

4

Steroid Receptors in Renal Cell Carcinoma

Evgeny Yakirevich, Andres Matoso,
David J. Morris and Murray B. Resnick
*Department of Pathology and Laboratory Medicine, Rhode Island Hospital and
Alpert Medical School of Brown University,
USA*

1. Introduction

Renal cell carcinomas (RCCs) are the most common epithelial neoplasms of adult kidney. It has been estimated that there will be about 60,920 new cases of kidney cancer in the United States in 2011 and about 13,120 people will die from this disease (Siegel et al. 2011). Currently, surgery remains the only effective treatment for RCC, since metastatic disease is highly resistant to radiotherapy and chemotherapy. Approximately 20 to 30% of patients with RCCs present with non-resectable metastatic disease and 20 to 40% of patients undergoing nephrectomy for clinically localized RCC will develop metastatic disease. In the past two decades significant advances in the diagnosis and treatment of patients with RCC have resulted in improved survival of a select group of patients. Prior to the availability of targeted therapies, Interferon-α (IFN) was the standard of care but was associated with a low response rate and significant toxicity (Interferon-alpha and survival in metastatic renal carcinoma: early results of a randomized controlled trial. Medical Research Council Renal Cancer Collaborators 1999). High dose interleukin-2 (IL-2) has a similar response rate as IFN, but can cure approximately 3-5% of patients (Yang, Sherry, et al. 2003). Targeted molecular therapies include inhibitors of angiogenesis (Yang, Haworth, et al. 2003), inhibitors of receptor tyrosine kinases with promiscuous targets including VEGFR1 and VEGFR2, PDGFR, C-Kit, Raf kinase, mammalian target of rapamycin (mTOR) (Atkins et al. 2004; Motzer et al. 2006; Porta et al. 2011) and combination treatment modalities (Escudier et al. 2007; Hudes et al. 2007; Motzer et al. 2007). These novel therapies have demonstrated improved outcomes and have become the first line of therapy in patients with advanced metastatic disease or second line of therapy in patients who have failed prior cytokine immunotherapy (Leveridge & Jewett 2011). As new treatment modalities become standard of care, clinical practices in diagnosis and treatment of the primary tumor will undergo revision. For instance, the role of cytoreductive surgery in patients selected for targeted therapy has not yet been established. This could increase the number of cases diagnosed and treated based on core needle biopsies alone, presenting new challenges to surgical pathologists who will likely have to use smaller amounts of tissue to accurately classify the tumor and provide molecular information aimed to personalize clinical care.

RCC is a heterogeneous neoplasm, which includes distinct histological subtypes (Table 1). Among the adult population, clear cell RCC constitutes the most prevalent subtype (70-80%)

Histological Subtype	Incidence	5-Year Survival	Cell of Origin
Clear Cell RCC	70-80%	45-76%	Proximal convoluted tubules
Papillary RCC	10-15%	82-90%	Shared phenotype of proximal and distal tubules
Chromophobe RCC	5%	78-92%	Intercalated cells of collecting tubules and ducts
Oncocytoma	5%	100%	Intercalated cells of collecting tubules and ducts

Table 1. Major Histological Subtypes of Renal Cell Neoplasms with Corresponding Incidence, Survival, and Cell of Origin

and has a relatively unfavorable prognosis (Amin et al. 2002; Eble et al. 2004). Papillary and chromophobe RCCs are less common, comprising 10-15% and 5%, respectively, and have a better prognosis compared to clear cell RCC (Amin et al. 2002). Oncocytoma is a benign renal cell tumor characterized by an extremely favorable prognosis. Renal epithelial tumors are thought to originate in cells of different compartments along the nephron. Clear cell RCC is believed to arise from the proximal tubules. Tumors that originate in the collecting tubules and ducts include chromophobe RCC, oncocytomas, and the more rare collecting duct and medullary carcinomas. The histogenesis of papillary carcinoma is controversial with some studies suggesting a proximal tubule origin while phenotyping by immunohistochemistry supports a distal nephron origin. Renal tumors with papillary growth include papillary RCC types 1 and 2, clear cell RCC with papillary features and the recently described clear cell papillary RCC (CPRCC) (Gobbo et al. 2008). CPRCC is a subtype of renal cell carcinoma characterized by cells with clear cytoplasm arranged in papillary structures which was first described in patients with end stage renal disease, but later also identified in kidneys unaffected by end stage renal disease (Fuzesi et al. 1999; Gobbo et al. 2008).

Immunohistochemistry is useful in distinguishing the different subtypes of renal neoplasms. Clear cell RCCs are frequently CD10 positive but AMACR and CK7 negative; papillary carcinoma, on the other hand, is positive for CK7 and AMACR and usually negative for CD10. Recent studies in CPRCC demonstrate positive immunoreactivity for CK7 but negative AMACR and CD10. These and other immunohistochemical markers are currently used routinely in diagnostic histopathology to help classify tumors. However, this is a constantly evolving field and new immunohistochemical and molecular markers are being investigated to address new clinical needs.

Steroid receptors are a family of ligand dependent transcription factors, which have important roles in control of growth and differentiation in many non-neoplastic and neoplastic cell types. The steroid receptor family is characterized by a unique modular structure, with receptors classically divided into three main domains and several

Steroid Receptor	Expression in Normal Kidney	Tumor Type	Clinical Relevance	References
GR	Proximal tubules, glomeruli	Clear cell RCC	Increased expression is a favorable marker	Yakirevich et al. 2011
MR	Distal tubules, loops of Henle and collecting ducts	Oncocytoma and chromophobe RCC	Diagnostic marker	Yakirevich et al. 2008
ER	Interstitial stromal cells	Cystic nephroma, mixed epithelial and stromal tumor, angiomyolipoma with epithelial cysts	Hormonal mechanism of pathogenesis	Adsay et al. 2000
PR	Interstitial stromal cells	Cystic nephroma, mixed epithelial and stromal tumor, angiomyolipoma with epithelial cysts, chromophobe RCC and oncocytoma	Hormonal mechanism of pathogenesis Diagnostic marker	Adsay et al. 2000 Tickoo et al. 2008 Mai et al. 2008
AR	Proximal and distal tubules	Clear cell, papillary, and chromophobe RCC	Increased expression is a favorable marker	Kimura et al 1993 Langner et al, 2004
VDR	Distal tubules and collecting ducts	Papillary RCC, chromophobe RCC, oncocytoma, collecting duct carcinoma	Diagnostic marker	Obara, Konda et al. 2007 Liu et al. 2006
RAR and RXR	Proximal tubules, interstitial cells	Clear cell RCC, chromophobe RCC (RAR-β)	Increased expression of RXR-γ is a favorable marker	Goelden et al. 2005 Obara, Konda et al. 2007

Table 2. Steroid Receptors in Renal Cell Neoplasms

subdomains or regions. In general, the receptor members share a variable amino-terminal transactivation domain, a central and well-conserved DNA-binding domain (DBD), and a moderately conserved carboxy-terminal domain responsible for ligand binding. The latter domain also contains activating functions. The well known members of the steroid receptor family includes glucocorticoid (GR), mineralocorticoid (MR), progesterone (PR), androgen (AR), estrogen (ER), vitamin D (VDR), thyroid, and retinoic acid (RAR)/retinoid X receptors (RXR) (Fuller 1991).

There is emerging evidence that steroid receptors can induce gene expression through both ligand-dependent and ligand-independent pathways, and distinct families of genes are likely to be regulated depending on the mechanism of nuclear receptor signaling. Until recently, the study of steroid receptors in renal cell neoplasm's (RCNs) has been limited to ER and PR. The employment of novel techniques for studying steroid receptors in RCCs, such as immunohistochemistry, tissue microarray technology, and quantitative real-time PCR has revealed the presence and biologic importance of several steroid receptors in RCNs, including GR, MR, VDR, and others (Table 2). This review will focus on histogenetic, diagnostic, and prognostic implications of steroid receptor expression in RCNs.

2. Glucocorticoid receptor

Glucocorticoids mediate their effects via their intracellular glucocorticoid receptors. Studies of GRs have revealed that there is only one GR gene, but several GR receptor isoforms resulting from alternative splicing or alternative translation initiation (Pujols et al. 2002; Revollo & Cidlowski 2009). Two main human isoforms, GR-α and GR-β, have a different distribution pattern and biologic activity in healthy and diseased human cells and tissues. It has been demonstrated that GR-α is the predominant isoform expressed in a large number of healthy human tissues including brain, liver, kidney, skeletal muscle, lung, and other organs. The GR- α isoform possesses steroid binding activity. In contrast, GR-β expression level is lower than that of the GR- α isoform and is relatively abundant in inflammatory blood cells (Pujols et al. 2002). In non-activated cells, the GR resides in the cytoplasm as a part of a large complex consisting of chaperone and cochaperone proteins including heat shock proteins hsp90, hsp70, immunophilins FKBP51 and FKBP52, and others (De Bosscher et al. 2003). Upon ligand binding, GR undergoes phosphorylation and activation and translocates from the cytoplasm to the nucleus where it converts to a DNA-binding form. Transcriptional responses triggered by activated GR include both positive and negative gene regulation. The direct positive transcriptional regulation of genes (transactivation) requires binding of the GR homodimer to glucocorticoid-response elements (GRE) in gene promoters. The indirect negative regulation (transrepression) is mediated through negative cross-talk with other transcription factors including AP-1, NF-kB and p53 (Beato et al. 1995). As a result, glucocorticoids modulate a variety of physiologic and pathologic processes, including among others cellular differentiation, growth, inflammation, immune response, and carbohydrate metabolism.

2.1 Expression of GR in the normal kidney

In normal human kidneys GRs contribute to the regulation of renal fluid and electrolyte homeostasis. Keeping with their physiologic function, GRs are differentially distributed along the kidney nephron. *In vitro* studies have implicated GRs in the regulation of ammoniagenesis, gluconeogenesis, GFR, Na-H exchange and Na-phosphate co-transport, all of which are proximal renal tubule processes (Baylis et al. 1990; Boross et al. 1986; Campen et al. 1983; Freiberg et al. 1982). Measurement of GRs in normal rat kidney cortical tubules enriched in proximal tubules yielded three to six fold higher GR content as compared to the distal tubules (Mishina et al. 1981). Predominant proximal tubule localization of GR was demonstrated by quantitation of GR mRNA levels in microdissected nephron segments from the rat kidney by a competitive polymerase chain reaction (PCR) technique (Todd-Turla et al. 1993). GR mRNA was twofold more abundant in glomeruli, proximal tubule, and thick ascending limb segments than in the collecting duct segments (Todd-Turla et al. 1993). In an additional study GR mRNA was localized by in-situ hybridization predominantly to renal proximal tubules and cortical collecting tubules with lower levels in distal collecting tubules of the rat kidney (Roland et al. 1995). In a recent study we provided immunohistochemical evidence of GR expression in the proximal tubular epithelium of normal human kidneys and in the epithelial cells of normal renal glomeruli (Yakirevich et al. 2011). However, several *in vitro* and *in vivo* studies have demonstrated that glucocorticoids can exert mineralocorticoid-like effects, such as Na+ reabsorption and K+ secretion, in the distal nephron (Morris & Souness 1992; Naray-Fejes-Toth & Fejes-Toth 1990; Thomas et al. 2006).

2.2 Expression of GR in kidney tumors

Initial studies of GR expression in RCCs based on ligand-binding assays in the early 1980's demonstrated the presence of GRs in kidney tumors (Bojar et al. 1979; Chen et al. 1980; Hemstreet et al. 1980; Liu et al. 1980). In these pioneer studies renal tumors were not subdivided into different histologic subtypes and were all designated as RCCs. Bojar et al. demonstrated GRs in 10 of 15 tumors studied (Bojar et al. 1979). The average dexamethasone binding capacity was calculated and found to be 7.1 fmol/mg of cytosol protein. The ligand specificity experiments clearly indicated that binding to GRs is not restricted to glucocorticoids alone. Progesterone and aldosterone turned out to be moderate competitors for dexamethasone binding. Medroxyprogesterone acetate, the compound widely used in hormone therapy of advanced renal cancer in man, was demonstrated to be one of the strongest inhibitors of [3H] dexamethasone. The binding of medroxyprogesterone acetate to GRs may represent the primary mechanism of action of the compound in causing tumor regression. Hemstreet et al. identified and measured the levels of GRs in 47 autologous pairs of normal and neoplastic renal tissue (Hemstreet et al. 1980). Glucocorticoid receptors were demonstrated in this study in normal and neoplastic tissues of both sexes. The levels of GRs were higher in the tumors (mean 31.3 fmol/mg) than in the normal tissue (18.5 fmol/mg). In an additional study conducted at the same time, Liu et al. reported high concentrations of GRs in four of seven RCC cases (Liu et al. 1980). The levels of GRs in RCCs were comparable to those in the glucocorticoid-responsive rat liver. Furthermore, the GR levels in RCCs were comparable to human acute lymphocytic leukemia cells sensitive (0.03 pmol/mg cytosol protein), in contrast to those that have become resistant (0.015 pmol/mg cytosol protein) to glucocorticoids. Chen et al. detected GRs in cytosol of RCCs (Chen et al. 1980). Competition experiments demonstrated that progestin competed for the GR sites in all renal tumors tested, whereas diethylstilbestrol and testosterone were weak or not competitive.

Development of antibodies against human GR enabled immunohistochemical and Western blot assessment of GR protein expression. In addition, molecular studies utilizing reverse transcriptase polymerase chain reaction (RT-PCR) revealed that most commonly used RCC cell lines express high levels of GR. In a study by Arai et al., two RCC cell lines OUR-10 and NC65 expressed high levels of GR, whereas Caki-1 cell exhibited low levels of GR expression by Western blot (Arai et al. 2008). Iwai et al. demonstrated GR mRNA expression in the A498, RCC270, Caki1, and ACHN renal carcinoma cells. A498 and RCC270 expressed especially high levels of the GR gene (Iwai et al. 2004). Recently, using tissue microarray technology and real-time RT-PCR we described the immunohistochemical and mRNA expression of GRs in different histologic subtypes of RCNs including clear cell RCC, papillary RCC, chromophobe RCC, and oncocytoma (Yakirevich et al. 2011). We found that GRs are strongly expressed in the majority of clear cell RCCs (66%), in 26% of papillary RCCs, and in only 6% of chromophobe RCC and 14% of oncocytomas. Within the clear cell carcinoma group, most positive cases (87%) demonstrated strong expression, whereas only 1 papillary RCC, 1 chromophobe RCC and none of the oncocytomas demonstrated strong immunoreactivity. In this study we used commercially available rabbit-antihuman GR polyclonal antibody PA1-511A from Affinity Bioreagents (Golden, CO) which recognizes both the -α and -β isoforms of GR. In order to recognize specific isoform expressed in RCC, we measured both isoforms by quantitative real-time PCR and demonstrated that RCCs express GR-α isoform. We found that GR expression is associated with tumors of low nuclear grade (Fuhrman grade 1 and 2) and low stage (stage 1 and 2). Although GR expression was demonstrated predominantly in clear cell RCC group, the loss of GR expression in high-grade tumors and overlap with other histologic subtypes of RCCs limit the diagnostic utility of this marker. GR appears to be a marker of less aggressive behavior in RCC as there is significant correlation between GR expression and overall survival in RCC. By the end of follow-up 86% of CRCC patients with tumors expressing GRs were alive as compared to 54% of patients whose tumors were negative.

Since GRs are cytoplasmic receptors, which are translocated to the nuclei upon activation, the predominantly nuclear immunoreactivity of GRs suggests that these receptors are activated in RCCs. Association of GR expression with less aggressive behavior also suggests the tumor-suppressive role of GRs. Signaling through GRs in renal cancer cells involves suppression of other transcription factors, including nuclear factor kB, AP-1, CREB, CCAAT enhancer binding protein (C/EBP), signal transduction activator of transcription (STAT), p53, Smad, *etc* (De Bosscher et al. 2003). Treatment of RCC cell lines with glucocorticoids (dexamethasone) inhibits the activation of nuclear factor kB and its downstream products including IL-2, IL-6, IL-8, and vascular endothelial growth factor which have been demonstrated to promote growth of RCC cell lines (Arai et al. 2008; Iwai et al. 2004; Miki et al. 1989; Takenawa et al. 1995). Glucocorticoids have long been used as anti-inflammatory drugs, and have been beneficial in the treatment of hematopoietic neoplasms (multiple myeloma) and solid malignancies such as hormone-refractory prostate cancer (Greenstein et al. 2002; Storlie et al. 1995). Although glucocorticoids have not been implicated in the treatment of patients with renal cancer, there are few case reports describing the beneficial effects of incidental glucocorticoid treatment in metastatic RCC (Christophersen et al. 2006; Omland & Fossa 1989; Tanaka et al. 2003). Palliation treatment with oral dexamethasone was associated with complete regression of pulmonary and brain metastases (Omland & Fossa 1989). In another case, multiple lung and bone metastases of RCC completely regressed after palliative treatment with betamethasone (Tanaka et al. 2003). A 10 year complete remission of metastatic RCC to the liver and retroperitoneal lymph nodes was described in a patient who received palliative cortisone therapy (Christophersen et al. 2006). The mechanism of metastases regression in these cases is unknown and is not likely to be immune related, because glucocorticoids are known to suppress the immune system. These observations suggest that GR and its agonists may have a potential role in novel anti-cancer hormonal therapies in clear cell RCC.

3. Mineralocorticoid receptor

The mineralocorticoid receptor (MR) has long been considered as a secondary glucocorticoid receptor, even though specific roles of its natural ligand, aldosterone, have been well established since the purification of electrocortin more than 50 years ago. Aldosterone was initially restricted to the control of sodium reabsorption in the kidney, thereby being recognized as a major regulator of volume status and blood pressure. The cloning of a specific receptor for aldosterone (Arriza et al. 1987) definitively moved MR out of the shadow of GR and opened a new era of exciting biological, biochemical, and genetic studies that have provided important insights into the complexity of MR action. The MR is closely related to GR and is 94% homologous in the DNA binding domain and 57% homologous in the ligand binding domain, but only 15% homologous in the N-terminal region (Evans 1988). The MR has a similar affinity for the mineralocorticoid aldosterone and the glucocorticoids corticosterone and cortisol (Krozowski & Funder 1983). Although rats and mice synthesize only corticosterone, cortisol is the predominant glucocorticoid in humans and many other mammals, including rodents. Since the circulating levels of glucocorticoids are several orders of magnitude higher than those of aldosterone, the primary mineralocorticoid, glucocorticoid activation of MR may be functionally significant. Specificity is conferred by the enzyme 11β-hydroxysteroid dehydrogenase type II (11β-HSD2) which converts the cortisol to the less active compound cortisone, thus allowing aldosterone binding to MR. In the absence of ligand, MRs are located in both the cytosol and nucleus bound by a variety of chaperone proteins, including hsp90. Upon exposure to either aldosterone or corticosterone, most MRs are found in the nucleus, where they bind to hormone-response elements and mediate gene expression of signaling proteins regulating water and electrolyte transport including K-ras, serine-threonine kinase Sgk1, and corticosteroid hormone-induced factor (Connell & Davies 2005). The most recent role of aldosterone in renal and cardiac fibrosis has indicated a pro-fibrotic role for MR and the product of 11β-HSD2, cortisone or 11-dehydro-corticosterone in the regulation of this process (Brem et al.).

3.1 Expression of MR in the normal kidney

In contrast to GRs which are expressed in a broad variety of cells, expression of MRs is restricted to fewer cell types. The MR is expressed in so-called "classical" aldosterone target tissues, which are sodium-transporting epithelia (kidney, colon, pancreas, salivary, and sweat glands) and in a variety of non-epithelial target tissues such as the central nervous system, mononuclear lymphocytes, large blood vessels, and the heart (Arriza et al. 1987; Sasano et al. 1992). A general agreement exists that the distal nephron is an aldosterone-specific target site. Specific nuclear binding sites for aldosterone exist from the thick ascending limb of Henle's loop (cortical part) to the distal collecting duct in rabbit and rat kidneys (Farman & Bonvalet 1983; Farman et al. 1982). MR is expressed in the distal tubules, the connecting tubules, and along the collecting ducts at the mRNA level in rat and rabbit kidneys (Escoubet et al. 1996; Todd-Turla et al. 1993) and at the protein level in rabbit kidneys (Lombes et al. 1990). Immunohistochemical studies showed that in normal human kidney MR is expressed in the distal convoluted tubules, collecting ducts, and loops of Henle with predominant nuclear localization (Hirasawa et al. 1997; Sasano et al. 1992; Yakirevich et al. 2008).

3.2 Expression of MR in kidney tumors

More than 30 years ago Rafestin-Oblin et al. demonstrated the presence of high-affinity sites for aldosterone in normal human kidneys using a ligand-binding assay. In RCCs the cytosol and nuclear aldosterone binding was significantly lower than in normal tissues (Rafestin-Oblin et al. 1979). However, this study focused exclusively on clear cell RCCs. Recently using immunohistochemistry we analyzed tissue microarray specimens from patients with different histologic subtypes of renal cell neoplasms, and in addition, we quantitated MR mRNA by real time RT-PCR (Yakirevich et al. 2008). Most of the chromophobe RCC (90%) and oncocytomas (93%) strongly expressed MR. No MR immunoreactivity was detected in clear cell RCC, including clear cell carcinoma with predominantly granular cytoplasm, or in papillary RCC. The MR+ immunophenotype of chromophobe carcinoma and oncocytoma reflects their histogenetic origin from phenotypically similar distal convoluted tubules and collecting ducts, whereas absence of immunoreactivity in clear cell RCC is consistent with its origin from proximal convoluted tubules. As we described in the previous section, proximal tubules and histogenetically related clear cell RCCs express high levels of GR. MR appears to be a sensitive and specific marker of the distal nephron and its related neoplasms (chromophobe RCC and oncocytoma) and may be considered in the immunohistochemical panel to more accurately subtype renal cell tumors.

4. Estrogen receptor

The effects of estrogens are mediated by estrogen receptors (ERs). ERs were discovered in the 1960's by Jensen and Jacobson (Jensen et al. 2010). The basic structure of ER protein is similar to other steroid receptors and contains a DNA binding domain, transcription modulating domain, and steroid hormone binding domain. There are two ER types encoded on different chromosomes: ER-α cloned in 1986 and ER-β, which was discovered in 1996 (Greene et al. 1986; Kuiper et al. 1996). ER-α is expressed in a variety of human organs, mainly reproductive, including the mammary gland, ovary, uterus, and vagina (Muramatsu & Inoue 2000). ER-β is expressed in genitourinary human tissues such as prostate, ovary, testis, bladder, uterus, and renal pelvis, in the central nervous system, and is especially increased compared to ER-α in various fetal tissues such as adrenals (Gustafsson 1999). The affinity of ER-β to bind estradiol-17β is similar to the ER-α form. However, ER-β binds both androgens and phytoestrogens with greater affinity. The main physiologic role of ERs is implicated in the control of proliferation, differentiation, and development of many tissues. In contrast to the beneficial physiologic effects, ERs may also promote the development and growth of variety of cancers, including breast, endometrial and ovarian carcinomas in humans (Speirs et al. 1999) and renal tumors in Syrian hamsters (Li et al. 2001).

4.1 Expression of ER in the normal kidney

Expression of ERs was extensively studied in hamster kidneys; however, the distribution of ER in normal hamster kidney is controversial. In a study by Bhat et al. who treated hamsters with estradiol to induce tumors, ER immunolocalization in normal kidneys of estrogen-treated hamsters or in untreated controls was identified only in the renal glomerular pododcytes, mesangial and parietal cells and in several interstitial cell types but not in the tubular epithelia of the cortex (Bhat et al. 1993). In addition, arterial cells, including pericytes and endothelial cells of the arteriolae rectae and endothelial cells of the arterial vasa recta, strongly expressed ER. The receptor distribution in kidneys of untreated female hamsters matched that of males, but the intensity of staining was higher than in male kidneys. Another study confirmed immunohistochemical expression of ER in interstitial cells and localized these cells to the corticomedullary junction (Li et al. 2001). The authors found that estrogen treatment causes a significant increase in ER-α positive interstitial cells compared to untreated controls and hypothesized that renal tumors arise from a subset of multipotential interstitial cells driven to proliferate by estrogens. However, in contrast to the study by Bhat et al., in this study ER expression was consistently demonstrated in nuclei of proximal tubules and disappeared after estrogen treatment.

4.2 Expression of ER in kidney tumors

Initial biochemical studies of ER status in renal tumors were performed in early 1980s by the dextran-coated charcoal method and the sucrose gradient centrifugation assay. These biochemical assays were based on cytosol preparations containing high, but unknown levels of plasma contamination. Furthermore, there was significant inconsistency in the number of tumor cells present within the specimens (Karr et al. 1983). Therefore, the level and frequency of ER expression in human kidney tumors were highly variable. Hemstreet et al. reported detectable ERs in 30% of the tumors compared to 40% of normals, whereas in other studies utilizing similar biochemical techniques ERs were not detected or detected in a rather low percentage of 4-9% of tumors (Hemstreet et al. 1980; Karr et al. 1983; Pearson et al. 1981). In a more recent immunohistochemical analysis of steroid hormone expression in tissue microarrays containing 182 RCCs of different histologic subtypes, Langer et al. demonstrated ER immunoreactivity in less than 10% of tumor cells in only 2 of 182 of patients (1.1%), including one clear cell RCC and one chromophobe RCC (Langner et al. 2004). Thus, the biochemical and immunohistochemical results provide evidence that ER is not expressed or very rare expressed in low levels in RCCs.

Recently, several benign renal tumors, characterized by the presence of stroma that resembles ovarian, endometrial, and mullerian-like, have been described, including cystic nephroma, mixed epithelial and stromal tumor (MEST) and angiomyolipomas with epithelial cysts (AMLEC) (Fine et al. 2006; Turbiner et al. 2007). Adsay et al. detected ERs in nuclei of the spindle cells in seven of 12 MESTs (Adsay et al. 2000). The staining was strong and diffuse and was present predominantly in the areas with long, slender, fibrocyte-like cells. In three of these cases, the epithelial cells also exhibited a cytoplasmic reaction with antibody to ER. Distinctive clinical and pathologic features characterize these lesions. Most of the patients in study of Adsay et al. were middle-aged (perimenopausal) females (mean age, 56 years) who had a long-term history of estrogen use. The only male patient also had a history of diethylstilbestrol exposure for 7 years followed by 4 years of lupron therapy for prostatic adenocarcinoma. These clinical findings, combined with frequent ER expression detected by immunohistochemistry raise the possibility of hormonal mechanism of pathogenesis of these tumors. It is plausible that the spindle cells of these tumors arise from a "periductal fetal mesenchyma" present in epithelial structures of organs such as kidney, pancreas, and liver. The primitive mesenchyme may have the capacity to interact with epithelia. Alterations of hormonal milieu (perimenopausal changes or therapeutic hormones with unopposed estrogens) may induce proliferation of this mesenchyme, which in turn activates the growth of epithelial component.

5. Progesterone receptor

The progesterone receptor (PR) has two predominant isoforms: PR-α, and PR-β, which are produced from a single gene by alternative promoter usage (Jeltsch et al. 1986). These isoforms have similar steroid hormone and DNA binding activities, but PR-β has a much higher transcriptional activating potential. Clinically, PR expression is routinely assessed by immunohistochemistry using an antibody that recognizes both PR-α and PR-β.

5.1 Expression of PR in the normal kidney

No detectable PR staining was seen in renal sections from untreated castrated male hamsters in a study by Bhat et al. (Bhat et al. 1993). However, after estrogen treatment, PR expression was detected in single interstitial cells. The pattern of PR immunoreactivity was largely confined to interstitial cells located at the renal corticomedullary region, similar to ER expressing cells described above. PRs were identified in normal human kidneys by biochemical and more recently immunohistochemical techniques (Hemstreet et al. 1980; McDonald et al. 1983). Interesting, in normal human kidneys PRs were detected by immunohistochemistry in interstitial stromal cells, some tubules, and mesangial cells of glomeruli in two of seven cases (Tickoo et al. 2008).

5.2 Expression of PR in kidney tumors

Expression of PR in kidney tumors was studied in parallel with ER analysis. The level and frequency of PR in human kidney tumors is highly variable when analyzed biochemically varying from 0 to 23% (Hemstreet et al. 1980; Karr et al. 1983; Pearson et al. 1981). Immunohistochemical analysis of steroid hormone expression in tissue microarrays containing 182 RCCs of different histologic subtypes demonstrated PR immunoreactivity in less than 10% of tumor cells in only two of 182 patients, including one clear cell RCC and one papillary RCC (Langner et al. 2004). PRs were found in stromal cells of renal neoplasms with ovarian-like stroma, although less frequently as compared to ER (Adsay et al. 2000). More recently Mai et al. identified PR immunoreactivity of tumor cells and stromal cells within the neoplasm and/or surrounding capsule in renal oncocytoma and chromophobe RCC (Mai et al. 2008). This immunoreactivity was not seen in other tumors with oncocytic/eosinophilic cytoplasm, such as papillary RCC with eosinophilc cytoplasm or clear cell RCC with eosinophilic cytoplasm. PR appears to be a sensitive and highly specific marker for renal oncocytoma and a highly specific marker for chromophobe RCC. It was demonstrated that PR immunoreactivity is more extensive in oncocytoma than in chromophobe RCC, therefore, the extent of PR immunoreactivity could be useful in distinguishing oncocytoma from chromophobe RCC. The presence of PR in oncocytoma and chromophobe RCC provides additional support to the histopathogenetic relationship between renal oncocytoma and chromophobe RCC.

6. Androgen receptor

Androgens are essential for differentiation and growth of male reproductive organs and for various biological effects in the kidney, brain, liver, muscle, bone and skin. Androgens include testosterone and dihydrotestosterone and mediate their biologic effect through the androgen receptor (AR). The AR gene is located on chromosome Xq11-12 (Brown et al. 1989; Lubahn et al. 1988). Males have a single copy of the gene allowing phenotypic manifestation of any genetic alteration. Transcription of the AR gene is cell-specific and modified by age, androgen and other steroid hormones (Gelmann 2002). Androgen is best known to influence development and growth of prostate cancer. However, its metabolic role in cancer is not limited to the prostate and a number of studies utilizing animal models combined with clinical and epidemiologic data suggest a role for androgen in RCC (Concolino, Marocchi, Conti et al. 1978; Karr et al. 1983).

6.1 Expression of AR in the normal kidney

AR is ubiquitously expressed in the whole body with studies showing detectable levels of protein and mRNA in adrenal glands, uterus, aorta, adipose tissue, kidney, spleen, heart, lung, large intestine, stomach, small intestine and liver (Kimura et al. 1993; Ruizeveld de Winter et al. 1991; Takeda et al. 1990). In normal kidneys AR expression was consistently demonstrated to be present in the nuclei of distal tubule cells (Kimura et al. 1993; Li et al. 2010). Additionally, a study by Takeda et al. showed AR immunoreactivity not only in the distal tubule but also in the proximal tubule and focal parietal expression in the Bowman's capsule (Takeda et al. 1990).

6.2 Expression of AR in kidney tumors

The hormone dependence of RCC has been established in animal models and in humans for many years (Bloom 1973; Concolino, Marocchi, Conti et al. 1978; Concolino, Marocchi, Tenaglia et al. 1978; Li et al. 1977). In humans, extensive research on AR in RCC has shown variable results (Concolino et al. 1981; Jakse & Muller-Holzner 1988; Karr et al. 1983; Klotzl et al. 1987; Nakano et al. 1984; Noronha & Rao 1985) In a case series study by Brown et al., that included 12 primary clear cell RCCs and 5 clear cell RCCs metastatic to the central nervous system, AR immunoreactivity was present in five primary and one metastatic RCC (Brown et al. 1998). A more recent study by Langner et al. demonstrated that AR immunoreactivity was not detectable in non-tumoral kidney tissue (Langner et al. 2004). However, AR was found in 15% of patients with RCC and inversely correlated with histopathologic stage, with 27% of pT1 tumors being positive versus 4% of pT3 tumors. Furthermore, expression of AR was higher in pT1a tumors compared to pT1b (32% vs. 17%). Additionally, AR expression inversely correlated with nuclear grade with 21% positivity in nuclear grades 1 and 2 and 7% in nuclear grades 3 and 4. Univariate analysis showed a longer disease free survival in patients with AR positive tumors compared to patients with

AR negative tumors (Langner et al. 2004). These results reflect similar trends observed with GRs in RCC (Yakirevich et al. 2011), however, the diagnostic, prognostic or therapeutic utility of AR analysis in RCC is uncertain and might require further investigations.

7. Vitamin D receptor

Vitamin D is a lipid-soluble compound whose major function is the maintenance of adequate plasma levels of calcium and phosphorus, important for bone mineralization, neuromuscular transmission and general cellular metabolism. Vitamin D receptor (VDR) is present in various tissues that do not participate in calcium metabolism and regulates the expression of hundreds of genes that control cell proliferation, differentiation and angiogenesis. Low levels of vitamin D have been associated with increased incidence of colon, prostate and breast cancer (Thacher & Clarke 2011). Recent studies suggest that vitamin D may be inversely associated with the risk of RCC. (Bosetti et al. 2007; Ikuyama et al. 2002; Karami et al. 2008; Obara, Suzuki et al. 2007). Vitamin D receptor is expressed in malignant tumors, including RCC, and mediates the biological actions of $1,25(OH)_2D_3$ (Lamprecht & Lipkin 2003). In this section, we will review the current literature on the relevance of vitamin D and its receptor in RCC.

7.1 Expression of VDR in the normal kidney

The kidney is a major organ for vitamin D metabolism and calcium homeostasis. Activation of vitamin D involves conversion of 7-dehydrocholesterol to cholecalciferol by UVB radiation in the skin. Cholecalciferol is metabolized by the 25-hydroxylases (CYP2R1 and CYP27A1) in the liver to 25-hydroxycholecalciferol ($25(OH)D_3$). $25(OH)D_3$ then undergoes glomerular filtration and is subsequently converted to the active form calcitriol ($1,25(OH)_2D_3$) by the 1α-hydroxylase (CYP27B1) located primarily in the proximal tubule. Calcitriol binds to an intracellular receptor (VDR), a ligand dependent transcription factor belonging to the class II nuclear receptor subfamily. The effect of calcitriol is negatively controlled by CYP24A1 (Fleet 2008; Nykjaer et al. 1999). Immunohistochemistry studies of non-tumoral kidney show expression of VDR predominantly in the distal tubules and collecting ducts with only faint or lack of stain in the proximal tubule cells (Blomberg Jensen et al. 2010; Liu et al. 2006; Obara, Konda et al. 2007). This expression pattern is consistent with studies that demonstrate that vitamin-D induced calcium re-absorption occurs in the distal tubules (Li & Christakos 1991).

7.2 Expression of VDR in kidney tumors

In keeping with absence of VDR expression in the proximal tubule, a study by Liu et al. showed that clear cell RCC is generally negative for VDR by immunohistochemistry and showed decreased mRNA level compared to non-tumoral kidney control tissue by RT-PCR (Liu et al. 2006). When whole sections of tumors were stained, expression of VDR was present only focally in the peripheral region of the tumor. Previously, a study by Madej et al. showed that expression of VDR in clear cell RCC was similar to control tissue by Western and Northern blot analysis (Madej et al. 2003). This discrepancy could be due to a difference in the degree of differentiation of the tumors analyzed in each study. While the expression level seems not to be affected by the Fuhrman nuclear grade, increased VDR immunoreactivity was observed in sarcomatous and poorly differentiated areas of RCC and in metastatic tumors or in intravascular tumor islands (Liu et al. 2006).

A different study by Blomberg Jensen et al. showed that VDR mRNA was detected in all normal kidney samples while almost undetectable in clear cell RCC with similar results confirmed by Western blot (Blomberg Jensen et al. 2010). Additionally, in this study, the authors investigated the expression of Vitamin D activating enzymes including CYP2R1, CYP27A1, and CYP27B1. The 1 α-hydroxylase (CYP27B1) was present in all normal samples with varying degrees of expression levels, the lowest expression in atrophic kidneys. By immunohistochemistry and in-situ hybridization, expression of CYP2R1 and CYP27A1 was localized to the distal tubule, collecting ducts and minimal expression in the proximal tubule. Expression of CYP27B1 was more prominent in the proximal tubule. Expression of these enzymes was diminished in clear cell RCC along with decreased expression of VDR (Blomberg Jensen et al. 2010). Papillary RCC is positive for VDR in the great majority of cases. This recapitulates more closely the phenotype of distal tubules. Similarly, chromophobe carcinoma and oncocytomas are also positive for VDR. Staining of chromophobe carcinoma accentuates the cell membrane while in oncocytomas it is stronger in the perinuclear area (Liu et al. 2006). Collecting duct carcinoma is thought to derive from the principal cells of the collecting duct of Bellini. Consistent with other tumors of origin from the distal nephron, three out of three collecting duct carcinomas tested were positive for VDR by immunohistochemistry (Liu et al. 2006).

Currently, immunohistochemistry for vitamin D is not routinely used for diagnostic purposes. However, several findings described above could eventually prove to have diagnostic utility in anatomic pathology. Because almost all clear cell RCC proved to be negative by immunohistochemistry (with the exception of some high grade tumors, or tumor present within vascular lumens), a positive VDR immunohistochemistry result should alert the pathologist about a potential problem in the classification of a tumor thought to be clear cell RCC (Liu et al. 2006).

A frequent problem in the diagnosis of renal tumors is the distinction between oncocytomas and eosinophilic chromophobe carcinoma (Takahashi et al. 2003; Young et al. 2001). This distinction is critical as these tumors have completely different prognostic and therapeutic clinical implications. Results reported in the literature indicate that both tumors are immunoreactive for VDR with a difference in the localization of the stain. While oncocytomas stained preferably in the perinuclear area, chromophobe carcinoma showed accentuated stain of the cell membrane (Liu et al. 2006).

Positive stain for VDR in papillary RCC could help differentiate this tumor from clear cell RCC with papillary features, which will be negative in the great majority of cases. VDR expression in CPRCC has not been tested; however, since these tumors are CK7 positive, it is likely that they are VDR positive as well, consistent with distal nephron phenotype. Only three cases of collecting duct carcinoma have been tested for VDR immunoreactivity and all of them turned positive. Differential diagnosis of these tumors could be challenging due to their infrequent presentations. Main differential diagnoses include adenocarcinoma or urothelial carcinoma with glandular differentiation. Although there is lack of information in the literature regarding expression of VDR receptor in urothelial carcinoma with glandular differentiation, studies on normal urothelium and urothelial neoplasms have shown consistent positivity for VDR for which it seems unlikely that it would have utility in the differential diagnosis on this context (Hermann & Andersen 1997; Konety et al. 2001).

The anti-cancer effect of vitamin D includes inhibition of cell proliferation and induction of apoptosis (Blutt et al. 2000; Rashid et al. 2001; Zhuang & Burnstein 1998). Expression of VDR as detected by immunohistochemistry was not associated with survival in a cohort of 68 RCC patients (Obara, Konda et al. 2007). This could be due to a small number of patients studied or secondary to other possible alterations within the signaling pathway that could interfere with the normal function of the receptor. Different studies have shown consistently that VDR-DNA complexes are decreased in RCC, even in the presence of exogenous vitamin D (Madej et al. 2003; Trydal et al. 1988). This functional impairment could be secondary to suboptimal VDR heterodimerization with its partners in tumor cells. Before binding to DNA, VDR heterodimerizes with retinoid X receptor (RXR), its obligate partner (Barsony & Prufer 2002; Prufer & Barsony 2002). Retinoid X receptors are part of the retinoic acid receptor systems and share with retinoic acid part of the signaling pathways. Notably, positive RXR-γ staining in RCC correlates with prolonged overall 5-years survival (Obara, Konda et al. 2007).

Calcitriol has anti-proliferative properties in a variety of malignant cell types (Getzenberg et al. 1997; Reichel et al. 1989). The anti-neoplastic activity of VDR ligands was first described in 1981 in a study showing differentiating properties of calcitriol in mouse myeloid leukemia cells (Abe et al. 1981). Since then, a number of studies have demonstrated the in-vitro and in-vivo anti-cancer potential of vitamin D in models of bladder, breast, colon, endometrium, lung, pancreas, prostate and squamous cell carcinoma, sarcomas of the soft tissues and bone, neuroblastoma, glioma, melanoma, and other malignancies (Beer & Myrthue 2004; Trump et al. 2004; Trump et al. 2006).

Calcitriol treatment of cells inhibited cell growth and clonogenicity of the RCC cell line derived from a pulmonary metastasis of RCC, (Nagakura et al. 1986). In a different study, BALB/c mice were inoculated with murine renal cancer Renca and graded doses of calcitriol were given intraperitoneally. Vitamin D inhibited tumor growth and prolonged the life span of Renca-bearing mice in a dose-dependent manner. Furthermore, vitamin D treated mice showed reduced pulmonary and hepatic metastates (Fujioka et al. 1998). Despite these and other promising results in cell culture and in murine models, the utility of vitamin D therapy in humans has been challenged by its hypercalcemic toxic effect (Fakih et al. 2007; Muindi et al. 2009). To try to bypass this toxicity, researchers have explored alternative vitamin D like molecules. A recent published study investigated the in-vitro and in-vivo effect of 1,25-dihydroxyvitamin D3-3-bromoacetate [1,25(OH)$_2$D3-3-BE], an alkylating derivative of 1,25(OH)$_2$D3 (Lambert et al. 2010). This study reports that 1,25(OH)$_2$D3-3-BE is significantly more potent than an equivalent concentration of 1,25(OH)$_2$D3 in inhibiting growth of A498 and Caki 1 human kidney cancer cells. The mechanisms behind cell growth inhibition of cell-cycle progression include downregulating cyclin A and induction of apoptosis through caspase activity. When compared to calcitriol, 1,25(OH)$_2$D3-3-BE was more potent at reducing tumor size, which was accompanied by an increase in apoptosis and reduction of cyclin A staining in the tumors. These results show a promising potential of vitamin D derived compounds as targeted therapy for RCC patients (Lambert et al. 2010).

8. Retinoic acid receptors

Retinoids are a family of molecules related to vitamin A that include retinoic acid (RA) and all-trans retinoid. Retinoids participate in diverse functions in many organ systems during development and in adulthood including vision, neural function and immune response. Extensive research also supports a role of retinoids in cell proliferation and differentiation through cell cycle signaling promoting block in G1 phase of cell cycle, by directly or indirectly modulating cyclins, CDKs, and cell-cycle inhibitors (Mongan & Gudas 2007; Tang & Gudas 2011). There are two distinct retinoid nuclear receptor systems, the RARs types -α, -β and -γ, and RXRs types -α, -β and -γ (Pemrick et al. 1994). RARs form heterodimers with RXRs and act by binding to retinoic acid response elements (RARE) located in the promoter regions of RA-target genes and modulate transcription rates (Altucci & Gronemeyer 2001). In addition to its role in senescence and cell differentiation, retinoic acid can follow an alternative pathway by binding to a so-called orphan nuclear receptor, PPAR-β/-δ to promote cell survival under certain conditions (Schug et al. 2007).

8.1 Expression of retinoic acid receptors in the normal kidney

Studies evaluating the expression of RARs and RXRs indicate that expression of a given receptor subtype is cell type specific and that retinoic acid effect in different cell types are linked to specific receptor type (Geradts et al. 1993; Kakizuka et al. 1991; Moasser et al. 1994; Moasser et al. 1995; Sheikh et al. 1994; Swisshelm et al. 1994). Information on expression of RARs in normal kidney derives primarily from normal controls used in studies for various purposes. RAR-β mRNA has consistently been found to be expressed in normal kidney tissue samples (Goelden et al. 2005; Vanderleede et al. 1995). Additionally, expression of RARs and RXRs were studied in podocytes, which expressed most isoforms of retinoic acid receptors (RAR) and RXRs with the exception of RXR-γ (He et al. 2007). Obara et al. detected expression of RXR-α and-γ in nuclei of proximal tubule cells, while RXR-β expression was present in proximal tubule cells and interstitial cells (Obara, Konda et al. 2007).

8.2 Expression of retinoic acid receptors in kidney tumors

Dysregulation of each RA receptor has been found in association with different types of cancer. RAR-α is dysregulated in acute promyelocytic leukemia (APL). Majority of APL cases present a chromosomal translocation that fuses the promyelocytic leukemia gene, *PML* and the *RAR-α* genes [t(15;17)(22;q11.2-12)] which can be effectively treated and cured with a combination of retinoid and chemotherapy. In contrast to RAR-α, RAR-β is involved in solid tumorigenesis including RCC (Argiles et al. 1994; Berg et al. 1999; Goelden et al. 2005; Hoffman et al. 1996). The RAR-β gene maps on the short arm of chromosome 3, a region frequently deleted in cancer (Houle et al. 1993). Several studies demonstrated decreased or undetectable levels of RAR-β mRNA in tissue or cell lines derived from different tumors including lung (Suh et al. 2002; Zhang et al. 1994), prostate (Nakayama et al. 2001), breast (Swisshelm et al. 1994), ovary (Sabichi et al. 1998), colon (Cote et al. 1998), head and neck

(Xu et al. 1994) and cervix (Geisen et al. 1997). RAR-β mRNA was decreased or not detectable in 11 of 12 RCC cell lines (Hoffman et al. 1996). These cell lines were either resistant or minimally inhibited when treated with 13-*cis*-RA (13-CRA). Conversely, chromophobe RCC shows much higher levels of expression of RAR-β with a ratio of tumor/normal of over 36 (Goelden et al. 2005). In clear cell RCC, immunoreactivity for RXR-α was observed in up to 70% of the cases, RXR-β was present in 47% of cases, and RXR-γ stain was seen in 85% of cases, in a study that included 49 CRCCs (Obara, Konda et al. 2007). Only expression of RXR-γ was found to correlate inversely with pathological and clinical stage. While all subtypes of RXRs showed variable nuclear or cytoplasmic stain, subcellular location did not correlate with any prognostic variables. Additionally, this study suggests a prolonged overall 5-year survival of patients with tumors that are RXR-γ positive (Obara, Konda et al. 2007).

In clinical trials, the effect of RA in RCC patients has been tested in patients with metastatic disease. A randomized clinical trial of 284 patients evaluated response to treatment with IFNα2a plus 13-cis-retinoic acid (13-CRA) or treatment with IFNα2a alone (Motzer et al. 2000). This study showed no difference in the overall survival but median duration of response (complete and partial combined) in the group treated with the combination was 33 months versus 22 months for the second group. Nineteen percent of patients treated with IFNα2a plus 13-CRA were progression-free at 24 months, compared with 10% of patients treated with IFNα2a alone (Motzer et al. 2000). However, a separate clinical trial that involved 320 patients concluded that progression-free and overall survival for patients with progressive metastatic RCC treated with IFNα2a plus 13-CRA were significantly longer compared with patients on IFN alone (Aass et al. 2005). Another clinical trial that included three different treatment regimens: *a*) triple combination of IL-2, IFNα2a, and fluorouracil; *b*) triple combination of group *a* and additional 13-CRA; *c*) control group treated with IFN-α and vinblastine. Progression-free and overall survival were significantly longer in groups *a* and *b* but there was no significant survival advantage for patients receiving 13-CRA (Atzpodien et al. 2004). These studies suggest that there is some beneficial effect of retinoids treatment, in at least a subset of patients with RCC.

9. Conclusion

Steroid receptors are differentially expressed in the normal kidney and in renal cell neoplasms. Several steroid receptors, such as MR, PR, and vitamin D receptor may be included in diagnostic immunohistochemical panels in order to more accurately subtype renal cell tumors. Although ER is not detected in significant amounts in RCCs, it is expressed by stromal cells in several benign renal neoplasms and may be involved in their pathogenesis. GR and AR appear to be markers of less aggressive behavior in clear cell RCC. Finally, steroid receptors and their downstream signaling mechanisms may have a potential role in novel anticancer hormonal therapies in RCCs.

10. References

Aass, N., De Mulder, P. H., Mickisch, G. H., Mulders, P., van Oosterom, A. T., van Poppel, H., Fossa, S. D., de Prijck, L., and Sylvester, R. J. 2005. Randomized phase II/III trial of interferon Alfa-2a with and without 13-cis-retinoic acid in patients with progressive metastatic renal cell Carcinoma: the European Organisation for Research and Treatment of Cancer Genito-Urinary Tract Cancer Group (EORTC 30951). *J Clin Oncol* 23 (18):4172-8.

Abe, E., Miyaura, C., Sakagami, H., Takeda, M., Konno, K., Yamazaki, T., Yoshiki, S., and Suda, T. 1981. Differentiation of mouse myeloid leukemia cells induced by 1 alpha,25-dihydroxyvitamin D3. *Proc Natl Acad Sci U S A* 78 (8):4990-4.

Adsay, N. V., Eble, J. N., Srigley, J. R., Jones, E. C., and Grignon, D. J. 2000. Mixed epithelial and stromal tumor of the kidney. *Am J Surg Pathol* 24 (7):958-70.

Altucci, L., and Gronemeyer, H. 2001. The promise of retinoids to fight against cancer. *Nat Rev Cancer* 1 (3):181-93.

Amin, M. B., Tamboli, P., Javidan, J., Stricker, H., de-Peralta Venturina, M., Deshpande, A., and Menon, M. 2002. Prognostic impact of histologic subtyping of adult renal epithelial neoplasms: an experience of 405 cases. *Am J Surg Pathol* 26 (3):281-91.

Arai, Y., Nonomura, N., Nakai, Y., Nishimura, K., Oka, D., Shiba, M., Nakayama, M., Takayama, H., Mizutani, Y., Miki, T., and Okuyama, A. 2008. The growth-inhibitory effects of dexamethasone on renal cell carcinoma in vivo and in vitro. *Cancer Invest* 26 (1):35-40.

Argiles, A., Ootaka, T., Hill, P. A., Nikolic-Paterson, D. J., Hutchinson, P., Kraft, N. E., and Atkins, R. C. 1994. Regulation of human renal adenocarcinoma cell growth by retinoic acid and its interactions with epidermal growth factor. *Kidney Int* 45 (1):23-31.

Arriza, J. L., Weinberger, C., Cerelli, G., Glaser, T. M., Handelin, B. L., Housman, D. E., and Evans, R. M. 1987. Cloning of human mineralocorticoid receptor complementary DNA: structural and functional kinship with the glucocorticoid receptor. *Science* 237 (4812):268-75.

Atkins, M. B., Hidalgo, M., Stadler, W. M., Logan, T. F., Dutcher, J. P., Hudes, G. R., Park, Y., Liou, S. H., Marshall, B., Boni, J. P., Dukart, G., and Sherman, M. L. 2004. Randomized phase II study of multiple dose levels of CCI-779, a novel mammalian target of rapamycin kinase inhibitor, in patients with advanced refractory renal cell carcinoma. *J Clin Oncol* 22 (5):909-18.

Atzpodien, J., Kirchner, H., Jonas, U., Bergmann, L., Schott, H., Heynemann, H., Fornara, P., Loening, S. A., Roigas, J., Muller, S. C., Bodenstein, H., Pomer, S., Metzner, B., Rebmann, U., Oberneder, R., Siebels, M., Wandert, T., Puchberger, T., and Reitz, M. 2004. Interleukin-2- and interferon alfa-2a-based immunochemotherapy in advanced renal cell carcinoma: a Prospectively Randomized Trial of the German Cooperative Renal Carcinoma Chemoimmunotherapy Group (DGCIN). *J Clin Oncol* 22 (7):1188-94.

Barsony, J., and Prufer, K. 2002. Vitamin D receptor and retinoid X receptor interactions in motion. *Vitam Horm* 65:345-76.

Baylis, C., Handa, R. K., and Sorkin, M. 1990. Glucocorticoids and control of glomerular filtration rate. *Semin Nephrol* 10 (4):320-9.

Beato, M., Herrlich, P., and Schutz, G. 1995. Steroid hormone receptors: many actors in search of a plot. *Cell* 83 (6):851-7.

Beer, T. M., and Myrthue, A. 2004. Calcitriol in cancer treatment: from the lab to the clinic. *Mol Cancer Ther* 3 (3):373-81.

Berg, W. J., Nanus, D. M., Leung, A., Brown, K. T., Hutchinson, B., Mazumdar, M., Xu, X. C., Lotan, R., Reuter, V. E., and Motzer, R. J. 1999. Up-regulation of retinoic acid receptor beta expression in renal cancers in vivo correlates with response to 13-cis-retinoic acid and interferon-alpha-2a. *Clin Cancer Res* 5 (7):1671-5.

Bhat, H. K., Hacker, H. J., Bannasch, P., Thompson, E. A., and Liehr, J. G. 1993. Localization of estrogen receptors in interstitial cells of hamster kidney and in estradiol-induced renal tumors as evidence of the mesenchymal origin of this neoplasm. *Cancer Res* 53 (22):5447-51.

Blomberg Jensen, M., Andersen, C. B., Nielsen, J. E., Bagi, P., Jorgensen, A., Juul, A., and Leffers, H. 2010. Expression of the vitamin D receptor, 25-hydroxylases, 1alpha-hydroxylase and 24-hydroxylase in the human kidney and renal clear cell cancer. *J Steroid Biochem Mol Biol* 121 (1-2):376-82.

Bloom, H. J. 1973. Proceedings: Hormone-induced and spontaneous regression of metastatic renal cancer. *Cancer* 32 (5):1066-71.

Blutt, S. E., McDonnell, T. J., Polek, T. C., and Weigel, N. L. 2000. Calcitriol-induced apoptosis in LNCaP cells is blocked by overexpression of Bcl-2. *Endocrinology* 141 (1):10-7.

Bojar, H., Maar, K., and Staib, W. 1979. The endocrine background of human renal cell carcinoma. IV. Glucocorticoid receptors as possible mediators of progestogen action. *Urol Int* 34 (5):330-8.

Boross, M., Kinsella, J., Cheng, L., and Sacktor, B. 1986. Glucocorticoids and metabolic acidosis-induced renal transports of inorganic phosphate, calcium, and NH4. *Am J Physiol* 250 (5 Pt 2):F827-33.

Bosetti, C., Scotti, L., Maso, L. D., Talamini, R., Montella, M., Negri, E., Ramazzotti, V., Franceschi, S., and La Vecchia, C. 2007. Micronutrients and the risk of renal cell cancer: a case-control study from Italy. *Int J Cancer* 120 (4):892-6.

Brem, A. S., Morris, D. J., Ge, Y., Dworkin, L. D., Tolbert, E., and Gong, R. 2010. Direct Fibrogenic Effects of Aldosterone on Normotensive Kidney: An Effect Modified by 11{beta}-HSD Activity. *Am J Physiol Renal Physiol.* 298: F1178–87.

Brown, C. J., Goss, S. J., Lubahn, D. B., Joseph, D. R., Wilson, E. M., French, F. S., and Willard, H. F. 1989. Androgen receptor locus on the human X chromosome: regional localization to Xq11-12 and description of a DNA polymorphism. *Am J Hum Genet* 44 (2):264-9.

Brown, D. F., Dababo, M. A., Hladik, C. L., Eagan, K. P., White, C. L., 3rd, and Rushing, E. J. 1998. Hormone receptor immunoreactivity in hemangioblastomas and clear cell renal cell carcinomas. *Mod Pathol* 11 (1):55-9.

Campen, T. J., Vaughn, D. A., and Fanestil, D. D. 1983. Mineralo- and glucocorticoid effects on renal excretion of electrolytes. *Pflugers Arch* 399 (2):93-101.

Chen, L., Weiss, F. R., Chaichik, S., and Keydar, I. 1980. Steroid receptors in human renal carcinoma. *Isr J Med Sci* 16 (11):756-60.

Christophersen, A. O., Lie, A. K., and Fossa, S. D. 2006. Unexpected 10 years complete remission after cortisone mono-therapy in metastatic renal cell carcinoma. *Acta Oncol* 45 (2):226-8.

Concolino, G., Marocchi, A., Conti, C., Tenaglia, R., Di Silverio, F., and Bracci, U. 1978. Human renal cell carcinoma as a hormone-dependent tumor. *Cancer Res* 38 (11 Pt 2):4340-4.

Concolino, G., Marocchi, A., Tenaglia, R., Di Silverio, F., and Sparano, F. 1978. Specific progesterone receptor in human renal cancer. *J Steroid Biochem* 9 (5):399-402.

Concolino, G., Marocchi, A., Toscano, V., and Di Silverio, F. 1981. Nuclear androgen receptor as marker of responsiveness to medroxyprogesterone acetate in human renal cell carcinoma. *J Steroid Biochem* 15:397-402.

Connell, J. M., and Davies, E. 2005. The new biology of aldosterone. *J Endocrinol* 186 (1):1-20.

Cote, S., Sinnett, D., and Momparler, R. L. 1998. Demethylation by 5-aza-2'-deoxycytidine of specific 5-methylcytosine sites in the promoter region of the retinoic acid receptor beta gene in human colon carcinoma cells. *Anticancer Drugs* 9 (9):743-50.

De Bosscher, K., Vanden Berghe, W., and Haegeman, G. 2003. The interplay between the glucocorticoid receptor and nuclear factor-kappaB or activator protein-1: molecular mechanisms for gene repression. *Endocr Rev* 24 (4):488-522.

Eble, J. N., Sauter, G. , Epstein, J. I., and Sesterhenn, I., eds. 2004. *World Health Organization classification of tumours: pathology and genetics of tumours of the urinary system and male genital organs*. Lyon, France: IARC Press.

Escoubet, B., Coureau, C., Blot-Chabaud, M., Bonvalet, J. P., and Farman, N. 1996. Corticosteroid receptor mRNA expression is unaffected by corticosteroids in rat kidney, heart, and colon. *Am J Physiol* 270 (5 Pt 1):C1343-53.

Escudier, B., Pluzanska, A., Koralewski, P., Ravaud, A., Bracarda, S., Szczylik, C., Chevreau, C., Filipek, M., Melichar, B., Bajetta, E., Gorbunova, V., Bay, J. O., Bodrogi, I., Jagiello-Gruszfeld, A., and Moore, N. 2007. Bevacizumab plus interferon alfa-2a for treatment of metastatic renal cell carcinoma: a randomised, double-blind phase III trial. *Lancet* 370 (9605):2103-11.

Evans, R. M. 1988. The steroid and thyroid hormone receptor superfamily. *Science* 240 (4854):889-95.

Fakih, M. G., Trump, D. L., Muindi, J. R., Black, J. D., Bernardi, R. J., Creaven, P. J., Schwartz, J., Brattain, M. G., Hutson, A., French, R., and Johnson, C. S. 2007. A phase I pharmacokinetic and pharmacodynamic study of intravenous calcitriol in combination with oral gefitinib in patients with advanced solid tumors. *Clin Cancer Res* 13 (4):1216-23.

Farman, N., and Bonvalet, J. P. 1983. Aldosterone binding in isolated tubules. III. Autoradiography along the rat nephron. *Am J Physiol* 245 (5 Pt 1):F606-14.

Farman, N., Vandewalle, A., and Bonvalet, J. P. 1982. Aldosterone binding in isolated tubules I. Biochemical determination in proximal and distal parts of the rabbit nephron. *Am J Physiol* 242 (1):F63-8.

Fine, S. W., Reuter, V. E., Epstein, J. I., and Argani, P. 2006. Angiomyolipoma with epithelial cysts (AMLEC): a distinct cystic variant of angiomyolipoma. *Am J Surg Pathol* 30 (5):593-9.

Fleet, J. C. 2008. Molecular actions of vitamin D contributing to cancer prevention. *Mol Aspects Med* 29 (6):388-96.

Freiberg, J. M., Kinsella, J., and Sacktor, B. 1982. Glucocorticoids increase the Na+-H+ exchange and decrease the Na+ gradient-dependent phosphate-uptake systems in renal brush border membrane vesicles. *Proc Natl Acad Sci U S A* 79 (16):4932-6.

Fujioka, T., Hasegawa, M., Ishikura, K., Matsushita, Y., Sato, M., and Tanji, S. 1998. Inhibition of tumor growth and angiogenesis by vitamin D3 agents in murine renal cell carcinoma. *J Urol* 160 (1):247-51.

Fuller, P. J. 1991. The steroid receptor superfamily: mechanisms of diversity. *FASEB J* 5 (15):3092-9.

Fuzesi, L., Gunawan, B., Bergmann, F., Tack, S., Braun, S., and Jakse, G. 1999. Papillary renal cell carcinoma with clear cell cytomorphology and chromosomal loss of 3p. *Histopathology* 35 (2):157-61.

Geisen, C., Denk, C., Gremm, B., Baust, C., Karger, A., Bollag, W., and Schwarz, E. 1997. High-level expression of the retinoic acid receptor beta gene in normal cells of the uterine cervix is regulated by the retinoic acid receptor alpha and is abnormally down-regulated in cervical carcinoma cells. *Cancer Res* 57 (8):1460-7.

Gelmann, E. P. 2002. Molecular biology of the androgen receptor. *J Clin Oncol* 20 (13):3001-15.

Geradts, J., Chen, J. Y., Russell, E. K., Yankaskas, J. R., Nieves, L., and Minna, J. D. 1993. Human lung cancer cell lines exhibit resistance to retinoic acid treatment. *Cell Growth Differ* 4 (10):799-809.

Getzenberg, R. H., Light, B. W., Lapco, P. E., Konety, B. R., Nangia, A. K., Acierno, J. S., Dhir, R., Shurin, Z., Day, R. S., Trump, D. L., and Johnson, C. S. 1997. Vitamin D inhibition of prostate adenocarcinoma growth and metastasis in the Dunning rat prostate model system. *Urology* 50 (6):999-1006.

Gobbo, S., Eble, J. N., Grignon, D. J., Martignoni, G., MacLennan, G. T., Shah, R. B., Zhang, S., Brunelli, M., and Cheng, L. 2008. Clear cell papillary renal cell carcinoma: a distinct histopathologic and molecular genetic entity. *Am J Surg Pathol* 32 (8):1239-45.

Goelden, U., Ukena, S. N., Pfoertner, S., Hofmann, R., Buer, J., and Schrader, A. J. 2005. RAR-beta(1) overexpression in chromophobe renal cell carcinoma: a novel target for therapeutic intervention? *Exp Oncol* 27 (3):220-4.

Greene, G. L., Gilna, P., Waterfield, M., Baker, A., Hort, Y., and Shine, J. 1986. Sequence and expression of human estrogen receptor complementary DNA. *Science* 231 (4742):1150-4.

Greenstein, S., Ghias, K., Krett, N. L., and Rosen, S. T. 2002. Mechanisms of glucocorticoid-mediated apoptosis in hematological malignancies. *Clin Cancer Res* 8 (6):1681-94.

Gustafsson, J. A. 1999. Estrogen receptor beta--a new dimension in estrogen mechanism of action. *J Endocrinol* 163 (3):379-83.

He, J. C., Lu, T. C., Fleet, M., Sunamoto, M., Husain, M., Fang, W., Neves, S., Chen, Y., Shankland, S., Iyengar, R., and Klotman, P. E. 2007. Retinoic acid inhibits HIV-1-induced podocyte proliferation through the cAMP pathway. *J Am Soc Nephrol* 18 (1):93-102.

Hemstreet, G. P., 3rd, Wittliff, J. L., Sarrif, A. M., Hall, M. L., 3rd, McRae, L. J., and Durant, J. R. 1980. Comparison of steroid receptor levels in renal-cell carcinoma and autologous normal kidney. *Int J Cancer* 26 (6):769-75.

Hermann, G. G., and Andersen, C. B. 1997. Transitional cell carcinoma express vitamin D receptors. *Scand J Urol Nephrol* 31 (2):161-6.

Hirasawa, G., Sasano, H., Takahashi, K., Fukushima, K., Suzuki, T., Hiwatashi, N., Toyota, T., Krozowski, Z. S., and Nagura, H. 1997. Colocalization of 11 beta-hydroxysteroid dehydrogenase type II and mineralocorticoid receptor in human epithelia. *J Clin Endocrinol Metab* 82 (11):3859-63.

Hoffman, A. D., Engelstein, D., Bogenrieder, T., Papandreou, C. N., Steckelman, E., Dave, A., Motzer, R. J., Dmitrovsky, E., Albino, A. P., and Nanus, D. M. 1996. Expression of retinoic acid receptor beta in human renal cell carcinomas correlates with sensitivity to the antiproliferative effects of 13-cis-retinoic acid. *Clin Cancer Res* 2 (6):1077-82.

Houle, B., Rochette-Egly, C., and Bradley, W. E. 1993. Tumor-suppressive effect of the retinoic acid receptor beta in human epidermoid lung cancer cells. *Proc Natl Acad Sci U S A* 90 (3):985-9.

Hudes, G., Carducci, M., Tomczak, P., Dutcher, J., Figlin, R., Kapoor, A., Staroslawska, E., Sosman, J., McDermott, D., Bodrogi, I., Kovacevic, Z., Lesovoy, V., Schmidt-Wolf, I. G., Barbarash, O., Gokmen, E., O'Toole, T., Lustgarten, S., Moore, L., and Motzer, R. J. 2007. Temsirolimus, interferon alfa, or both for advanced renal-cell carcinoma. *N Engl J Med* 356 (22):2271-81.

Ikuyama, T., Hamasaki, T., Inatomi, H., Katoh, T., Muratani, T., and Matsumoto, T. 2002. Association of vitamin D receptor gene polymorphism with renal cell carcinoma in Japanese. *Endocr J* 49 (4):433-8.

Interferon-alpha and survival in metastatic renal carcinoma: early results of a randomised controlled trial. Medical Research Council Renal Cancer Collaborators. 1999. *Lancet* 353 (9146):14-7.

Iwai, A., Fujii, Y., Kawakami, S., Takazawa, R., Kageyama, Y., Yoshida, M. A., and Kihara, K. 2004. Down-regulation of vascular endothelial growth factor in renal cell carcinoma cells by glucocorticoids. *Mol Cell Endocrinol* 226 (1-2):11-7.

Jakse, G., and Muller-Holzner, E. 1988. Hormone receptors in renal cancer: an overview. *Semin Surg Oncol* 4 (3):161-4.

Jeltsch, J. M., Krozowski, Z., Quirin-Stricker, C., Gronemeyer, H., Simpson, R. J., Garnier, J. M., Krust, A., Jacob, F., and Chambon, P. 1986. Cloning of the chicken progesterone receptor. *Proc Natl Acad Sci U S A* 83 (15):5424-8.

Jensen, E. V., Jacobson, H. I., Walf, A. A., and Frye, C. A. 2010. Estrogen action: a historic perspective on the implications of considering alternative approaches. *Physiol Behav* 99 (2):151-62.

Kakizuka, A., Miller, W. H., Jr., Umesono, K., Warrell, R. P., Jr., Frankel, S. R., Murty, V. V., Dmitrovsky, E., and Evans, R. M. 1991. Chromosomal translocation t(15;17) in human acute promyelocytic leukemia fuses RAR alpha with a novel putative transcription factor, PML. *Cell* 66 (4):663-74.

Karami, S., Brennan, P., Hung, R. J., Boffetta, P., Toro, J., Wilson, R. T., Zaridze, D., Navratilova, M., Chatterjee, N., Mates, D., Janout, V., Kollarova, H., Bencko, V., Szeszenia-Dabrowska, N., Holcatova, I., Moukeria, A., Welch, R., Chanock, S., Rothman, N., Chow, W. H., and Moore, L. E. 2008. Vitamin D receptor polymorphisms and renal cancer risk in Central and Eastern Europe. *J Toxicol Environ Health A* 71 (6):367-72.

Karr, J. P., Pontes, J. E., Schneider, S., Sandberg, A. A., and Murphy, G. P. 1983. Clinical aspects of steroid hormone receptors in human renal cell carcinoma. *J Surg Oncol* 23 (2):117-24.

Kimura, N., Mizokami, A., Oonuma, T., Sasano, H., and Nagura, H. 1993. Immunocytochemical localization of androgen receptor with polyclonal antibody in paraffin-embedded human tissues. *J Histochem Cytochem* 41 (5):671-8.

Klotzl, G., Otto, U., Becker, H., and Klosterhalfen, H. 1987. Determination of androgen, progestin and estrogen receptors with two different assays in renal cell carcinoma. *Urol Int* 42 (2):100-4.

Konety, B. R., Lavelle, J. P., Pirtskalaishvili, G., Dhir, R., Meyers, S. A., Nguyen, T. S., Hershberger, P., Shurin, M. R., Johnson, C. S., Trump, D. L., Zeidel, M. L., and Getzenberg, R. H. 2001. Effects of vitamin D (calcitriol) on transitional cell carcinoma of the bladder in vitro and in vivo. *J Urol* 165 (1):253-8.

Krozowski, Z. S., and Funder, J. W. 1983. Renal mineralocorticoid receptors and hippocampal corticosterone-binding species have identical intrinsic steroid specificity. *Proc Natl Acad Sci U S A* 80 (19):6056-60.

Kuiper, G. G., Enmark, E., Pelto-Huikko, M., Nilsson, S., and Gustafsson, J. A. 1996. Cloning of a novel receptor expressed in rat prostate and ovary. *Proc Natl Acad Sci U S A* 93 (12):5925-30.

Lambert, J. R., Eddy, V. J., Young, C. D., Persons, K. S., Sarkar, S., Kelly, J. A., Genova, E., Lucia, M. S., Faller, D. V., and Ray, R. 2010. A vitamin D receptor-alkylating derivative of 1alpha,25-dihydroxyvitamin D3 inhibits growth of human kidney cancer cells and suppresses tumor growth. *Cancer Prev Res (Phila)* 3 (12):1596-607.

Lamprecht, S. A., and Lipkin, M. 2003. Chemoprevention of colon cancer by calcium, vitamin D and folate: molecular mechanisms. *Nat Rev Cancer* 3 (8):601-14.

Langner, C., Ratschek, M., Rehak, P., Schips, L., and Zigeuner, R. 2004. Steroid hormone receptor expression in renal cell carcinoma: an immunohistochemical analysis of 182 tumors. *J Urol* 171 (2 Pt 1):611-4.

Leveridge, M. J., and Jewett, M. A. 2011. Recent developments in kidney cancer. *Can Urol Assoc J* 5 (3):195-203.

Li, H., and Christakos, S. 1991. Differential regulation by 1,25-dihydroxyvitamin D3 of calbindin-D9k and calbindin-D28k gene expression in mouse kidney. *Endocrinology* 128 (6):2844-52.

Li, J. J., Weroha, S. J., Davis, M. F., Tawfik, O., Hou, X., and Li, S. A. 2001. ER and PR in renomedullary interstitial cells during Syrian hamster estrogen-induced tumorigenesis: evidence for receptor-mediated oncogenesis. *Endocrinology* 142 (9):4006-14.

Li, J. Y., Zhou, T., Gao, X., Xu, C., Sun, Y., Peng, Y., Chang, Z., Zhang, Y., Jiang, J., Wang, L., and Hou, J. 2010. Testosterone and androgen receptor in human nephrolithiasis. *J Urol* 184 (6):2360-3.

Li, S. A., Li, J. J., and Villee, C. A. 1977. Significance of the progesterone receptor in the estrogen-induced and -dependent renal tumor of the Syrian golden hamster. *Ann N Y Acad Sci* 286:369-83.

Liu, S. H., Otal-Brun, M., and Webb, T. E. 1980. Glucocorticoid receptors in human tumors. *Cancer Lett* 10 (3):269-75.

Liu, W., Tretiakova, M., Kong, J., Turkyilmaz, M., Li, Y. C., and Krausz, T. 2006. Expression of vitamin D3 receptor in kidney tumors. *Hum Pathol* 37 (10):1268-78.

Lombes, M., Farman, N., Oblin, M. E., Baulieu, E. E., Bonvalet, J. P., Erlanger, B. F., and Gasc, J. M. 1990. Immunohistochemical localization of renal mineralocorticoid receptor by using an anti-idiotypic antibody that is an internal image of aldosterone. *Proc Natl Acad Sci U S A* 87 (3):1086-8.

Lubahn, D. B., Joseph, D. R., Sullivan, P. M., Willard, H. F., French, F. S., and Wilson, E. M. 1988. Cloning of human androgen receptor complementary DNA and localization to the X chromosome. *Science* 240 (4850):327-30.

Madej, A., Puzianowska-Kuznicka, M., Tanski, Z., Nauman, J., and Nauman, A. 2003. Vitamin D receptor binding to DNA is altered without the change in its expression in human renal clear cell cancer. *Nephron Exp Nephrol* 93 (4):e150-7.

Mai, K. T., Teo, I., Belanger, E. C., Robertson, S. J., Marginean, E. C., and Islam, S. 2008. Progesterone receptor reactivity in renal oncocytoma and chromophobe renal cell carcinoma. *Histopathology* 52 (3):277-82.

McDonald, M. W., Diokno, A. C., Seski, J. C., and Menon, K. M. 1983. Measurement of progesterone receptor in human renal cell carcinoma and normal renal tissue. *J Surg Oncol* 22 (3):164-6.

Miki, S., Iwano, M., Miki, Y., Yamamoto, M., Tang, B., Yokokawa, K., Sonoda, T., Hirano, T., and Kishimoto, T. 1989. Interleukin-6 (IL-6) functions as an in vitro autocrine growth factor in renal cell carcinomas. *FEBS Lett* 250 (2):607-10.

Mishina, T., Scholer, D. W., and Edelman, I. S. 1981. Glucocorticoid receptors in rat kidney cortical tubules enriched in proximal and distal segments. *Am J Physiol* 240 (1):F38-45.

Moasser, M. M., DeBlasio, A., and Dmitrovsky, E. 1994. Response and resistance to retinoic acid are mediated through the retinoic acid nuclear receptor gamma in human teratocarcinomas. *Oncogene* 9 (3):833-40.

Moasser, M. M., Reuter, V. E., and Dmitrovsky, E. 1995. Overexpression of the retinoic acid receptor gamma directly induces terminal differentiation of human embryonal carcinoma cells. *Oncogene* 10 (8):1537-43.

Mongan, N. P., and Gudas, L. J. 2007. Diverse actions of retinoid receptors in cancer prevention and treatment. *Differentiation* 75 (9):853-70.

Morris, D. J., and Souness, G. W. 1992. Protective and specificity-conferring mechanisms of mineralocorticoid action. *Am J Physiol* 263 (5 Pt 2):F759-68.

Motzer, R. J., Hudes, G. R., Curti, B. D., McDermott, D. F., Escudier, B. J., Negrier, S., Duclos, B., Moore, L., O'Toole, T., Boni, J. P., and Dutcher, J. P. 2007. Phase I/II trial of temsirolimus combined with interferon alfa for advanced renal cell carcinoma. *J Clin Oncol* 25 (25):3958-64.

Motzer, R. J., Michaelson, M. D., Redman, B. G., Hudes, G. R., Wilding, G., Figlin, R. A., Ginsberg, M. S., Kim, S. T., Baum, C. M., DePrimo, S. E., Li, J. Z., Bello, C. L., Theuer, C. P., George, D. J., and Rini, B. I. 2006. Activity of SU11248, a multitargeted inhibitor of vascular endothelial growth factor receptor and platelet-derived growth factor receptor, in patients with metastatic renal cell carcinoma. *J Clin Oncol* 24 (1):16-24.

Motzer, R. J., Murphy, B. A., Bacik, J., Schwartz, L. H., Nanus, D. M., Mariani, T., Loehrer, P., Wilding, G., Fairclough, D. L., Cella, D., and Mazumdar, M. 2000. Phase III trial of interferon alfa-2a with or without 13-cis-retinoic acid for patients with advanced renal cell carcinoma. *J Clin Oncol* 18 (16):2972-80.

Muindi, J. R., Johnson, C. S., Trump, D. L., Christy, R., Engler, K. L., and Fakih, M. G. 2009. A phase I and pharmacokinetics study of intravenous calcitriol in combination with oral dexamethasone and gefitinib in patients with advanced solid tumors. *Cancer Chemother Pharmacol* 65 (1):33-40.

Muramatsu, M., and Inoue, S. 2000. Estrogen receptors: how do they control reproductive and nonreproductive functions? *Biochem Biophys Res Commun* 270 (1):1-10.

Nagakura, K., Abe, E., Suda, T., Hayakawa, M., Nakamura, H., and Tazaki, H. 1986. Inhibitory effect of 1 alpha,25-dihydroxyvitamin D3 on the growth of the renal carcinoma cell line. *Kidney Int* 29 (4):834-40.

Nakano, E., Tada, Y., Fujioka, H., Matsuda, M., Osafune, M., Kotake, T., Sato, B., Takaha, M., and Sonoda, T. 1984. Hormone receptor in renal cell carcinoma and correlation with clinical response to endocrine therapy. *J Urol* 132 (2):240-5.

Nakayama, T., Watanabe, M., Yamanaka, M., Hirokawa, Y., Suzuki, H., Ito, H., Yatani, R., and Shiraishi, T. 2001. The role of epigenetic modifications in retinoic acid receptor beta2 gene expression in human prostate cancers. *Lab Invest* 81 (7):1049-57.

Naray-Fejes-Toth, A., and Fejes-Toth, G. 1990. Glucocorticoid receptors mediate mineralocorticoid-like effects in cultured collecting duct cells. *Am J Physiol* 259 (4 Pt 2):F672-8.

Noronha, R. F., and Rao, B. R. 1985. Increased dihydrotestosterone receptor levels in high-stage renal adenocarcinoma. *Cancer* 56 (1):134-7.

Nykjaer, A., Dragun, D., Walther, D., Vorum, H., Jacobsen, C., Herz, J., Melsen, F., Christensen, E. I., and Willnow, T. E. 1999. An endocytic pathway essential for renal uptake and activation of the steroid 25-(OH) vitamin D3. *Cell* 96 (4):507-15.

Obara, W., Konda, R., Akasaka, S., Nakamura, S., Sugawara, A., and Fujioka, T. 2007. Prognostic significance of vitamin D receptor and retinoid X receptor expression in renal cell carcinoma. *J Urol* 178 (4 Pt 1):1497-503.

Obara, W., Suzuki, Y., Kato, K., Tanji, S., Konda, R., and Fujioka, T. 2007. Vitamin D receptor gene polymorphisms are associated with increased risk and progression of renal cell carcinoma in a Japanese population. *Int J Urol* 14 (6):483-7.

Omland, H., and Fossa, S. D. 1989. Spontaneous regression of cerebral and pulmonary metastases in renal cell carcinoma. *Scand J Urol Nephrol* 23 (2):159-60.

Pearson, J., Friedman, M. A., and Hoffman, P. G., Jr. 1981. Hormone receptors in renal cell carcinoma. Their utility as predictors of response to endocrine therapy. *Cancer Chemother Pharmacol* 6 (2):151-4.

Pemrick, S. M., Lucas, D. A., and Grippo, J. F. 1994. The retinoid receptors. *Leukemia* 8 Suppl 3:S1-10.

Porta, C., Tortora, G., Linassier, C., Papazisis, K., Awada, A., Berthold, D., Maroto, J. P., Powles, T., and De Santis, M. 2011. Maximising the duration of disease control in metastatic renal cell carcinoma with targeted agents: an expert agreement. *Med Oncol*.

Prufer, K., and Barsony, J. 2002. Retinoid X receptor dominates the nuclear import and export of the unliganded vitamin D receptor. *Mol Endocrinol* 16 (8):1738-51.

Pujols, L., Mullol, J., Roca-Ferrer, J., Torrego, A., Xaubet, A., Cidlowski, J. A., and Picado, C. 2002. Expression of glucocorticoid receptor alpha- and beta-isoforms in human cells and tissues. *Am J Physiol Cell Physiol* 283 (4):C1324-31.

Rafestin-Oblin, M. E., Roth-Meyer, C., Claire, M., Michaud, A., Baviera, E., Brisset, J. M., and Corvol, P. 1979. Are mineralocorticoid receptors present in human renal adenocarcinoma? *Clin Sci (Lond)* 57 (5):421-5.

Rashid, S. F., Moore, J. S., Walker, E., Driver, P. M., Engel, J., Edwards, C. E., Brown, G., Uskokovic, M. R., and Campbell, M. J. 2001. Synergistic growth inhibition of prostate cancer cells by 1 alpha,25 Dihydroxyvitamin D(3) and its 19-nor-hexafluoride analogs in combination with either sodium butyrate or trichostatin A. *Oncogene* 20 (15):1860-72.

Reichel, H., Koeffler, H. P., and Norman, A. W. 1989. The role of the vitamin D endocrine system in health and disease. *N Engl J Med* 320 (15):980-91.

Revollo, J. R., and Cidlowski, J. A. 2009. Mechanisms generating diversity in glucocorticoid receptor signaling. *Ann N Y Acad Sci* 1179:167-78.

Roland, B. L., Krozowski, Z. S., and Funder, J. W. 1995. Glucocorticoid receptor, mineralocorticoid receptors, 11 beta-hydroxysteroid dehydrogenase-1 and -2 expression in rat brain and kidney: in situ studies. *Mol Cell Endocrinol* 111 (1):R1-7.

Ruizeveld de Winter, J. A., Trapman, J., Vermey, M., Mulder, E., Zegers, N. D., and van der Kwast, T. H. 1991. Androgen receptor expression in human tissues: an immunohistochemical study. *J Histochem Cytochem* 39 (7):927-36.

Sabichi, A. L., Hendricks, D. T., Bober, M. A., and Birrer, M. J. 1998. Retinoic acid receptor beta expression and growth inhibition of gynecologic cancer cells by the synthetic retinoid N-(4-hydroxyphenyl) retinamide. *J Natl Cancer Inst* 90 (8):597-605.

Sasano, H., Fukushima, K., Sasaki, I., Matsuno, S., Nagura, H., and Krozowski, Z. S. 1992. Immunolocalization of mineralocorticoid receptor in human kidney, pancreas, salivary, mammary and sweat glands: a light and electron microscopic immunohistochemical study. *J Endocrinol* 132 (2):305-10.

Schug, T. T., Berry, D. C., Shaw, N. S., Travis, S. N., and Noy, N. 2007. Opposing effects of retinoic acid on cell growth result from alternate activation of two different nuclear receptors. *Cell* 129 (4):723-33.

Sheikh, M. S., Shao, Z. M., Li, X. S., Dawson, M., Jetten, A. M., Wu, S., Conley, B. A., Garcia, M., Rochefort, H., and Fontana, J. A. 1994. Retinoid-resistant estrogen receptor-negative human breast carcinoma cells transfected with retinoic acid receptor-alpha acquire sensitivity to growth inhibition by retinoids. *J Biol Chem* 269 (34):21440-7.

Siegel, R., Ward, E., Brawley, O., and Jemal, A. 2011. Cancer statistics, 2011: The impact of eliminating socioeconomic and racial disparities on premature cancer deaths. *CA Cancer J Clin* 61 (4):212-36.

Speirs, V., Parkes, A. T., Kerin, M. J., Walton, D. S., Carleton, P. J., Fox, J. N., and Atkin, S. L. 1999. Coexpression of estrogen receptor alpha and beta: poor prognostic factors in human breast cancer? *Cancer Res* 59 (3):525-8.

Storlie, J. A., Buckner, J. C., Wiseman, G. A., Burch, P. A., Hartmann, L. C., and Richardson, R. L. 1995. Prostate specific antigen levels and clinical response to low dose dexamethasone for hormone-refractory metastatic prostate carcinoma. *Cancer* 76 (1):96-100.

Suh, Y. A., Lee, H. Y., Virmani, A., Wong, J., Mann, K. K., Miller, W. H., Jr., Gazdar, A., and Kurie, J. M. 2002. Loss of retinoic acid receptor beta gene expression is linked to aberrant histone H3 acetylation in lung cancer cell lines. *Cancer Res* 62 (14):3945-9.

Swisshelm, K., Ryan, K., Lee, X., Tsou, H. C., Peacocke, M., and Sager, R. 1994. Down-regulation of retinoic acid receptor beta in mammary carcinoma cell lines and its up-regulation in senescing normal mammary epithelial cells. *Cell Growth Differ* 5 (2):133-41.

Takahashi, M., Yang, X. J., Sugimura, J., Backdahl, J., Tretiakova, M., Qian, C. N., Gray, S. G., Knapp, R., Anema, J., Kahnoski, R., Nicol, D., Vogelzang, N. J., Furge, K. A., Kanayama, H., Kagawa, S., and Teh, B. T. 2003. Molecular subclassification of kidney tumors and the discovery of new diagnostic markers. *Oncogene* 22 (43):6810-8.

Takeda, H., Chodak, G., Mutchnik, S., Nakamoto, T., and Chang, C. 1990. Immunohistochemical localization of androgen receptors with mono- and polyclonal antibodies to androgen receptor. *J Endocrinol* 126 (1):17-25.

Takenawa, J., Kaneko, Y., Okumura, K., Yoshida, O., Nakayama, H., and Fujita, J. 1995. Inhibitory effect of dexamethasone and progesterone in vitro on proliferation of human renal cell carcinomas and effects on expression of interleukin-6 or interleukin-6 receptor. *J Urol* 153 (3 Pt 1):858-62.

Tanaka, M., Fukuda, H., and Higashi, Y. 2003. [A case of complete regression of metastatic renal cell carcinoma following corticosteroid treatment]. *Hinyokika Kiyo* 49 (4):225-8.

Tang, X. H., and Gudas, L. J. 2011. Retinoids, retinoic acid receptors, and cancer. *Annu Rev Pathol* 6:345-64.

Thacher, T. D., and Clarke, B. L. 2011. Vitamin D insufficiency. *Mayo Clin Proc* 86 (1):50-60.

Thomas, C. P., Liu, K. Z., and Vats, H. S. 2006. Medroxyprogesterone acetate binds the glucocorticoid receptor to stimulate alpha-ENaC and sgk1 expression in renal collecting duct epithelia. *Am J Physiol Renal Physiol* 290 (2):F306-12.

Tickoo, S. K., Gopalan, A., Tu, J. J., Harik, L. R., Al-Ahmadie, H. A., Fine, S. W., Olgac, S., and Reuter, V. E. 2008. Estrogen and progesterone-receptor-positive stroma as a non-tumorous proliferation in kidneys: a possible metaplastic response to obstruction. *Mod Pathol* 21 (1):60-5.

Todd-Turla, K. M., Schnermann, J., Fejes-Toth, G., Naray-Fejes-Toth, A., Smart, A., Killen, P. D., and Briggs, J. P. 1993. Distribution of mineralocorticoid and glucocorticoid receptor mRNA along the nephron. *Am J Physiol* 264 (5 Pt 2):F781-91.

Trump, D. L., Hershberger, P. A., Bernardi, R. J., Ahmed, S., Muindi, J., Fakih, M., Yu, W. D., and Johnson, C. S. 2004. Anti-tumor activity of calcitriol: pre-clinical and clinical studies. *J Steroid Biochem Mol Biol* 89-90 (1-5):519-26.

Trump, D. L., Muindi, J., Fakih, M., Yu, W. D., and Johnson, C. S. 2006. Vitamin D compounds: clinical development as cancer therapy and prevention agents. *Anticancer Res* 26 (4A):2551-6.

Trydal, T., Bakke, A., Aksnes, L., and Aarskog, D. 1988. 1,25-Dihydroxyvitamin D3 receptor measurement in primary renal cell carcinomas and autologous normal kidney tissue. *Cancer Res* 48 (9):2458-61.

Turbiner, J., Amin, M. B., Humphrey, P. A., Srigley, J. R., De Leval, L., Radhakrishnan, A., and Oliva, E. 2007. Cystic nephroma and mixed epithelial and stromal tumor of kidney: a detailed clinicopathologic analysis of 34 cases and proposal for renal epithelial and stromal tumor (REST) as a unifying term. *Am J Surg Pathol* 31 (4):489-500.

Vanderleede, B., Opdenoordt, T., Vandenbrink, C., Ebert, T., and Vandersaag, P. 1995. Implication of retinoic Acid receptor-Beta in renal-cell carcinoma. *Int J Oncol* 6 (2):391-400.

Xu, X. C., Ro, J. Y., Lee, J. S., Shin, D. M., Hong, W. K., and Lotan, R. 1994. Differential expression of nuclear retinoid receptors in normal, premalignant, and malignant head and neck tissues. *Cancer Res* 54 (13):3580-7.

Yakirevich, E., Matoso, A., Sabo, E., Wang, L. J., Tavares, R., Meitner, P., Morris, D. J., Pareek, G., Delellis, R. A., and Resnick, M. B. 2011. Expression of the glucocorticoid receptor in renal cell neoplasms: an immunohistochemical and quantitative reverse transcriptase polymerase chain reaction study. *Hum Pathol.* 42 (11):1684-92.

Yakirevich, E., Morris, D. J., Tavares, R., Meitner, P. A., Lechpammer, M., Noble, L., de Rodriguez, A. F., Gomez-Sanchez, C. E., Wang, L. J., Sabo, E., Delellis, R. A., and Resnick, M. B. 2008. Mineralocorticoid receptor and 11beta-hydroxysteroid dehydrogenase type II expression in renal cell neoplasms: a tissue microarray and quantitative RT-PCR study. *Am J Surg Pathol* 32 (6):874-83.

Yang, J. C., Sherry, R. M., Steinberg, S. M., Topalian, S. L., Schwartzentruber, D. J., Hwu, P., Seipp, C. A., Rogers-Freezer, L., Morton, K. E., White, D. E., Liewehr, D. J., Merino, M. J., and Rosenberg, S. A. 2003. Randomized study of high-dose and low-dose interleukin-2 in patients with metastatic renal cancer. *J Clin Oncol* 21 (16):3127-32.

Yang, J. C., Haworth, L., Sherry, R. M., Hwu, P., Schwartzentruber, D. J., Topalian, S. L., Steinberg, S. M., Chen, H. X., Rosenberg, S. A. 2003. A randomized trial of bevacizumab, an anti-vascular endothelial growth factor antibody, for metastatic renal cancer. *N Engl J Med* 349 (5):427-34.

Young, A. N., Amin, M. B., Moreno, C. S., Lim, S. D., Cohen, C., Petros, J. A., Marshall, F. F., and Neish, A. S. 2001. Expression profiling of renal epithelial neoplasms: a method for tumor classification and discovery of diagnostic molecular markers. *Am J Pathol* 158 (5):1639-51.

Zhang, X. K., Liu, Y., Lee, M. O., and Pfahl, M. 1994. A specific defect in the retinoic acid response associated with human lung cancer cell lines. *Cancer Res* 54 (21):5663-9.

Zhuang, S. H., and Burnstein, K. L. 1998. Antiproliferative effect of 1alpha,25-dihydroxyvitamin D3 in human prostate cancer cell line LNCaP involves reduction of cyclin-dependent kinase 2 activity and persistent G1 accumulation. *Endocrinology* 139 (3):1197-207.

5

The VHL-HIF Signaling in Renal Cell Carcinoma: Promises and Pitfalls

Christudas Morais[1*], David W. Johnson[1,2] and Glenda C. Gobe[1]
*[1]Centre for Kidney Disease Research, School of Medicine, The University of Queensland,
[2]Department of Renal Medicine, The University of Queensland at
Princess Alexandra Hospital, Brisbane,
Australia*

1. Introduction

Renal cell carcinoma (RCC) is the third most common genitourinary cancer behind prostate and bladder cancer, accounting for 3% of all adult malignancies (Curti, 2004). It is a highly metastatic and heterogeneous disease with at least 16 histologic subtypes (Eble et al., 2001; Lopez-Beltran et al., 2006), among which clear cell (70-80%), papillary (10-15%) and chromophobe (5%) are the most common (Curti, 2004). Up to 25% of patients with RCC have distant metastases at presentation. Another 50% develop metastases or local recurrence during follow-up, despite treatment of the primary tumor (Thyavihally et al., 2005). The average survival, following metastatic RCC, is about 4 months, and only 10% of patients survive for one year. The global incidence of RCC per year is close to 300000, with a male to female ratio of 3:2 and an estimated mortality of approximately 100000 (Arai&Kanai, 2010; Ferlay et al., 2010). The incidence of RCC has been rising steadily, probably because of incidental findings from imaging techniques performed for other reasons. It can occur at any age, but is most frequently diagnosed in the 40-70 year old group (Eble et al., 2001; Pascual & Borque, 2008; Arai&Kanai, 2010).

Well before the advent of the modern era of genetics and molecular biology, surgeons and pathologists were aware of the hyper-vascular nature of RCC (Corn, 2007). The subsequent isolation of the von Hippel-Lindau (VHL) gene in 1993 led to the important discoveries that aberrant VHL is the most important risk for RCC and that VHL negatively regulates the hypoxia inducible factor (HIF) and thus the downstream angiogenesis pathway thereby engendering increased vascularity. In this chapter, we will focus on the role of the VHL-HIF pathway in RCC, advancements in novel therapeutics targeting this pathway and future directions.

2. Von Hippel-Lindau syndrome

VHL disease, commonly known as the VHL syndrome, is named after the German ophthalmologist Eugene von Hippel, and the Swedish neuropathologist Arvid Lindau, who

* Corresponding Author

in the early 1900s, described highly vascularised tumors of the retina and the central nervous system (Kim&Kaelin, 2004; Ohh, 2006). VHL syndrome is the result of germ line mutations in VHL, a tumor-suppressor gene located on chromosome 3p25 (Seizinger et al., 1988; Kim&Kaelin, 2004; Clark, 2009; Gossage&Eisen, 2010). It affects 1 in 35,000 individuals and is associated with the development of tumors in multiple organs, including the brain, spinal cord, pancreas, adrenal gland, epididymis (in males), broad ligament (in women) and kidneys (Lonser et al., 2003; Kim&Kaelin, 2004; Grubb et al., 2005; Clark, 2009). Individuals with VHL syndrome carry one wild type VHL allele and one faulty allele. Tumors develop only after the spontaneous somatic loss (loss of heterzygosity [LoH]) or inactivation, or both, of the remaining wild type. Thus, at cellular level, VHL syndrome can be considered as an autosomal recessive disease, whilst clinically, it manifests more like an autosomal dominant disease because the inactivation of the wild type allele is almost guaranteed (Ohh&Kaelin, 2003; Ohh, 2006). Apart from LoH and mutations, hypermethylation of the VHL promoter regions can prevent the wild-type VHL gene from expressing its functional tumor suppressor protein pVHL (Kim&Kaelin, 2004). The VHL gene is mutated in 50-80% (Weiss&Lin, 2006; Arai&Kanai, 2010) and hypermethylated in 19% (Herman et al., 1994; Arai&Kanai, 2010) of sporadic clear cell RCC. Clear cell RCC is the leading cause of death in patients with VHL mutation (Maher et al., 1990; Clark, 2009; Gossage&Eisen, 2010).

The VHL gene, which was isolated in 1993 (Latif et al., 1993), has three exons and encodes for two mRNA transcripts that are translated into three types of pVHL (Ohh&Kaelin, 2003; Ohh, 2006). The first VHL mRNA transcript that contains all three exons, is translated into a larger 213 amino acid protein of approximately 24-30 kDa (pVHL$_{30}$), and a smaller 160 amino acid protein of approximately 18-19 kDa (pVHL$_{19}$) due to alternative translation initiation (Iliopoulos et al., 1998; Schoenfeld et al., 1998; Blankenship et al., 1999; Safran&Kaelin, 2003). In the early days, both pVHL$_{30}$ and pVHL$_{19}$ were considered to be tumor suppressors (Iliopoulos et al., 1995; Ohh, 2006). However, further studies have cast doubt on the tumor suppressive role of pVHL$_{19}$ (Ohh, 2006). Generally, the term 'pVHL' is used to refer to both isoforms (Kim&Kaelin, 2004; Kaelin, 2007). The second VHL mRNA transcript lacks exon 2 due to alternative splicing. Literature on this isoform is scant, although RCCs that exclusively produce this shorter VHL mRNA transcript have been identified (Gnarra et al., 1996; Safran&Kaelin, 2003; Ohh, 2006).

pVHL consists of α and β domains (Fig.1), which are essential for its tumor suppressor activities (Stebbins et al., 1999; Kaelin, 2002). pVHL forms complexes with elonginB, elonginC, Rbx1, and Cullin 2 to form an E3 ubiquitin ligase complex (Stebbins et al., 1999; Ohh et al., 2000; Tanimoto et al., 2000; Kaelin, 2002; Kaelin, 2005a; Kaelin, 2005b; Gossage&Eisen, 2010). The α domain binds to elongin C and the β domain interacts with hydroxylated prolines of HIF (Fig.1). This complex has multiple functions, which can be broadly classified into HIF-independent and HIF-dependent. The HIF-independent functions include maintenance of primary cilia (Hergovich et al., 2003; Baldewijns et al., 2010), assembly of extracellular fibronectin matrix (Guo et al., 2009), regulation of apoptosis (Guo et al., 2009), epithelial mesenchymal transition (EMT) (Koochekpour et al., 1999; Hara et al., 2006), and transcriptional regulation (Yuen et al., 2007; Mikhaylova et al., 2008; Baldewijns et al., 2010). The best studied role is its HIF-dependent function in RCC, which is the degradation of HIF (Ohh, 2006; Baldewijns et al., 2010; Gossage&Eisen, 2010).

3. Hypoxia-inducible factor

A hypoxic tumor microenvironment is one of the characteristics of solid tumors. Cells undergo a variety of adaptive changes that will facilitate their survival under hypoxic conditions. One such change at the molecular level is the activation of the hypoxia-sensitive transcription factor, HIF. HIF is a heterodimer consisting of two subunits: α and β (Wang et al., 1995; Kaluz et al., 2008). The β subunit, also known as aryl hydrocarbon receptor nuclear translocator (ARNT), is constitutively expressed and is independent of intracellular oxygen tension. The oxygen-sensitive α subunit, which has three further subunits, HIF-1α, HIF-2α, and HIF-3α, is also constitutively expressed, but is rapidly degraded under normoxic conditions (Semenza, 1999; Huang&Bunn, 2003; Maynard et al., 2003; Maynard&Ohh, 2004; Kaluz et al., 2008; Baldewijns et al., 2010). At least two mechanisms that negatively regulate the stability of HIF-α under normoxia have been recognized: oxygen-dependent prolyl hydroxylation and asparaginyl hydroxylation (Lando et al., 2002a; Lando et al., 2002b; Ohh, 2006).

HIF-1α and HIF-2α contain an N-terminal transactivation domain (NTAD), a C-terminal transactivation domain (CTAD) and an oxygen-dependent degradation domain (ODDD) [Fig.1] (Pugh et al., 1997; Sang et al., 2002; Baldewijns et al., 2010). The ODDD has a stretch of proline residues. HIF-3α lacks the transactivation domain and has many splice variants. Under normoxic conditions, the proline residues within the ODDD of HIF-α are hydroxylated by prolyl hydroxylases (PH) at positions 402 and 564 (Ivan et al., 2001; Jaakkola et al., 2001; Schofield&Ratcliffe, 2005; Koivunen et al., 2007; Kaluz et al., 2008; Baldewijns et al., 2010). The pVHL-E3 ubiquitin ligase complex binds to the hydroxylated HIF-α through the β domain of pVHL and enables polyubiquitination. The polyubiquitinated HIF-α is degraded by the 26S proteasome (Maxwell et al., 1999; Ohh et al., 2000; Tanimoto et al., 2000; Jaakkola et al., 2001; Baldewijns et al., 2010). While the prolyl hydroxylation enables the binding of pVHL to HIF-α and its eventual degradation, the asparaginyl hydroxylation prevents the transcriptional activation of HIF target genes (Dames et al., 2002; Freedman et al., 2002). For transcriptional activity, HIF-α requires the recruitment of p300/CBP transcriptional coactivators (Arany et al., 1996). The CTAD has a conserved C-terminal asparagine. In normoxia, the factor inhibiting HIF-1 (FIH-1), an oxygenase, hydroxylates asparagine at position 803, which diminishes the recruitment of p300/CBP to HIF-α (Freedman et al., 2002) leading to the transcriptional downregulation of HIF responsive elements (Mahon et al., 2001; Dames et al., 2002; Lando et al., 2002a; Lando et al., 2002b).

In hypoxia, the activity of prolyl hydroxylases and FIH-1 are reduced, leading to the inhibition of proline and asparginyl hydroxylation, respectively. In the absence of a functional pVHL, the binding of the pVHL-E3 ubiquitin ligase complex to HIF-α and the subsequent polyubiquitination and degradation of HIF-α are inhibited even under normoxic conditions. Both events lead to the stabilization and accumulation of HIF-α in cells. As a result, HIF-α is translocated to the nucleus, where it dimerizes with HIF-β. The HIF-α/HIF-β heterodimer binds to hypoxia-responsive elements (HRE) of the DNA, recruits p300/CBP to the CTAD and transactivates over 60 hypoxia-inducible genes of which, vascular endothelial growth factor (VEGF) (angiogenesis), transforming growth factor alpha (TGF-α) and epidermal growth factor receptor (EGFR) (proliferation), carbonic anhydrase IX (CAIX) (pH regulation), erythropoietin (EPO) (erythropoiesis), e-cadherin (EMT) and glucose transporter-1 (GLUT-1) (glucose metabolism) have attracted much attention (Ohh, 2006; Clark, 2009; Baldewijns et al., 2010). Because of the defective VHL-HIF-VEGF pathway, RCC is considered to be one of the most hypervascularized tumors. Hence, it is not surprising that considerable research in the past decade has focused on the angiogenic pathway, which led to the development of some promising novel therapeutics.

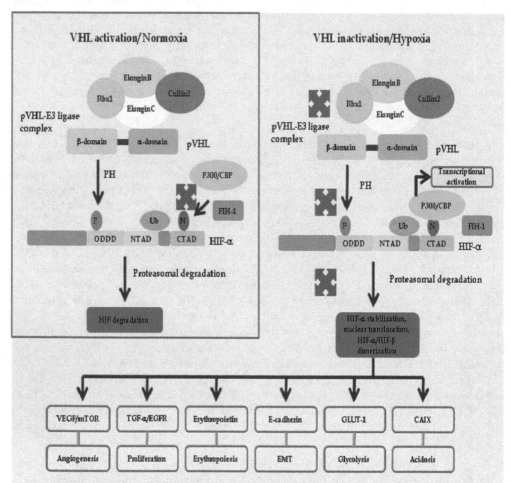

Fig. 1. The von Hippel-Lindau-Hypoxia Inducible Factor (VHL-HIF) pathway. The details are given in text. In brief, under active VHL and normoxic conditions, HIF is degraded. When the VHL gene is inactive due to mutations or hypermethylation, HIF is stabilized, translocated to the nucleus and activates the transcription of over 60 hypoxia-responsive molecules that are involved in oncogenesis and tumor progression. Only selected molecules and their alleged roles in tumor progression that are discussed in this chapter are shown. X, represents inhibition or inactivation. N, asparagine; P, proline; PH, prolyl hydroxylases; Ub, ubiquitination.

4. VHL inactivation and HIF-induced hypoxia responsive genes

4.1 Vascular endothelial growth factor – mammalian target of rapamycin

Of the many HIF-regulated angiogenic molecules, VEGF is perhaps the most studied - not only in RCC but also cancers in general. In humans, the VEGF system consists of five secreted ligands, namely VEGF-A, VEGF-B, VEGF-C, VEGF-D and placenta growth factor-1 (PlGF) and three receptor tyrosine kinases, VEGF-R1 (flt-1), VEGF-R2 (flk1 in the mouse, KDR in the human), and VEGF-R3 (flt4) (Carmeliet, 2005; Hicklin&Ellis, 2005; Tammela et al., 2005; Cebe-Suarez et al., 2006; Donovan&Kummar, 2006; Roy et al., 2006; Thurston&Kitajewski, 2008; Clark, 2009; Stuttfeld&Ballmer-Hofer, 2009; Bates, 2010). VEGF-R1 and VEGF-R2 are predominantly expressed in vascular endothelial cells and VEGF-R3 in lymphatic endothelial cells (Tammela et al., 2005; Thurston&Kitajewski, 2008). Hence, VEGF-R1 and VEGF-R2 are thought to be more important for angiogenesis and VEGF-R3 for lymphangiogenesis (Donovan&Kummar, 2006; Clark, 2009). The binding of the ligands to the receptors is an essential step in the initiation of the VEGF signaling. Generally, VEGF-R1 binds to VEGF-A, VEGF-B and PlGF; VEGF-R2 binds to VEGF-A, VEGF-C and VEGF-D and VEGF-R3 to VEGF-C and VEGF-D (Cebe-Suarez et al., 2006; Stuttfeld&Ballmer-Hofer, 2009). The receptor-ligand binding promotes conformational changes, followed by phosphorylation of specific tyrosine residues of the receptor (Cebe-Suarez et al., 2006; Stuttfeld&Ballmer-Hofer, 2009). Subsequently, a variety of downstream signaling pathways is activated, of which the most studied are the RAF-MEK-ERK series of kinases and the phosphatidylinositol-3 kinase-protein kinase B-mammalian target of rapamycin (PI3K-AKT-mTOR) pathway (Clark, 2009; Banumathy&Cairns, 2010). Increased mTOR, which itself is the result of HIF activation secondary to VHL loss, can in turn lead to an increase in HIF thereby maintaining a positive feedback loop that exacerbates the deleterious effects of VHL inactivation (Cho et al., 2007; Clark, 2009; Banumathy&Cairns, 2010). Both pathways predominantly up-regulate a variety of pro-angiogenic factors, thereby imparting a hyper-angiogenic phenotype to RCC.

There is considerable evidence demonstrating that VEGF is significantly elevated in RCC, with some studies reporting its up-regulation in up to 96% of RCC (Takahashi et al., 1994). There is a direct correlation between VEGF expression, tumor microvascular density, disease progression and metastasis of RCC (Takahashi et al., 1994; Zhang et al., 2002; Fukata et al., 2005; Baldewijns et al., 2007; Rioux-Leclercq et al., 2007; Patard et al., 2009). Apart from VEGF, RCC is reported to over-express several potent pro-angiogenic factors, including basic fibroblast growth factor (bFGF) (Cenni et al., 2007), PlGF (Takahashi et al., 1994), platelet-derived growth factor (PDGF) (Xu et al., 2005a), epidermal growth factor (EGF) (Kedar et al., 2002), the interleukins IL-6 (Angelo et al., 2002) and IL-8 (Konig et al., 1999), leptin (Horiguchi et al., 2006b; Horiguchi et al., 2006a) and various chemokines (Slaton et al., 2001; Fukata et al., 2005).

Hence, it is not surprising that the past decade has placed much emphasis on HIF-regulated downstream pathways, especially angiogenesis. This has resulted in the development of many clinically available novel chemotherapeutic agents. They can be broadly categorized as VEGF inhibitors, multiple tyrosine kinase inhibitors and mTOR inhibitors. The most successful VEGF inhibitor is the humanized VEGF-neutralizing antibody, bevacizumab. Bevacizumab is thought to exert its anti-angiogenic activity by acting against the angiogenic endothelial cells surrounding the tumor rather than the tumor *per se* thus blocking the supply of oxygen and nutrients to the tumors (Ellis&Hicklin, 2008; Ainsworth et al., 2009; Banumathy&Cairns, 2010). The clinically available multiple tyrosine kinase inhibitors are sunitinib, sorafenib, pazopanib and axitinib. As summarized in Table 1, they target multiple tyrosine kinase receptors neutralizing the downstream signaling pathways activated by ligand-receptor binding, as discussed above. Two of the most successful mTOR inhibitors are temsirolimus and everolimus. Both are rapamycin analogues and bind to FK506-binding protein 12 (FKBP12), which in turn binds to mTOR leading to the inhibition of the PI3K/Akt/mTOR pathway (Thomas et al., 2006; Abraham&Gibbons, 2007; Ainsworth et al., 2009; Banumathy&Cairns, 2010). In addition, temsirolimus has been shown to have a direct inhibitory effect on HIF-α and VEGF (Del Bufalo et al., 2006; Motzer et al., 2008; Banumathy&Cairns, 2010; Houghton, 2010).

Drug	Target receptors	Reference
Sunitinib	VEGFR1, VEGFR2, VEGFR3, PDGFR-α, PDGFR-β, FLT3, c-KIT, RET	(Mendel et al., 2003; Faivre et al., 2006; Ainsworth et al., 2009; Banumathy&Cairns, 2010)
Sorafenib	VEGFR-2, PDGFR-β, c-KIT, Raf-1	(Wilhelm&Chien, 2002; Wilhelm et al., 2004; Ainsworth et al., 2009)
Pazopanib	VEGFR1, VEGFR2, VEGFR3, PDGFR-α, PDGFR-β, c-KIT	(Kumar et al., 2007; Ainsworth et al., 2009; Banumathy&Cairns, 2010; Sternberg et al., 2010)
Axitinib	VEGFR1, VEGFR2, VEGFR3, PDGFR-β, c-KIT,	(Rugo et al., 2005; Rixe et al., 2007)

Table 1. Clinically available multiple tyrosine kinase inhibitors for metastatic RCC (Bullock et al., 2010)

4.2 Transforming growth factor-α and epidermal growth factor receptor

TGF-α is an autocrine mitogen for fibroblasts and epithelial cells. It has structural and functional homology to EGF (Derynck, 1986; Everitt et al., 1997). TGF-α is thought to mediate its biological effects through the binding of EGFR, which is a family of four closely related cell membrane receptors, EGFR (HER1; ErbB1), HER2 (ErbB2), HER3 (ErbB3), and HER4 (ErbB4) (Higashiyama et al., 2008; Pu et al., 2009). These receptors are transmembrane glycoproteins with an extracellular ligand-binding domain and an intracellular tyrosine kinase domain (Higashiyama et al., 2008; Pu et al., 2009). Ligand-binding to the extracellular domain of EGFR activates tyrosine kinase, resulting in autophosphorylation of EGFR and subsequent signal transduction leading to cell cycle progression, inhibition of apoptosis, induction of angiogenesis, promotion of invasion and metastasis, and other oncogenic activities (Derynck, 1986; Everitt et al., 1997; Gunaratnam et al., 2003; Black&Dinney, 2008; Lee et al., 2008; Uberall et al., 2008; Pu et al., 2009). TGF-α/EGFR activation in RCC is either independent of, or dependent on the VHL status. While the mechanisms behind VHL-independent activation have not been fully elucidated, the VHL-dependent TGF-α/EGFR follows the classical pattern of HIF-1 up-regulation secondary to loss of VHL function (de

Paulsen et al., 2001; Gunaratnam et al., 2003; Lee et al., 2008). It has been suggested that TGF-α overproduction secondary to VHL deficiency is the consequence of HIF activation and that such activation establishes an autocrine TGF-α/EGFR stimulatory system leading to the oncogenic transformation of normal renal epithelial cells and the formation of RCC (Ishikawa et al., 1990; Atlas et al., 1992; Yoshida et al., 1994; Everitt et al., 1997; de Paulsen et al., 2001; Gunaratnam et al., 2003; Pelletier et al., 2009; Pu et al., 2009). For example, transgenic expression of TGF-α in mice leads to the formation of multiple renal cysts reminiscent of pre-neoplastic lesions of the human kidney, whilst the re-introduction of wild type VHL inhibits TGF-α expression and cyst formation (Lowden et al., 1994; Everitt et al., 1997; Knebelmann et al., 1998; de Paulsen et al., 2001; Kaelin, 2002; Gunaratnam et al., 2003).

Many studies have reported the over expression of TGF-α and EGFR in RCC (Freeman et al., 1989; Gomella et al., 1989; Mydlo et al., 1989; Sargent et al., 1989; Petrides et al., 1990; Lager et al., 1994; Yoshida et al., 1994; Uhlman et al., 1995; Everitt et al., 1997; Yoshida et al., 1997; Ramp et al., 2000; Merseburger et al., 2005; Lee et al., 2008; Pelletier et al., 2009; Pu et al., 2009). The expression pattern of TGF-α in RCC is such that it has been identified as an ideal candidate for immunotherapy (Pelletier et al., 2009). The prognostic association between over-expression of EGFR in RCC, and development of the cancer is controversial. Two distinct patterns of EGFR expression have been observed: a) cytoplasmic in normal renal cells, and b) membranous in RCC. These observations suggest that it is not just the over expression of EGFR, but the location of its over-expression that determines prognosis. Accordingly, RCC patients with positive membranous EGFR expression may have a poorer survival outcome when compared with those with negative expression of membranous EGFR (Pu et al., 2009). However, a previous study casts doubt on this hypothesis (Kallio et al., 2003).

Some studies have explored the therapeutic efficiency of EGFR inhibitors, either as single agents or in combination, with a success rate of around 10% (Motzer et al., 2003; Dawson et al., 2004; Rowinsky et al., 2004; Jermann et al., 2006; Ravaud et al., 2008; Gordon et al., 2009; Pu et al., 2009). Interestingly however, results of anti-EGFR therapy in other cancers show a lack of correlation between EGFR expression and response to therapy, suggesting that differential intracellular signaling events rather than the mere expression of EGFR may also play significant roles in predicting response to anti-EGFR therapy (Marks et al., 2008; Gordon et al., 2009). Furthermore, RCC cells with wild type VHL have been shown to be more sensitive to anti-EGFR treatment than those with mutated VHL (Perera et al., 2000; Gordon et al., 2009).

4.3 Erythropoietin

Paraneoplastic erythrocytosis is a salient feature of many cancers, including RCC in which about 5% of patients are polycythemic (Wiesener et al., 2002; Wiesener et al., 2007; Papworth et al., 2009). In adults, the kidney is the major source of EPO. EPO regulates erythropoiesis and is the only hematopoietic cytokine whose production is regulated by hypoxia (Lacombe&Mayeux, 1999; Fandrey, 2004; Michael et al., 2007; Wiesener et al., 2007). Although RCC is thought to arise from proximal tubular epithelial cells (PTEC), normal PTEC do not express detectable levels of EPO even under hypoxic conditions (Wiesener et al., 2002; Wiesener et al., 2007). This pointed towards the role of molecular mechanisms that transform a non-EPO expressing PTEC to an EPO-expressing RCC , leading to the identification of the link between VHL mutation and the subsequent HIF-mediated EPO upregulation in RCC (Da Silva et al., 1990; Noguchi et al., 1999; Wiesener et al., 2002; Pastore et al., 2003; Lee et al., 2005; Wiesener et al., 2007; Rad et al., 2008; Papworth et al., 2009). Enhanced expression of EPO and its receptor EPOR has been reported in cultured RCC cells and in patient samples, the reported prevalence ranges from 33 - 84% (Murphy et al., 1970; Hagiwara et al., 1984; Da Silva et al., 1990; Ljungberg et al., 1992; Noguchi et al., 1999; Wiesener et al., 2002; Sakamoto et al., 2003; Lee et al., 2005; Michael et al., 2007; Wiesener et al., 2007; Papworth et al., 2009).

Although 33-84% of the RCC patients have elevated plasma level of EPO, only 5% of them are polycythemic (Kazal&Erslev, 1975; Ljungberg et al., 1992; Michael et al., 2007; Wiesener et al., 2007; Papworth et al., 2009). The lack of correlation between paraneoplastic EPO production and paraneoplastic erythrocytosis has led to the suggestion that other cancer-related factors can counterbalance the effect of increased EPO. One of the well studied factors is the reduced iron availability and the resultant anemia in cancer patients. Since recombinant human EPO (rhEPO) is frequently used to treat anemia in patients with cancer, the presence of EPOR in RCC has raised concern (Lai&Grandis, 2006; Papworth et al., 2009). As EPOR is over-expressed in RCC, and EPO exerts its effects through its binding of EPOR, exogenous rhEPO could enhance tumor aggressiveness as reported in breast and head and neck cancers (Henke et al., 2003; Leyland-Jones et al., 2005; Wiesener et al., 2007). Furthermore, EPO has been shown to reduce cisplatin-induced apoptosis in cultured RCC cells (Li et al., 2007). In contrast, EPO sensitized RCC cell lines to vinblastin and daunorubicin-induced apoptosis (Carvalho et al., 2005).

4.4 E-cadherin

Cell-cell adherence, mediated by intercellular junctional complexes, plays an important role in tissue formation and maintenance of cell phenotypes. Intercellular junctional complexes are composed of tight junctions, adherence junctions and desmosomes (Cavallaro & Christofori, 2004; Krishnamachary et al., 2006; Migita et al., 2008). E-cadherin, a transmembrane glycoprotein, is the principal component of adherence junctions and desmosomes in epithelial cells (Cavallaro&Christofori, 2004; Krishnamachary et al., 2006). The extracellular domain of E-cadherin mediates cell-cell adherence through homophilic interaction with the E-cadherin of adjacent cells, whereas the intracellular domain binds with the cytoskeleton *via* a protein complex containing α-, ß- and γ -catenins (Behrens et al., 1989; Cavallaro&Christofori, 2004; Krishnamachary et al., 2006; Russell&Ohh, 2007). EMT is the hallmark of many cancers, in which E-cadherin-mediated cell-cell adherence is lost and the cells attain hyper-proliferative, invasive and metastatic properties (Behrens et al., 1989; Thiery, 2002; Krishnamachary et al., 2006). While the reasons for loss of E-cadherin in cancers are undoubtedly multifactoral, many studies have shown a direct role of VHL in regulating E-cadherin expression in RCC (Esteban et al., 2006; Krishnamachary et al., 2006; Evans et al., 2007; Russell&Ohh, 2007).

The loss of VHL in turn leads to a loss or significant downregulation of E-cadherin and its re-introduction restores E-cadherin expression in RCC (Esteban et al., 2006; Krishnamachary et al., 2006; Russell&Ohh, 2007). Further reports of E-cadherin loss in pre-malignant foci of VHL patients has led to the suggestion that E-cadherin loss is an early step in the pathogenesis of RCC, attributed to VHL inactivation (Esteban et al., 2006; Russell&Ohh,

2007). In line with these observations, tissue microarray of human RCC samples has shown the lack of E-cadherin immunoreactivity in VHL-deficient samples (Gervais et al., 2007). This study also found that low Fuhrman grade samples were positive for E-cadherin and VHL immunostaining and had a better prognosis. Conversely, high-grade tumors were negative for E-cadherin and VHL immunoreactivity and had a worse prognosis. However, these observations have been contradicted by another report, which found no association between E-cadherin expression, tumor grade and prognosis in RCC (Ronkainen et al., 2010).

4.5 Glucose transporter-1

Glucose is the major substrate for energy production in mammalian cells. The intracellular transport of glucose and its oxidative metabolism are vital for normal functioning of cells. Intracellular glucose transport is facilitated by a family of 14 glucose transporters (GLUT), of which GLUT-1 is the most studied (Macheda et al., 2005; Ozcan et al., 2007; Suganuma et al., 2007; Lidgren et al., 2008). Due to rapid proliferative rate relative to vascular support of cancer cells, the tumor microenvironment is in a constant state of hypoxia (Ozcan et al., 2007). In order to counteract the deleterious effects of hypoxia, such as apoptosis and necrosis, malignant cells undergo adaptive and genetic changes. One such change is increased uptake of glucose when compared with normal cells through accelerated glycolysis – often referred to as 'glycolytic switch' or 'Warburg effect' (Warburg, 1956; Airley&Mobasheri, 2007; Singer et al., 2011). This is largely mediated by the up-regulation of GLUT especially GLUT-1 (Binder et al., 1997; Smith, 1999; Medina&Owen, 2002; Airley&Mobasheri, 2007; Ozcan et al., 2007; Suganuma et al., 2007). It is now well established that accelerated glycolysis and increased glucose uptake mediated by GLUT-1 are the hallmarks of many malignant tumors and that these adaptive changes in glucose metabolism favor survival, proliferation and metastasis of tumor cells, even under hypoxic conditions (Airley&Mobasheri, 2007; Ozcan et al., 2007; Singer et al., 2011).

The link between VHL-HIF and GLUT-1 has been well established. GLUT-1 is over-expressed in VHL-mutated mice and the GLUT-1 promoter region has an HRE (Ebert et al., 1995; Park et al., 2007; Lidgren et al., 2008). While the basal level of expression of GLUT-1 in normal PTEC is a subject of debate (Nagase et al., 1995; Ozcan et al., 2007), the over-expression of GLUT-1 in RCC has been demonstrated by many studies (Nagase et al., 1995; Miyakita et al., 2002; Ozcan et al., 2007; Suganuma et al., 2007; Lidgren et al., 2008; Singer et al., 2011). All of these studies concluded that GLUT-1 is over-expressed markedly in clear cell RCC compared with other RCC subtypes, confirming the link between VHL aberration and the subsequent HIF up-regulation. Lactate is one of the byproducts of glycolysis. Due to the enhanced glycolysis, RCC patients are reported to have increased glycolytic enzymes and higher levels of lactate in their serum (Gao et al., 2008). Increased dependence of cancer cells on glycolysis suggests that glycolysis inhibition may be a therapeutic option. Although not well-documented in RCC, experimental glycolysis inhibition has produced anti-cancer effects in certain cancer cell lines (Xu et al., 2005b; Pelicano et al., 2006).

4.6 Carbonic anhydrase IX

CAIX is a membrane-bound glycoprotein belonging to the carbonic anhydrase (CA) family of enzymes and is thought to promote cell proliferation, oncogenesis and tumor progression in response to hypoxia (Grabmaier et al., 2000; Ivanov et al., 2001; Bui et al., 2003; Lawrentschuk et al., 2011). There are at least 15 isoforms of CA. These enzymes play an important role in the regulation of pH of cells by catalyzing one of the vital reactions of biological systems - the reversible hydration of CO_2 into bicarbonate and hydrogen ions, $CO_2+H_2O \Leftrightarrow HCO_3^- + H^+$ (Opavsky et al., 1996; Pastorekova et al., 2008; Stillebroer et al., 2010). As discussed above, enhanced glycolysis is a hallmark of cancer cells, which results in accumulation of lactate and a hypoxic acidic microenvironment. CO_2 is a significant source of hypoxia and acidity in tumors (Pastorekova et al., 2008). Enhanced CAIX expression and the resultant rapid reversible conversion of CO_2 to H^+ helps to maintain an acidic, hypoxic microenvironment thereby sustaining tumor progression (Opavsky et al., 1996; Dorai et al., 2006; Pastorekova et al., 2008; Patard et al., 2008; Stillebroer et al., 2010). CAIX is regulated by HIF and the correlation between VHL-HIF-CAIX is well-established (Wykoff et al., 2000; Grabmaier et al., 2004; Patard et al., 2008; Kaluz et al., 2009; Lawrentschuk et al., 2011). Enhanced expression of CAIX has been well documented in RCC (Bui et al., 2003; Zavada et al., 2003; Atkins et al., 2005; Al-Ahmadie et al., 2008; Jensen et al., 2008; Li et al., 2008; Patard et al., 2008; Patard et al., 2009; Stillebroer et al., 2010; Zhou et al., 2010). However, in contrast to other cancers, enhanced CAIX in RCC is associated with a better prognosis. Furthermore, metastatic patients with higher tumoral CAIX expression showed a better response to interleukin-2 treatment (Atkins et al., 2005). Based on the VHL-CAIX status of RCC, Patard and colleagues (Patard et al., 2008) stratified RCC patients into three distinct groups: patients with both VHL mutation and high CAIX expression had the most favourable prognosis; patients with either VHL mutation or high CAIX expression had an intermediate prognosis; and patients with neither VHL mutation nor high CAIX expression had the worst prognosis.

5. Promises, pitfalls and future directions

The past decade has witnessed an unprecedented increase in the understanding of molecular mechanisms of RCC, of which, the VHL-HIF pathway arguably is the most explored. Not surprisingly, this has resulted in promising, clinically available novel therapeutic agents. Patients were reported to have progression-free survival with these novel therapeutic agents, and many new drugs are under clinical trial, offering hope for better treatment strategies in the future. However, progression-free survival, which occurs in approximately 10% of selected patients, is generally measured in months, rather than years. Moreover, there is currently no compound, either singly or in combination, which is capable of producing a complete response in metastatic RCC. Systemic toxicity and resistance of RCC in response to currently available VEGF/mTOR inhibitors are starting to emerge. Also, the rising costs of therapy associated with these novel drugs are another barrier to effective treatment. These highlight the need for more effective therapeutic agents for metastatic RCC. One approach would be simultaneous targeting of multiple molecular pathways. Pertinent to the molecular mechanism of VHL-HIF, there are at least 60 HIF-regulated molecules that are engaged in tumor development and progression. This means that targeting the VEGF/mTOR pathway could be potentially abrogated by the opposing actions of numerous molecules favoring tumor progression. Therefore, given the heterogeneity of RCC, individualized, targeted treatment based on a preceding 'molecular map' of each tumor might represent an innovative therapeutic approach to achieving improved clinical outcomes. With the rapid advancements in technology, especially microarrays and bioinformatics, the availability of clinically feasible platforms to generate molecular maps of individual tumors and customized treatment strategies may become a reality in the near future.

6. References

Abraham, R.T. & Gibbons, J.J. (2007). The mammalian target of rapamycin signaling pathway: twists and turns in the road to cancer therapy. *Clin Cancer Res* Vol.13, No.11, (Jun 1), pp.3109-14

Ainsworth, N.L., Lee, J.S. & Eisen, T. (2009). Impact of anti-angiogenic treatments on metastatic renal cell carcinoma. *Expert Rev Anticancer Ther* Vol.9, No.12, (Dec), pp.1793-805

Airley, R.E. & Mobasheri, A. (2007). Hypoxic regulation of glucose transport, anaerobic metabolism and angiogenesis in cancer: novel pathways and targets for anticancer therapeutics. *Chemotherapy* Vol.53, No.4, pp.233-56

Al-Ahmadie, H.A., Alden, D., Qin, L.X., Olgac, S., Fine, S.W., Gopalan, A., Russo, P., Motzer, R.J., Reuter, V.E. & Tickoo, S.K. (2008). Carbonic anhydrase IX expression in clear cell renal cell carcinoma: an immunohistochemical study comparing 2 antibodies. *Am J Surg Pathol* Vol.32, No.3, (Mar), pp.377-82

Angelo, L.S., Talpaz, M. & Kurzrock, R. (2002). Autocrine interleukin-6 production in renal cell carcinoma: evidence for the involvement of p53. *Cancer Res* Vol.62, No.3, (Feb 1), pp.932-40

Arai, E. & Kanai, Y. (2010). Genetic and epigenetic alterations during renal carcinogenesis. *Int J Clin Exp Pathol* Vol.4, No.1, pp.58-73

Arany, Z., Huang, L.E., Eckner, R., Bhattacharya, S., Jiang, C., Goldberg, M.A., Bunn, H.F. & Livingston, D.M. (1996). An essential role for p300/CBP in the cellular response to hypoxia. *Proc Natl Acad Sci U S A* Vol.93, No.23, (Nov 12), pp.12969-73

Atkins, M., Regan, M., McDermott, D., Mier, J., Stanbridge, E., Youmans, A., Febbo, P., Upton, M., Lechpammer, M. & Signoretti, S. (2005). Carbonic anhydrase IX expression predicts outcome of interleukin 2 therapy for renal cancer. *Clin Cancer Res* Vol.11, No.10, (May 15), pp.3714-21

Atlas, I., Mendelsohn, J., Baselga, J., Fair, W.R., Masui, H. & Kumar, R. (1992). Growth regulation of human renal carcinoma cells: role of transforming growth factor alpha. *Cancer Res* Vol.52, No.12, (Jun 15), pp.3335-9

Baldewijns, M.M., Thijssen, V.L., Van den Eynden, G.G., Van Laere, S.J., Bluekens, A.M., Roskams, T., van Poppel, H., De Bruine, A.P., Griffioen, A.W. & Vermeulen, P.B. (2007). High-grade clear cell renal cell carcinoma has a higher angiogenic activity than low-grade renal cell carcinoma based on histomorphological quantification and qRT-PCR mRNA expression profile. *Br J Cancer* Vol.96, No.12, (Jun 18), pp.1888-95

Baldewijns, M.M., van Vlodrop, I.J., Vermeulen, P.B., Soetekouw, P.M., van Engeland, M. & de Bruine, A.P. (2010). VHL and HIF signalling in renal cell carcinogenesis. *J Pathol* Vol.221, No.2, (Jun), pp.125-38

Banumathy, G. & Cairns, P. (2010). Signaling pathways in renal cell carcinoma. *Cancer Biol Ther* Vol.10, No.7, (Oct), pp.658-64

Bates, D.O. (2010). Vascular endothelial growth factors and vascular permeability. *Cardiovasc Res* Vol.87, No.2, (Jul 15), pp.262-71

Behrens, J., Mareel, M.M., Van Roy, F.M. & Birchmeier, W. (1989). Dissecting tumor cell invasion: epithelial cells acquire invasive properties after the loss of uvomorulin-mediated cell-cell adhesion. *J Cell Biol* Vol.108, No.6, (Jun), pp.2435-47

Binder, C., Binder, L., Marx, D., Schauer, A. & Hiddemann, W. (1997). Deregulated simultaneous expression of multiple glucose transporter isoforms in malignant cells and tissues. *Anticancer Res* Vol.17, No.6D, (Nov-Dec), pp.4299-304

Black, P.C. & Dinney, C.P. (2008). Growth factors and receptors as prognostic markers in urothelial carcinoma. *Curr Urol Rep* Vol.9, No.1, (Jan), pp.55-61

Blankenship, C., Naglich, J.G., Whaley, J.M., Seizinger, B. & Kley, N. (1999). Alternate choice of initiation codon produces a biologically active product of the von Hippel Lindau gene with tumor suppressor activity. *Oncogene* Vol.18, No.8, (Feb 25), pp.1529-35

Bui, M.H., Seligson, D., Han, K.R., Pantuck, A.J., Dorey, F.J., Huang, Y., Horvath, S., Leibovich, B.C., Chopra, S., Liao, S.Y., Stanbridge, E., Lerman, M.I., Palotie, A., Figlin, R.A. & Belldegrun, A.S. (2003). Carbonic anhydrase IX is an independent predictor of survival in advanced renal clear cell carcinoma: implications for prognosis and therapy. *Clin Cancer Res* Vol.9, No.2, (Feb), pp.802-11

Bullock, A., McDermott, D.F. & Atkins, M.B. (2010). Management of metastatic renal cell carcinoma in patients with poor prognosis. *Cancer Manag Res* Vol.2, pp.123-32

Carmeliet, P. (2005). VEGF as a key mediator of angiogenesis in cancer. *Oncology* Vol.69 Suppl 3, pp.4-10

Carvalho, G., Lefaucheur, C., Cherbonnier, C., Metivier, D., Chapel, A., Pallardy, M., Bourgeade, M.F., Charpentier, B., Hirsch, F. & Kroemer, G. (2005). Chemosensitization by erythropoietin through inhibition of the NF-kappaB rescue pathway. *Oncogene* Vol.24, No.5, (Jan 27), pp.737-45

Cavallaro, U. & Christofori, G. (2004). Cell adhesion and signalling by cadherins and Ig-CAMs in cancer. *Nat Rev Cancer* Vol.4, No.2, (Feb), pp.118-32

Cebe-Suarez, S., Zehnder-Fjallman, A. & Ballmer-Hofer, K. (2006). The role of VEGF receptors in angiogenesis; complex partnerships. *Cell Mol Life Sci* Vol.63, No.5, (Mar), pp.601-15

Cenni, E., Perut, F., Granchi, D., Avnet, S., Amato, I., Brandi, M.L., Giunti, A. & Baldini, N. (2007). Inhibition of angiogenesis via FGF-2 blockage in primitive and bone metastatic renal cell carcinoma. *Anticancer Res* Vol.27, No.1A, (Jan-Feb), pp.315-9

Cho, D., Signoretti, S., Regan, M., Mier, J.W. & Atkins, M.B. (2007). The role of mammalian target of rapamycin inhibitors in the treatment of advanced renal cancer. *Clin Cancer Res* Vol.13, No.2 Pt 2, (Jan 15), pp.758s-63s

Clark, P.E. (2009). The role of VHL in clear-cell renal cell carcinoma and its relation to targeted therapy. *Kidney Int* Vol.76, No.9, (Nov), pp.939-45

Corn, P.G. (2007). Role of the ubiquitin proteasome system in renal cell carcinoma. *BMC Biochem* Vol.8 Suppl 1, pp.S4

Curti, B.D. (2004). Renal cell carcinoma. *Jama* Vol.292, No.1, (Jul 7), pp.97-100

Da Silva, J.L., Lacombe, C., Bruneval, P., Casadevall, N., Leporrier, M., Camilleri, J.P., Bariety, J., Tambourin, P. & Varet, B. (1990). Tumor cells are the site of erythropoietin synthesis in human renal cancers associated with polycythemia. *Blood* Vol.75, No.3, (Feb 1), pp.577-82

Dames, S.A., Martinez-Yamout, M., De Guzman, R.N., Dyson, H.J. & Wright, P.E. (2002). Structural basis for Hif-1 alpha /CBP recognition in the cellular hypoxic response. *Proc Natl Acad Sci U S A* Vol.99, No.8, (Apr 16), pp.5271-6

Dawson, N.A., Guo, C., Zak, R., Dorsey, B., Smoot, J., Wong, J. & Hussain, A. (2004). A phase II trial of gefitinib (Iressa, ZD1839) in stage IV and recurrent renal cell carcinoma. *Clin Cancer Res* Vol.10, No.23, (Dec 1), pp.7812-9

de Paulsen, N., Brychzy, A., Fournier, M.C., Klausner, R.D., Gnarra, J.R., Pause, A. & Lee, S. (2001). Role of transforming growth factor-alpha in von Hippel--Lindau (VHL)(-/-) clear cell renal carcinoma cell proliferation: a possible mechanism coupling VHL tumor suppressor inactivation and tumorigenesis. *Proc Natl Acad Sci U S A* Vol.98, No.4, (Feb 13), pp.1387-92

Del Bufalo, D., Ciuffreda, L., Trisciuoglio, D., Desideri, M., Cognetti, F., Zupi, G. & Milella, M. (2006). Antiangiogenic potential of the Mammalian target of rapamycin inhibitor temsirolimus. *Cancer Res* Vol.66, No.11, (Jun 1), pp.5549-54

Derynck, R. (1986). Transforming growth factor-alpha: structure and biological activities. *J Cell Biochem* Vol.32, No.4, pp.293-304

Donovan, E.A. & Kummar, S. (2006). Targeting VEGF in cancer therapy. *Curr Probl Cancer* Vol.30, No.1, (Jan-Feb), pp.7-32

Dorai, T., Sawczuk, I., Pastorek, J., Wiernik, P.H. & Dutcher, J.P. (2006). Role of carbonic anhydrases in the progression of renal cell carcinoma subtypes: proposal of a unified hypothesis. *Cancer Invest* Vol.24, No.8, (Dec), pp.754-79

Ebert, B.L., Firth, J.D. & Ratcliffe, P.J. (1995). Hypoxia and mitochondrial inhibitors regulate expression of glucose transporter-1 via distinct Cis-acting sequences. *J Biol Chem* Vol.270, No.49, (Dec 8), pp.29083-9

Eble, J., Sauter, G., Epstein, J. & Sesterhenn, I. (2001). *Pathology and genetics. Tumours of the urinary system and male genital organs*, (Editor ed.). Lyon: IARC Press.

Ellis, L.M. & Hicklin, D.J. (2008). VEGF-targeted therapy: mechanisms of anti-tumour activity. *Nat Rev Cancer* Vol.8, No.8, (Aug), pp.579-91

Esteban, M.A., Tran, M.G., Harten, S.K., Hill, P., Castellanos, M.C., Chandra, A., Raval, R., O'Brien T, S. & Maxwell, P.H. (2006). Regulation of E-cadherin expression by VHL and hypoxia-inducible factor. *Cancer Res* Vol.66, No.7, (Apr 1), pp.3567-75

Evans, A.J., Russell, R.C., Roche, O., Burry, T.N., Fish, J.E., Chow, V.W., Kim, W.Y., Saravanan, A., Maynard, M.A., Gervais, M.L., Sufan, R.I., Roberts, A.M., Wilson, L.A., Betten, M., Vandewalle, C., Berx, G., Marsden, P.A., Irwin, M.S., Teh, B.T., Jewett, M.A. & Ohh, M. (2007). VHL promotes E2 box-dependent E-cadherin transcription by HIF-mediated regulation of SIP1 and snail. *Mol Cell Biol* Vol.27, No.1, (Jan), pp.157-69

Everitt, J.I., Walker, C.L., Goldsworthy, T.W. & Wolf, D.C. (1997). Altered expression of transforming growth factor-alpha: an early event in renal cell carcinoma development. *Mol Carcinog* Vol.19, No.3, (Jul), pp.213-9

Faivre, S., Delbaldo, C., Vera, K., Robert, C., Lozahic, S., Lassau, N., Bello, C., Deprimo, S., Brega, N., Massimini, G., Armand, J.P., Scigalla, P. & Raymond, E. (2006). Safety, pharmacokinetic, and antitumor activity of SU11248, a novel oral multitarget tyrosine kinase inhibitor, in patients with cancer. *J Clin Oncol* Vol.24, No.1, (Jan 1), pp.25-35

Fandrey, J. (2004). Oxygen-dependent and tissue-specific regulation of erythropoietin gene expression. *Am J Physiol Regul Integr Comp Physiol* Vol.286, No.6, (Jun), pp.R977-88

Ferlay, J., Shin, H.R., Bray, F., Forman, D., Mathers, C. & Parkin, D.M. (2010). Estimates of worldwide burden of cancer in 2008: GLOBOCAN 2008. *Int J Cancer* Vol.127, No.12, (Dec 15), pp.2893-917

Freedman, S.J., Sun, Z.Y., Poy, F., Kung, A.L., Livingston, D.M., Wagner, G. & Eck, M.J. (2002). Structural basis for recruitment of CBP/p300 by hypoxia-inducible factor-1 alpha. *Proc Natl Acad Sci U S A* Vol.99, No.8, (Apr 16), pp.5367-72

Freeman, M.R., Washecka, R. & Chung, L.W. (1989). Aberrant expression of epidermal growth factor receptor and HER-2 (erbB-2) messenger RNAs in human renal cancers. *Cancer Res* Vol.49, No.22, (Nov 15), pp.6221-5

Fukata, S., Inoue, K., Kamada, M., Kawada, C., Furihata, M., Ohtsuki, Y. & Shuin, T. (2005). Levels of angiogenesis and expression of angiogenesis-related genes are prognostic for organ-specific metastasis of renal cell carcinoma. *Cancer* Vol.103, No.5, (Mar 1), pp.931-42

Gao, H., Dong, B., Liu, X., Xuan, H., Huang, Y. & Lin, D. (2008). Metabonomic profiling of renal cell carcinoma: high-resolution proton nuclear magnetic resonance spectroscopy of human serum with multivariate data analysis. *Anal Chim Acta* Vol.624, No.2, (Aug 29), pp.269-77

Gervais, M.L., Henry, P.C., Saravanan, A., Burry, T.N., Gallie, B.L., Jewett, M.A., Hill, R.P., Evans, A.J. & Ohh, M. (2007). Nuclear E-cadherin and VHL immunoreactivity are prognostic indicators of clear-cell renal cell carcinoma. *Lab Invest* Vol.87, No.12, (Dec), pp.1252-64

Gnarra, J.R., Zhou, S., Merrill, M.J., Wagner, J.R., Krumm, A., Papavassiliou, E., Oldfield, E.H., Klausner, R.D. & Linehan, W.M. (1996). Post-transcriptional regulation of vascular endothelial growth factor mRNA by the product of the VHL tumor suppressor gene. *Proc Natl Acad Sci U S A* Vol.93, No.20, (Oct 1), pp.10589-94

Gomella, L.G., Sargent, E.R., Wade, T.P., Anglard, P., Linehan, W.M. & Kasid, A. (1989). Expression of transforming growth factor alpha in normal human adult kidney and enhanced expression of transforming growth factors alpha and beta 1 in renal cell carcinoma. *Cancer Res* Vol.49, No.24 Pt 1, (Dec 15), pp.6972-5

Gordon, M.S., Hussey, M., Nagle, R.B., Lara, P.N., Jr., Mack, P.C., Dutcher, J., Samlowski, W., Clark, J.I., Quinn, D.I., Pan, C.X. & Crawford, D. (2009). Phase II study of erlotinib in patients with locally advanced or metastatic papillary histology renal cell cancer: SWOG S0317. *J Clin Oncol* Vol.27, No.34, (Dec 1), pp.5788-93

Gossage, L. & Eisen, T. (2010). Alterations in VHL as potential biomarkers in renal-cell carcinoma. *Nat Rev Clin Oncol* Vol.7, No.5, (May), pp.277-88

Grabmaier, K., MC, A.d.W., Verhaegh, G.W., Schalken, J.A. & Oosterwijk, E. (2004). Strict regulation of CAIX(G250/MN) by HIF-1alpha in clear cell renal cell carcinoma. *Oncogene* Vol.23, No.33, (Jul 22), pp.5624-31

Grabmaier, K., Vissers, J.L., De Weijert, M.C., Oosterwijk-Wakka, J.C., Van Bokhoven, A., Brakenhoff, R.H., Noessner, E., Mulders, P.A., Merkx, G., Figdor, C.G., Adema, G.J.

& Oosterwijk, E. (2000). Molecular cloning and immunogenicity of renal cell carcinoma-associated antigen G250. *Int J Cancer* Vol.85, No.6, (Mar 15), pp.865-70

Grubb, R.L., 3rd, Choyke, P.L., Pinto, P.A., Linehan, W.M. & Walther, M.M. (2005). Management of von Hippel-Lindau-associated kidney cancer. *Nat Clin Pract Urol* Vol.2, No.5, (May), pp.248-55

Gunaratnam, L., Morley, M., Franovic, A., de Paulsen, N., Mekhail, K., Parolin, D.A., Nakamura, E., Lorimer, I.A. & Lee, S. (2003). Hypoxia inducible factor activates the transforming growth factor-alpha/epidermal growth factor receptor growth stimulatory pathway in VHL(-/-) renal cell carcinoma cells. *J Biol Chem* Vol.278, No.45, (Nov 7), pp.44966-74

Guo, Y., Schoell, M.C. & Freeman, R.S. (2009). The von Hippel-Lindau protein sensitizes renal carcinoma cells to apoptotic stimuli through stabilization of BIM(EL). *Oncogene* Vol.28, No.16, (Apr 23), pp.1864-74

Hagiwara, M., Chen, I.L., McGonigle, R., Beckman, B., Kasten, F.H. & Fisher, J.W. (1984). Erythropoietin production in a primary culture of human renal carcinoma cells maintained in nude mice. *Blood* Vol.63, No.4, (Apr), pp.828-35

Hara, S., Nakashiro, K., Klosek, S.K., Ishikawa, T., Shintani, S. & Hamakawa, H. (2006). Hypoxia enhances c-Met/HGF receptor expression and signaling by activating HIF-1alpha in human salivary gland cancer cells. *Oral Oncol* Vol.42, No.6, (Jul), pp.593-8

Henke, M., Laszig, R., Rube, C., Schafer, U., Haase, K.D., Schilcher, B., Mose, S., Beer, K.T., Burger, U., Dougherty, C. & Frommhold, H. (2003). Erythropoietin to treat head and neck cancer patients with anaemia undergoing radiotherapy: randomised, double-blind, placebo-controlled trial. *Lancet* Vol.362, No.9392, (Oct 18), pp.1255-60

Hergovich, A., Lisztwan, J., Barry, R., Ballschmieter, P. & Krek, W. (2003). Regulation of microtubule stability by the von Hippel-Lindau tumour suppressor protein pVHL. *Nat Cell Biol* Vol.5, No.1, (Jan), pp.64-70

Herman, J.G., Latif, F., Weng, Y., Lerman, M.I., Zbar, B., Liu, S., Samid, D., Duan, D.S., Gnarra, J.R., Linehan, W.M. & et al. (1994). Silencing of the VHL tumor-suppressor gene by DNA methylation in renal carcinoma. *Proc Natl Acad Sci U S A* Vol.91, No.21, (Oct 11), pp.9700-4

Hicklin, D.J. & Ellis, L.M. (2005). Role of the vascular endothelial growth factor pathway in tumor growth and angiogenesis. *J Clin Oncol* Vol.23, No.5, (Feb 10), pp.1011-27

Higashiyama, S., Iwabuki, H., Morimoto, C., Hieda, M., Inoue, H. & Matsushita, N. (2008). Membrane-anchored growth factors, the epidermal growth factor family: beyond receptor ligands. *Cancer Sci* Vol.99, No.2, (Feb), pp.214-20

Horiguchi, A., Sumitomo, M., Asakuma, J., Asano, T., Zheng, R., Nanus, D.M. & Hayakawa, M. (2006a). Increased serum leptin levels and over expression of leptin receptors are associated with the invasion and progression of renal cell carcinoma. *J Urol* Vol.176, No.4 Pt 1, (Oct), pp.1631-5

Horiguchi, A., Sumitomo, M., Asakuma, J., Asano, T., Zheng, R., Nanus, D.M. & Hayakawa, M. (2006b). Leptin promotes invasiveness of murine renal cancer cells via extracellular signal-regulated kinases and rho dependent pathway. *J Urol* Vol.176, No.4 Pt 1, (Oct), pp.1636-41

Houghton, P.J. (2010). Everolimus. *Clin Cancer Res* Vol.16, No.5, (Mar 1), pp.1368-72

Huang, L.E. & Bunn, H.F. (2003). Hypoxia-inducible factor and its biomedical relevance. *J Biol Chem* Vol.278, No.22, (May 30), pp.19575-8

Iliopoulos, O., Kibel, A., Gray, S. & Kaelin, W.G., Jr. (1995). Tumour suppression by the human von Hippel-Lindau gene product. *Nat Med* Vol.1, No.8, (Aug), pp.822-6

Iliopoulos, O., Ohh, M. & Kaelin, W.G., Jr. (1998). pVHL19 is a biologically active product of the von Hippel-Lindau gene arising from internal translation initiation. *Proc Natl Acad Sci U S A* Vol.95, No.20, (Sep 29), pp.11661-6

Ishikawa, J., Maeda, S., Umezu, K., Sugiyama, T. & Kamidono, S. (1990). Amplification and overexpression of the epidermal growth factor receptor gene in human renal-cell carcinoma. *Int J Cancer* Vol.45, No.6, (Jun 15), pp.1018-21

Ivan, M., Kondo, K., Yang, H., Kim, W., Valiando, J., Ohh, M., Salic, A., Asara, J.M., Lane, W.S. & Kaelin, W.G., Jr. (2001). HIFalpha targeted for VHL-mediated destruction by proline hydroxylation: implications for O2 sensing. *Science* Vol.292, No.5516, (Apr 20), pp.464-8

Ivanov, S., Liao, S.Y., Ivanova, A., Danilkovitch-Miagkova, A., Tarasova, N., Weirich, G., Merrill, M.J., Proescholdt, M.A., Oldfield, E.H., Lee, J., Zavada, J., Waheed, A., Sly, W., Lerman, M.I. & Stanbridge, E.J. (2001). Expression of hypoxia-inducible cell-surface transmembrane carbonic anhydrases in human cancer. *Am J Pathol* Vol.158, No.3, (Mar), pp.905-19

Jaakkola, P., Mole, D.R., Tian, Y.M., Wilson, M.I., Gielbert, J., Gaskell, S.J., Kriegsheim, A., Hebestreit, H.F., Mukherji, M., Schofield, C.J., Maxwell, P.H., Pugh, C.W. & Ratcliffe, P.J. (2001). Targeting of HIF-alpha to the von Hippel-Lindau ubiquitylation complex by O2-regulated prolyl hydroxylation. *Science* Vol.292, No.5516, (Apr 20), pp.468-72

Jensen, H.K., Nordsmark, M., Donskov, F., Marcussen, N. & von der Maase, H. (2008). Immunohistochemical expression of carbonic anhydrase IX assessed over time and during treatment in renal cell carcinoma. *BJU Int* Vol.101 Suppl 4, (Jun), pp.41-4

Jermann, M., Stahel, R.A., Salzberg, M., Cerny, T., Joerger, M., Gillessen, S., Morant, R., Egli, F., Rhyner, K., Bauer, J.A. & Pless, M. (2006). A phase II, open-label study of gefitinib (IRESSA) in patients with locally advanced, metastatic, or relapsed renal-cell carcinoma. *Cancer Chemother Pharmacol* Vol.57, No.4, (Apr), pp.533-9

Kaelin, W.G. (2005a). The von Hippel-Lindau tumor suppressor protein: roles in cancer and oxygen sensing. *Cold Spring Harb Symp Quant Biol* Vol.70, pp.159-66

Kaelin, W.G., Jr. (2002). Molecular basis of the VHL hereditary cancer syndrome. *Nat Rev Cancer* Vol.2, No.9, (Sep), pp.673-82

Kaelin, W.G., Jr. (2005b). The von Hippel-Lindau protein, HIF hydroxylation, and oxygen sensing. *Biochem Biophys Res Commun* Vol.338, No.1, (Dec 9), pp.627-38

Kaelin, W.G., Jr. (2007). The von Hippel-Lindau tumor suppressor protein and clear cell renal carcinoma. *Clin Cancer Res* Vol.13, No.2 Pt 2, (Jan 15), pp.680s-4s

Kallio, J.P., Hirvikoski, P., Helin, H., Kellokumpu-Lehtinen, P., Luukkaala, T., Tammela, T.L. & Martikainen, P.M. (2003). Membranous location of EGFR immunostaining is associated with good prognosis in renal cell carcinoma. *Br J Cancer* Vol.89, No.7, (Oct 6), pp.1266-9

Kaluz, S., Kaluzova, M., Liao, S.Y., Lerman, M. & Stanbridge, E.J. (2009). Transcriptional control of the tumor- and hypoxia-marker carbonic anhydrase 9: A one transcription factor (HIF-1) show? *Biochim Biophys Acta* Vol.1795, No.2, (Apr), pp.162-72

Kaluz, S., Kaluzova, M. & Stanbridge, E.J. (2008). Does inhibition of degradation of hypoxia-inducible factor (HIF) alpha always lead to activation of HIF? Lessons learnt from the effect of proteasomal inhibition on HIF activity. *J Cell Biochem* Vol.104, No.2, (May 15), pp.536-44

Kazal, L.A. & Erslev, A.J. (1975). Erythropoietin production in renal tumors. *Ann Clin Lab Sci* Vol.5, No.2, (Mar-Apr), pp.98-109

Kedar, D., Baker, C.H., Killion, J.J., Dinney, C.P. & Fidler, I.J. (2002). Blockade of the epidermal growth factor receptor signaling inhibits angiogenesis leading to regression of human renal cell carcinoma growing orthotopically in nude mice. *Clin Cancer Res* Vol.8, No.11, (Nov), pp.3592-600

Kim, W.Y. & Kaelin, W.G. (2004). Role of VHL gene mutation in human cancer. *J Clin Oncol* Vol.22, No.24, (Dec 15), pp.4991-5004

Knebelmann, B., Ananth, S., Cohen, H.T. & Sukhatme, V.P. (1998). Transforming growth factor alpha is a target for the von Hippel-Lindau tumor suppressor. *Cancer Res* Vol.58, No.2, (Jan 15), pp.226-31

Koivunen, P., Tiainen, P., Hyvarinen, J., Williams, K.E., Sormunen, R., Klaus, S.J., Kivirikko, K.I. & Myllyharju, J. (2007). An endoplasmic reticulum transmembrane prolyl 4-hydroxylase is induced by hypoxia and acts on hypoxia-inducible factor alpha. *J Biol Chem* Vol.282, No.42, (Oct 19), pp.30544-52

Konig, B., Steinbach, F., Janocha, B., Drynda, A., Stumm, M., Philipp, C., Allhoff, E.P. & Konig, W. (1999). The differential expression of proinflammatory cytokines IL-6, IL-8 and TNF-alpha in renal cell carcinoma. *Anticancer Res* Vol.19, No.2C, (Mar-Apr), pp.1519-24

Koochekpour, S., Jeffers, M., Wang, P.H., Gong, C., Taylor, G.A., Roessler, L.M., Stearman, R., Vasselli, J.R., Stetler-Stevenson, W.G., Kaelin, W.G., Jr., Linehan, W.M., Klausner, R.D., Gnarra, J.R. & Vande Woude, G.F. (1999). The von Hippel-Lindau tumor suppressor gene inhibits hepatocyte growth factor/scatter factor-induced invasion and branching morphogenesis in renal carcinoma cells. *Mol Cell Biol* Vol.19, No.9, (Sep), pp.5902-12

Krishnamachary, B., Zagzag, D., Nagasawa, H., Rainey, K., Okuyama, H., Baek, J.H. & Semenza, G.L. (2006). Hypoxia-inducible factor-1-dependent repression of E-cadherin in von Hippel-Lindau tumor suppressor-null renal cell carcinoma mediated by TCF3, ZFHX1A, and ZFHX1B. *Cancer Res* Vol.66, No.5, (Mar 1), pp.2725-31

Kumar, R., Knick, V.B., Rudolph, S.K., Johnson, J.H., Crosby, R.M., Crouthamel, M.C., Hopper, T.M., Miller, C.G., Harrington, L.E., Onori, J.A., Mullin, R.J., Gilmer, T.M., Truesdale, A.T., Epperly, A.H., Boloor, A., Stafford, J.A., Luttrell, D.K. & Cheung, M. (2007). Pharmacokinetic-pharmacodynamic correlation from mouse to human with pazopanib, a multikinase angiogenesis inhibitor with potent antitumor and antiangiogenic activity. *Mol Cancer Ther* Vol.6, No.7, (Jul), pp.2012-21

Lacombe, C. & Mayeux, P. (1999). The molecular biology of erythropoietin. *Nephrol Dial Transplant* Vol.14 Suppl 2, pp.22-8

Lager, D.J., Slagel, D.D. & Palechek, P.L. (1994). The expression of epidermal growth factor receptor and transforming growth factor alpha in renal cell carcinoma. *Mod Pathol* Vol.7, No.5, (Jun), pp.544-8

Lai, S.Y. & Grandis, J.R. (2006). Understanding the presence and function of erythropoietin receptors on cancer cells. *J Clin Oncol* Vol.24, No.29, (Oct 10), pp.4675-6

Lando, D., Peet, D.J., Gorman, J.J., Whelan, D.A., Whitelaw, M.L. & Bruick, R.K. (2002a). FIH-1 is an asparaginyl hydroxylase enzyme that regulates the transcriptional activity of hypoxia-inducible factor. *Genes Dev* Vol.16, No.12, (Jun 15), pp.1466-71

Lando, D., Peet, D.J., Whelan, D.A., Gorman, J.J. & Whitelaw, M.L. (2002b). Asparagine hydroxylation of the HIF transactivation domain a hypoxic switch. *Science* Vol.295, No.5556, (Feb 1), pp.858-61

Latif, F., Tory, K., Gnarra, J., Yao, M., Duh, F.M., Orcutt, M.L., Stackhouse, T., Kuzmin, I., Modi, W., Geil, L. & et al. (1993). Identification of the von Hippel-Lindau disease tumor suppressor gene. *Science* Vol.260, No.5112, (May 28), pp.1317-20

Lawrentschuk, N., Lee, F.T., Jones, G., Rigopoulos, A., Mountain, A., O'Keefe, G., Papenfuss, A.T., Bolton, D.M., Davis, I.D. & Scott, A.M. (2011). Investigation of hypoxia and carbonic anhydrase IX expression in a renal cell carcinoma xenograft model with oxygen tension measurements and (124)I-cG250 PET/CT. *Urol Oncol* Vol.29, No.4, (Jul-Aug), pp.411-20

Lee, S.J., Lattouf, J.B., Xanthopoulos, J., Linehan, W.M., Bottaro, D.P. & Vasselli, J.R. (2008). Von Hippel-Lindau tumor suppressor gene loss in renal cell carcinoma promotes oncogenic epidermal growth factor receptor signaling via Akt-1 and MEK-1. *Eur Urol* Vol.54, No.4, (Oct), pp.845-53

Lee, Y.S., Vortmeyer, A.O., Lubensky, I.A., Vogel, T.W., Ikejiri, B., Ferlicot, S., Benoit, G., Giraud, S., Oldfield, E.H., Linehan, W.M., Teh, B.T., Richard, S. & Zhuang, Z. (2005). Coexpression of erythropoietin and erythropoietin receptor in von Hippel-Lindau disease-associated renal cysts and renal cell carcinoma. *Clin Cancer Res* Vol.11, No.3, (Feb 1), pp.1059-64

Leyland-Jones, B., Semiglazov, V., Pawlicki, M., Pienkowski, T., Tjulandin, S., Manikhas, G., Makhson, A., Roth, A., Dodwell, D., Baselga, J., Biakhov, M., Valuckas, K., Voznyi, E., Liu, X. & Vercammen, E. (2005). Maintaining normal hemoglobin levels with epoetin alfa in mainly nonanemic patients with metastatic breast cancer receiving first-line chemotherapy: a survival study. *J Clin Oncol* Vol.23, No.25, (Sep 1), pp.5960-72

Li, G., Feng, G., Gentil-Perret, A., Genin, C. & Tostain, J. (2008). Serum carbonic anhydrase 9 level is associated with postoperative recurrence of conventional renal cell cancer. *J Urol* Vol.180, No.2, (Aug), pp.510-3; discussion 3-4

Li, J., Vesey, D.A., Johnson, D.W. & Gobe, G. (2007). Erythropoietin reduces cisplatin-induced apoptosis in renal carcinoma cells via a PKC dependent pathway. *Cancer Biol Ther* Vol.6, No.12, (Dec), pp.1944-50

Lidgren, A., Bergh, A., Grankvist, K., Rasmuson, T. & Ljungberg, B. (2008). Glucose transporter-1 expression in renal cell carcinoma and its correlation with hypoxia inducible factor-1 alpha. *BJU Int* Vol.101, No.4, (Feb), pp.480-4

Ljungberg, B., Rasmuson, T. & Grankvist, K. (1992). Erythropoietin in renal cell carcinoma: evaluation of its usefulness as a tumor marker. *Eur Urol* Vol.21, No.2, pp.160-3

Lonser, R.R., Glenn, G.M., Walther, M., Chew, E.Y., Libutti, S.K., Linehan, W.M. & Oldfield, E.H. (2003). von Hippel-Lindau disease. *Lancet* Vol.361, No.9374, (Jun 14), pp.2059-67

Lopez-Beltran, A., Scarpelli, M., Montironi, R. & Kirkali, Z. (2006). 2004 WHO classification of the renal tumors of the adults. *Eur Urol* Vol.49, No.5, (May), pp.798-805

Lowden, D.A., Lindemann, G.W., Merlino, G., Barash, B.D., Calvet, J.P. & Gattone, V.H., 2nd. (1994). Renal cysts in transgenic mice expressing transforming growth factor-alpha. *J Lab Clin Med* Vol.124, No.3, (Sep), pp.386-94

Macheda, M.L., Rogers, S. & Best, J.D. (2005). Molecular and cellular regulation of glucose transporter (GLUT) proteins in cancer. *J Cell Physiol* Vol.202, No.3, (Mar), pp.654-62

Maher, E.R., Yates, J.R., Harries, R., Benjamin, C., Harris, R., Moore, A.T. & Ferguson-Smith, M.A. (1990). Clinical features and natural history of von Hippel-Lindau disease. *Q J Med* Vol.77, No.283, (Nov), pp.1151-63

Mahon, P.C., Hirota, K. & Semenza, G.L. (2001). FIH-1: a novel protein that interacts with HIF-1alpha and VHL to mediate repression of HIF-1 transcriptional activity. *Genes Dev* Vol.15, No.20, (Oct 15), pp.2675-86

Marks, J.L., Broderick, S., Zhou, Q., Chitale, D., Li, A.R., Zakowski, M.F., Kris, M.G., Rusch, V.W., Azzoli, C.G., Seshan, V.E., Ladanyi, M. & Pao, W. (2008). Prognostic and therapeutic implications of EGFR and KRAS mutations in resected lung adenocarcinoma. *J Thorac Oncol* Vol.3, No.2, (Feb), pp.111-6

Maxwell, P.H., Wiesener, M.S., Chang, G.W., Clifford, S.C., Vaux, E.C., Cockman, M.E., Wykoff, C.C., Pugh, C.W., Maher, E.R. & Ratcliffe, P.J. (1999). The tumour suppressor protein VHL targets hypoxia-inducible factors for oxygen-dependent proteolysis. *Nature* Vol.399, No.6733, (May 20), pp.271-5

Maynard, M.A. & Ohh, M. (2004). Von Hippel-Lindau tumor suppressor protein and hypoxia-inducible factor in kidney cancer. *Am J Nephrol* Vol.24, No.1, (Jan-Feb), pp.1-13

Maynard, M.A., Qi, H., Chung, J., Lee, E.H., Kondo, Y., Hara, S., Conaway, R.C., Conaway, J.W. & Ohh, M. (2003). Multiple splice variants of the human HIF-3 alpha locus are targets of the von Hippel-Lindau E3 ubiquitin ligase complex. *J Biol Chem* Vol.278, No.13, (Mar 28), pp.11032-40

Medina, R.A. & Owen, G.I. (2002). Glucose transporters: expression, regulation and cancer. *Biol Res* Vol.35, No.1, pp.9-26

Mendel, D.B., Laird, A.D., Xin, X., Louie, S.G., Christensen, J.G., Li, G., Schreck, R.E., Abrams, T.J., Ngai, T.J., Lee, L.B., Murray, L.J., Carver, J., Chan, E., Moss, K.G., Haznedar, J.O., Sukbuntherng, J., Blake, R.A., Sun, L., Tang, C., Miller, T., Shirazian, S., McMahon, G. & Cherrington, J.M. (2003). In vivo antitumor activity of SU11248, a novel tyrosine kinase inhibitor targeting vascular endothelial growth factor and platelet-derived growth factor receptors: determination of a pharmacokinetic/pharmacodynamic relationship. *Clin Cancer Res* Vol.9, No.1, (Jan), pp.327-37

Merseburger, A.S., Hennenlotter, J., Simon, P., Kruck, S., Koch, E., Horstmann, M., Kuehs, U., Kufer, R., Stenzl, A. & Kuczyk, M.A. (2005). Membranous expression and prognostic implications of epidermal growth factor receptor protein in human renal cell cancer. *Anticancer Res* Vol.25, No.3B, (May-Jun), pp.1901-7

Michael, A., Politi, E., Havranek, E., Corbishley, C., Karapanagiotou, L., Anderson, C., Relph, K., Syrigos, K.N. & Pandha, H. (2007). Prognostic significance of erythropoietin expression in human renal cell carcinoma. *BJU Int* Vol.100, No.2, (Aug), pp.291-4

Migita, T., Oda, Y., Masuda, K., Hirata, A., Kuwano, M., Naito, S. & Tsuneyoshi, M. (2008). Inverse relationship between E-cadherin and p27Kip1 expression in renal cell carcinoma. *Int J Oncol* Vol.33, No.1, (Jul), pp.41-7

Mikhaylova, O., Ignacak, M.L., Barankiewicz, T.J., Harbaugh, S.V., Yi, Y., Maxwell, P.H., Schneider, M., Van Geyte, K., Carmeliet, P., Revelo, M.P., Wyder, M., Greis, K.D., Meller, J. & Czyzyk-Krzeska, M.F. (2008). The von Hippel-Lindau tumor suppressor protein and Egl-9-Type proline hydroxylases regulate the large subunit of RNA polymerase II in response to oxidative stress. *Mol Cell Biol* Vol.28, No.8, (Apr), pp.2701-17

Miyakita, H., Tokunaga, M., Onda, H., Usui, Y., Kinoshita, H., Kawamura, N. & Yasuda, S. (2002). Significance of 18F-fluorodeoxyglucose positron emission tomography (FDG-PET) for detection of renal cell carcinoma and immunohistochemical glucose transporter 1 (GLUT-1) expression in the cancer. *Int J Urol* Vol.9, No.1, (Jan), pp.15-8

Motzer, R.J., Amato, R., Todd, M., Hwu, W.J., Cohen, R., Baselga, J., Muss, H., Cooper, M., Yu, R., Ginsberg, M.S. & Needle, M. (2003). Phase II trial of antiepidermal growth factor receptor antibody C225 in patients with advanced renal cell carcinoma. *Invest New Drugs* Vol.21, No.1, (Feb), pp.99-101

Motzer, R.J., Escudier, B., Oudard, S., Hutson, T.E., Porta, C., Bracarda, S., Grunwald, V., Thompson, J.A., Figlin, R.A., Hollaender, N., Urbanowitz, G., Berg, W.J., Kay, A., Lebwohl, D. & Ravaud, A. (2008). Efficacy of everolimus in advanced renal cell carcinoma: a double-blind, randomised, placebo-controlled phase III trial. *Lancet* Vol.372, No.9637, (Aug 9), pp.449-56

Murphy, G.P., Kenny, G.M. & Mirand, E.A. (1970). Erythropoietin levels in patients with renal tumors or cysts. *Cancer* Vol.26, No.1, (Jul), pp.191-4

Mydlo, J.H., Michaeli, J., Cordon-Cardo, C., Goldenberg, A.S., Heston, W.D. & Fair, W.R. (1989). Expression of transforming growth factor alpha and epidermal growth factor receptor messenger RNA in neoplastic and nonneoplastic human kidney tissue. *Cancer Res* Vol.49, No.12, (Jun 15), pp.3407-11

Nagase, Y., Takata, K., Moriyama, N., Aso, Y., Murakami, T. & Hirano, H. (1995). Immunohistochemical localization of glucose transporters in human renal cell carcinoma. *J Urol* Vol.153, No.3 Pt 1, (Mar), pp.798-801

Noguchi, Y., Goto, T., Yufu, Y., Uike, N., Hasegawa, Y., Fukuda, T., Jimi, A. & Funakoshi, A. (1999). Gene expression of erythropoietin in renal cell carcinoma. *Intern Med* Vol.38, No.12, (Dec), pp.991-4

Ohh, M. (2006). Ubiquitin pathway in VHL cancer syndrome. *Neoplasia* Vol.8, No.8, (Aug), pp.623-9

Ohh, M. & Kaelin, W.G., Jr. (2003). VHL and kidney cancer. *Methods Mol Biol* Vol.222, pp.167-83

Ohh, M., Park, C.W., Ivan, M., Hoffman, M.A., Kim, T.Y., Huang, L.E., Pavletich, N., Chau, V. & Kaelin, W.G. (2000). Ubiquitination of hypoxia-inducible factor requires direct binding to the beta-domain of the von Hippel-Lindau protein. *Nat Cell Biol* Vol.2, No.7, (Jul), pp.423-7

Opavsky, R., Pastorekova, S., Zelnik, V., Gibadulinova, A., Stanbridge, E.J., Zavada, J., Kettmann, R. & Pastorek, J. (1996). Human MN/CA9 gene, a novel member of the carbonic anhydrase family: structure and exon to protein domain relationships. *Genomics* Vol.33, No.3, (May 1), pp.480-7

Ozcan, A., Shen, S.S., Zhai, Q.J. & Truong, L.D. (2007). Expression of GLUT1 in primary renal tumors: morphologic and biologic implications. *Am J Clin Pathol* Vol.128, No.2, (Aug), pp.245-54

Papworth, K., Bergh, A., Grankvist, K., Ljungberg, B. & Rasmuson, T. (2009). Expression of erythropoietin and its receptor in human renal cell carcinoma. *Tumour Biol* Vol.30, No.2, pp.86-92

Park, S.K., Haase, V.H. & Johnson, R.S. (2007). von Hippel Lindau tumor suppressor regulates hepatic glucose metabolism by controlling expression of glucose transporter 2 and glucose 6-phosphatase. *Int J Oncol* Vol.30, No.2, (Feb), pp.341-8

Pascual, D. & Borque, A. (2008). Epidemiology of kidney cancer. *Adv Urol* pp.782381

Pastore, Y., Jedlickova, K., Guan, Y., Liu, E., Fahner, J., Hasle, H., Prchal, J.F. & Prchal, J.T. (2003). Mutations of von Hippel-Lindau tumor-suppressor gene and congenital polycythemia. *Am J Hum Genet* Vol.73, No.2, (Aug), pp.412-9

Pastorekova, S., Ratcliffe, P.J. & Pastorek, J. (2008). Molecular mechanisms of carbonic anhydrase IX-mediated pH regulation under hypoxia. *BJU Int* Vol.101 Suppl 4, (Jun), pp.8-15

Patard, J.J., Fergelot, P., Karakiewicz, P.I., Klatte, T., Trinh, Q.D., Rioux-Leclercq, N., Said, J.W., Belldegrun, A.S. & Pantuck, A.J. (2008). Low CAIX expression and absence of VHL gene mutation are associated with tumor aggressiveness and poor survival of clear cell renal cell carcinoma. *Int J Cancer* Vol.123, No.2, (Jul 15), pp.395-400

Patard, J.J., Rioux-Leclercq, N., Masson, D., Zerrouki, S., Jouan, F., Collet, N., Dubourg, C., Lobel, B., Denis, M. & Fergelot, P. (2009). Absence of VHL gene alteration and high VEGF expression are associated with tumour aggressiveness and poor survival of renal-cell carcinoma. *Br J Cancer* Vol.101, No.8, (Oct 20), pp.1417-24

Pelicano, H., Martin, D.S., Xu, R.H. & Huang, P. (2006). Glycolysis inhibition for anticancer treatment. *Oncogene* Vol.25, No.34, (Aug 7), pp.4633-46

Pelletier, S., Tanguay, S., Lee, S., Gunaratnam, L., Arbour, N. & Lapointe, R. (2009). TGF-alpha as a candidate tumor antigen for renal cell carcinomas. *Cancer Immunol Immunother* Vol.58, No.8, (Aug), pp.1207-18

Perera, A.D., Kleymenova, E.V. & Walker, C.L. (2000). Requirement for the von Hippel-Lindau tumor suppressor gene for functional epidermal growth factor receptor blockade by monoclonal antibody C225 in renal cell carcinoma. *Clin Cancer Res* Vol.6, No.4, (Apr), pp.1518-23

Petrides, P.E., Bock, S., Bovens, J., Hofmann, R. & Jakse, G. (1990). Modulation of pro-epidermal growth factor, pro-transforming growth factor alpha and epidermal growth factor receptor gene expression in human renal carcinomas. *Cancer Res* Vol.50, No.13, (Jul 1), pp.3934-9

Pu, Y.S., Huang, C.Y., Kuo, Y.Z., Kang, W.Y., Liu, G.Y., Huang, A.M., Yu, H.J., Lai, M.K., Huang, S.P., Wu, W.J., Chiou, S.J. & Hour, T.C. (2009). Characterization of membranous and cytoplasmic EGFR expression in human normal renal cortex and renal cell carcinoma. *J Biomed Sci* Vol.16, pp.82

Pugh, C.W., O'Rourke, J.F., Nagao, M., Gleadle, J.M. & Ratcliffe, P.J. (1997). Activation of hypoxia-inducible factor-1; definition of regulatory domains within the alpha subunit. *J Biol Chem* Vol.272, No.17, (Apr 25), pp.11205-14

Rad, F.H., Ulusakarya, A., Gad, S., Sibony, M., Juin, F., Richard, S., Machover, D. & Uzan, G. (2008). Novel somatic mutations of the VHL gene in an erythropoietin-producing renal carcinoma associated with secondary polycythemia and elevated circulating endothelial progenitor cells. *Am J Hematol* Vol.83, No.2, (Feb), pp.155-8

Ramp, U., Reinecke, P., Gabbert, H.E. & Gerharz, C.D. (2000). Differential response to transforming growth factor (TGF)-alpha and fibroblast growth factor (FGF) in human renal cell carcinomas of the clear cell and papillary types. *Eur J Cancer* Vol.36, No.7, (May), pp.932-41

Ravaud, A., Hawkins, R., Gardner, J.P., von der Maase, H., Zantl, N., Harper, P., Rolland, F., Audhuy, B., Machiels, J.P., Petavy, F., Gore, M., Schoffski, P. & El-Hariry, I. (2008). Lapatinib versus hormone therapy in patients with advanced renal cell carcinoma: a randomized phase III clinical trial. *J Clin Oncol* Vol.26, No.14, (May 10), pp.2285-91

Rioux-Leclercq, N., Fergelot, P., Zerrouki, S., Leray, E., Jouan, F., Bellaud, P., Epstein, J.I. & Patard, J.J. (2007). Plasma level and tissue expression of vascular endothelial growth factor in renal cell carcinoma: a prospective study of 50 cases. *Hum Pathol* Vol.38, No.10, (Oct), pp.1489-95

Rixe, O., Bukowski, R.M., Michaelson, M.D., Wilding, G., Hudes, G.R., Bolte, O., Motzer, R.J., Bycott, P., Liau, K.F., Freddo, J., Trask, P.C., Kim, S. & Rini, B.I. (2007). Axitinib treatment in patients with cytokine-refractory metastatic renal-cell cancer: a phase II study. *Lancet Oncol* Vol.8, No.11, (Nov), pp.975-84

Ronkainen, H., Kauppila, S., Hirvikoski, P. & Vaarala, M.H. (2010). Evaluation of myosin VI, E-cadherin and beta-catenin immunostaining in renal cell carcinoma. *J Exp Clin Cancer Res* Vol.29, pp.2

Rowinsky, E.K., Schwartz, G.H., Gollob, J.A., Thompson, J.A., Vogelzang, N.J., Figlin, R., Bukowski, R., Haas, N., Lockbaum, P., Li, Y.P., Arends, R., Foon, K.A., Schwab, G. & Dutcher, J. (2004). Safety, pharmacokinetics, and activity of ABX-EGF, a fully human anti-epidermal growth factor receptor monoclonal antibody in patients with metastatic renal cell cancer. *J Clin Oncol* Vol.22, No.15, (Aug 1), pp.3003-15

Roy, H., Bhardwaj, S. & Yla-Herttuala, S. (2006). Biology of vascular endothelial growth factors. *Febs Letters* Vol.580, No.12, (May 22), pp.2879-87

Rugo, H.S., Herbst, R.S., Liu, G., Park, J.W., Kies, M.S., Steinfeldt, H.M., Pithavala, Y.K., Reich, S.D., Freddo, J.L. & Wilding, G. (2005). Phase I trial of the oral antiangiogenesis agent AG-013736 in patients with advanced solid tumors: pharmacokinetic and clinical results. *J Clin Oncol* Vol.23, No.24, (Aug 20), pp.5474-83

Russell, R.C. & Ohh, M. (2007). The role of VHL in the regulation of E-cadherin: a new connection in an old pathway. *Cell Cycle* Vol.6, No.1, (Jan 1), pp.56-9

Safran, M. & Kaelin, W.G., Jr. (2003). HIF hydroxylation and the mammalian oxygen-sensing pathway. *J Clin Invest* Vol.111, No.6, (Mar), pp.779-83

Sakamoto, S., Igarashi, T., Osumi, N., Imamoto, T., Tobe, T., Kamiya, M. & Ito, H. (2003). Erythropoietin-producing renal cell carcinoma in chronic hemodialysis patients: a report of two cases. *Int J Urol* Vol.10, No.1, (Jan), pp.49-51

Sang, N., Fang, J., Srinivas, V., Leshchinsky, I. & Caro, J. (2002). Carboxyl-terminal transactivation activity of hypoxia-inducible factor 1 alpha is governed by a von Hippel-Lindau protein-independent, hydroxylation-regulated association with p300/CBP. *Mol Cell Biol* Vol.22, No.9, (May), pp.2984-92

Sargent, E.R., Gomella, L.G., Belldegrun, A., Linehan, W.M. & Kasid, A. (1989). Epidermal growth factor receptor gene expression in normal human kidney and renal cell carcinoma. *J Urol* Vol.142, No.5, (Nov), pp.1364-8

Schoenfeld, A., Davidowitz, E.J. & Burk, R.D. (1998). A second major native von Hippel-Lindau gene product, initiated from an internal translation start site, functions as a tumor suppressor. *Proc Natl Acad Sci U S A* Vol.95, No.15, (Jul 21), pp.8817-22

Schofield, C.J. & Ratcliffe, P.J. (2005). Signalling hypoxia by HIF hydroxylases. *Biochem Biophys Res Commun* Vol.338, No.1, (Dec 9), pp.617-26

Seizinger, B.R., Rouleau, G.A., Ozelius, L.J., Lane, A.H., Farmer, G.E., Lamiell, J.M., Haines, J., Yuen, J.W., Collins, D., Majoor-Krakauer, D. & et al. (1988). Von Hippel-Lindau disease maps to the region of chromosome 3 associated with renal cell carcinoma. *Nature* Vol.332, No.6161, (Mar 17), pp.268-9

Semenza, G.L. (1999). Regulation of mammalian O2 homeostasis by hypoxia-inducible factor 1. *Annu Rev Cell Dev Biol* Vol.15, pp.551-78

Singer, K., Kastenberger, M., Gottfried, E., Hammerschmied, C.G., Buttner, M., Aigner, M., Seliger, B., Walter, B., Schlosser, H., Hartmann, A., Andreesen, R., Mackensen, A. & Kreutz, M. (2011). Warburg phenotype in renal cell carcinoma: high expression of glucose-transporter 1 (GLUT-1) correlates with low CD8(+) T-cell infiltration in the tumor. *Int J Cancer* Vol.128, No.9, (May 1), pp.2085-95

Slaton, J.W., Inoue, K., Perrotte, P., El-Naggar, A.K., Swanson, D.A., Fidler, I.J. & Dinney, C.P. (2001). Expression levels of genes that regulate metastasis and angiogenesis correlate with advanced pathological stage of renal cell carcinoma. *Am J Pathol* Vol.158, No.2, (Feb), pp.735-43

Smith, T.A. (1999). Facilitative glucose transporter expression in human cancer tissue. *Br J Biomed Sci* Vol.56, No.4, pp.285-92

Stebbins, C.E., Kaelin, W.G., Jr. & Pavletich, N.P. (1999). Structure of the VHL-ElonginC-ElonginB complex: implications for VHL tumor suppressor function. *Science* Vol.284, No.5413, (Apr 16), pp.455-61

Sternberg, C.N., Davis, I.D., Mardiak, J., Szczylik, C., Lee, E., Wagstaff, J., Barrios, C.H., Salman, P., Gladkov, O.A., Kavina, A., Zarba, J.J., Chen, M., McCann, L., Pandite, L., Roychowdhury, D.F. & Hawkins, R.E. (2010). Pazopanib in locally advanced or metastatic renal cell carcinoma: results of a randomized phase III trial. *J Clin Oncol* Vol.28, No.6, (Feb 20), pp.1061-8

Stillebroer, A.B., Mulders, P.F., Boerman, O.C., Oyen, W.J. & Oosterwijk, E. (2010). Carbonic anhydrase IX in renal cell carcinoma: implications for prognosis, diagnosis, and therapy. *Eur Urol* Vol.58, No.1, (Jul), pp.75-83

Stuttfeld, E. & Ballmer-Hofer, K. (2009). Structure and function of VEGF receptors. *IUBMB Life* Vol.61, No.9, (Sep), pp.915-22

Suganuma, N., Segade, F., Matsuzu, K. & Bowden, D.W. (2007). Differential expression of facilitative glucose transporters in normal and tumour kidney tissues. *BJU Int* Vol.99, No.5, (May), pp.1143-9

Takahashi, A., Sasaki, H., Kim, S.J., Tobisu, K., Kakizoe, T., Tsukamoto, T., Kumamoto, Y., Sugimura, T. & Terada, M. (1994). Markedly increased amounts of messenger RNAs for vascular endothelial growth factor and placenta growth factor in renal cell carcinoma associated with angiogenesis. *Cancer Res* Vol.54, No.15, (Aug 1), pp.4233-7

Tammela, T., Enholm, B., Alitalo, K. & Paavonen, K. (2005). The biology of vascular endothelial growth factors. *Cardiovasc Res* Vol.65, No.3, (Feb 15), pp.550-63

Tanimoto, K., Makino, Y., Pereira, T. & Poellinger, L. (2000). Mechanism of regulation of the hypoxia-inducible factor-1 alpha by the von Hippel-Lindau tumor suppressor protein. *Embo J* Vol.19, No.16, (Aug 15), pp.4298-309

Thiery, J.P. (2002). Epithelial-mesenchymal transitions in tumour progression. *Nat Rev Cancer* Vol.2, No.6, (Jun), pp.442-54

Thomas, G.V., Tran, C., Mellinghoff, I.K., Welsbie, D.S., Chan, E., Fueger, B., Czernin, J. & Sawyers, C.L. (2006). Hypoxia-inducible factor determines sensitivity to inhibitors of mTOR in kidney cancer. *Nat Med* Vol.12, No.1, (Jan), pp.122-7

Thurston, G. & Kitajewski, J. (2008). VEGF and Delta-Notch: interacting signalling pathways in tumour angiogenesis. *Br J Cancer* Vol.99, No.8, (Oct 21), pp.1204-9

Thyavihally, Y.B., Mahantshetty, U., Chamarajanagar, R.S., Raibhattanavar, S.G. & Tongaonkar, H.B. (2005). Management of renal cell carcinoma with solitary metastasis. *World J Surg Oncol* Vol.3, (Jul 20), pp.48

Uberall, I., Kolar, Z., Trojanec, R., Berkovcova, J. & Hajduch, M. (2008). The status and role of ErbB receptors in human cancer. *Exp Mol Pathol* Vol.84, No.2, (Apr), pp.79-89

Uhlman, D.L., Nguyen, P., Manivel, J.C., Zhang, G., Hagen, K., Fraley, E., Aeppli, D. & Niehans, G.A. (1995). Epidermal growth factor receptor and transforming growth factor alpha expression in papillary and nonpapillary renal cell carcinoma: correlation with metastatic behavior and prognosis. *Clin Cancer Res* Vol.1, No.8, (Aug), pp.913-20

Wang, G.L., Jiang, B.H., Rue, E.A. & Semenza, G.L. (1995). Hypoxia-inducible factor 1 is a basic-helix-loop-helix-PAS heterodimer regulated by cellular O2 tension. *Proc Natl Acad Sci U S A* Vol.92, No.12, (Jun 6), pp.5510-4

Warburg, O. (1956). On the origin of cancer cells. *Science* Vol.123, No.3191, (Feb 24), pp.309-14

Weiss, R.H. & Lin, P.Y. (2006). Kidney cancer: identification of novel targets for therapy. *Kidney Int* Vol.69, No.2, (Jan), pp.224-32

Wiesener, M.S., Munchenhagen, P., Glaser, M., Sobottka, B.A., Knaup, K.X., Jozefowski, K., Jurgensen, J.S., Roigas, J., Warnecke, C., Grone, H.J., Maxwell, P.H., Willam, C. & Eckardt, K.U. (2007). Erythropoietin gene expression in renal carcinoma is considerably more frequent than paraneoplastic polycythemia. *Int J Cancer* Vol.121, No.11, (Dec 1), pp.2434-42

Wiesener, M.S., Seyfarth, M., Warnecke, C., Jurgensen, J.S., Rosenberger, C., Morgan, N.V., Maher, E.R., Frei, U. & Eckardt, K.U. (2002). Paraneoplastic erythrocytosis associated with an inactivating point mutation of the von Hippel-Lindau gene in a renal cell carcinoma. *Blood* Vol.99, No.10, (May 15), pp.3562-5

Wilhelm, S. & Chien, D.S. (2002). BAY 43-9006: preclinical data. *Curr Pharm Des* Vol.8, No.25, pp.2255-7

Wilhelm, S.M., Carter, C., Tang, L., Wilkie, D., McNabola, A., Rong, H., Chen, C., Zhang, X., Vincent, P., McHugh, M., Cao, Y., Shujath, J., Gawlak, S., Eveleigh, D., Rowley, B., Liu, L., Adnane, L., Lynch, M., Auclair, D., Taylor, I., Gedrich, R., Voznesensky, A., Riedl, B., Post, L.E., Bollag, G. & Trail, P.A. (2004). BAY 43-9006 exhibits broad spectrum oral antitumor activity and targets the RAF/MEK/ERK pathway and receptor tyrosine kinases involved in tumor progression and angiogenesis. *Cancer Res* Vol.64, No.19, (Oct 1), pp.7099-109

Wykoff, C.C., Beasley, N.J., Watson, P.H., Turner, K.J., Pastorek, J., Sibtain, A., Wilson, G.D., Turley, H., Talks, K.L., Maxwell, P.H., Pugh, C.W., Ratcliffe, P.J. & Harris, A.L. (2000). Hypoxia-inducible expression of tumor-associated carbonic anhydrases. *Cancer Res* Vol.60, No.24, (Dec 15), pp.7075-83

Xu, L., Tong, R., Cochran, D.M. & Jain, R.K. (2005a). Blocking platelet-derived growth factor D/platelet-derived growth factor receptor beta signaling inhibits human renal cell carcinoma progression in an orthotopic mouse model. *Cancer Res* Vol.65, No.13, (Jul 1), pp.5711-9

Xu, R.H., Pelicano, H., Zhou, Y., Carew, J.S., Feng, L., Bhalla, K.N., Keating, M.J. & Huang, P. (2005b). Inhibition of glycolysis in cancer cells: a novel strategy to overcome drug resistance associated with mitochondrial respiratory defect and hypoxia. *Cancer Res* Vol.65, No.2, (Jan 15), pp.613-21

Yoshida, K., Hosoya, Y., Sumi, S., Honda, M., Moriguchi, H., Yano, M. & Ueda, Y. (1997). Studies of the expression of epidermal growth factor receptor in human renal cell carcinoma: a comparison of immunohistochemical method versus ligand binding assay. *Oncology* Vol.54, No.3, (May-Jun), pp.220-5

Yoshida, K., Tosaka, A., Takeuchi, S. & Kobayashi, N. (1994). Epidermal growth factor receptor content in human renal cell carcinomas. *Cancer* Vol.73, No.7, (Apr 1), pp.1913-8

Yuen, J.S., Cockman, M.E., Sullivan, M., Protheroe, A., Turner, G.D., Roberts, I.S., Pugh, C.W., Werner, H. & Macaulay, V.M. (2007). The VHL tumor suppressor inhibits expression of the IGF1R and its loss induces IGF1R upregulation in human clear cell renal carcinoma. *Oncogene* Vol.26, No.45, (Oct 4), pp.6499-508

Zavada, J., Zavadova, Z., Zat'ovicova, M., Hyrsl, L. & Kawaciuk, I. (2003). Soluble form of carbonic anhydrase IX (CA IX) in the serum and urine of renal carcinoma patients. *Br J Cancer* Vol.89, No.6, (Sep 15), pp.1067-71

Zhang, X., Yamashita, M., Uetsuki, H. & Kakehi, Y. (2002). Angiogenesis in renal cell carcinoma: Evaluation of microvessel density, vascular endothelial growth factor and matrix metalloproteinases. *Int J Urol* Vol.9, No.9, (Sep), pp.509-14

Zhou, G.X., Ireland, J., Rayman, P., Finke, J. & Zhou, M. (2010). Quantification of carbonic
    anhydrase IX expression in serum and tissue of renal cell carcinoma patients using
    enzyme-linked immunosorbent assay: prognostic and diagnostic potentials.
    Urology Vol.75, No.2, (Feb), pp.257-61

6

Anticancer Target Molecules Against the SCF Ubiquitin E3 Ligase in RCC: Potential Approaches to the NEDD8 Pathway

Tomoaki Tanaka and Tatsuya Nakatani

Osaka City University Graduate School of Medicine, Department of Urology

Japan

1. Introduction

Several alternative treatments have recently been developed for metastatic renal cell carcinoma (RCC). Vascular endothelial growth factor (VEGF) is a potent pro-angiogenic protein, which is responsible for increased vasculature and tumor-growth in RCC. Fundamentally, a mutation in the von Hippel-Lindau (VHL) tumor suppressor gene induces overexpression of VEGF via accumulation of hypoxia-inducible factor (HIF)-1 in RCC. Several agents inhibiting the VEGF signaling cascade, such as sorafenib, sunitinib and bevacizumab, have been found to exert significant anti-tumor effects and provide meaningful clinical benefits. Furthermore, temsirolimus and everolimus, inhibitors of the mammalian target of rapamycin (mTOR), which block the phosphoinositide 3-kinase (PI3K)/AKT signaling pathway involved in numerous cellular functions including cell proliferation, survival and angiogenesis, have been found to be effective agents against advanced RCC in the clinical setting. Although molecular targeting therapies against the VEGF or mTOR signaling pathway have revolutionized the treatment of advanced RCC, no curative therapy has yet been established.

In this chapter, we focus on potent molecules and agents possibly suppressing the tumor growth of RCC via regulation of the ubiquitination-proteasome system. NEDD8, one of the ubiquitin-like proteins, reportedly forms conjugates with cullin family proteins and thereby activates the Skp1-Cullin-F-box (SCF) ubiquitin protein ligase complex that catalyzes the ubiquitination of many cell-cycle regulators, e.g. cyclin E, p21, p73 and p27. It is possible that negative regulation of NEDD8 and its conjugation system induces an antiproliferative action on RCC, secondary to inhibition of ubiqitin-proteasome activity. We previously showed that these negative regulator proteins, such as NEDD8 ultimate buster 1 (NUB1) and a dominant negative form (Ubc12 C111S) of NEDD8 E2 ligase, exhibited remarkable antitumor effects against some tumors, including RCC. Moreover, MLN4924, a potent and selective inhibitor of NEDD8-activating enzyme (NAE), was recently reported to disrupt SCF ubiquitin E3 ligase-induced protein turnover leading to apoptosis in tumor cells via deregulation of the cell cycle. This compound has already been applied in the clinical setting, e.g., malignant lymphoma. Thus, negative regulation of NEDD8 and its conjugation is an attractive anti-cancer strategy based on evidence obtained by basic research. We have developed a hypoxia-inducible factor-1 (HIF-1)-triggered expression vector for the purpose of selective gene therapy using NEDD8 negative regulator molecules, including NUB1 and the Ubc12 dominant negative form.

In this chapter, we summarize the data on potent molecules associated with the ubiquitin-proteasome system as anti-cancer targets on the basis of our reseach and discuss future perspectives in the treatment of RCC.

2. Mechanisms of ubiquitination pathway

Programmed destruction of regulatory proteins is crucial for homeostasis of cellular biological functions. The ubiquitination-proteasome pathway is a major scavenger system associated with regulated proteolysis inside cells. The pathway of protein destruction begins by conjugating a chain of polyubiquitin to a target molecule (Hershko & Ciechanover, 1998). The first step in the production of this chain is to connect a monoubiquitin molecule to E1(ubiquitin-activating enzyme) through a thioester bond in an ATP-dependent manner. Next, E2 (ubiquitin-conjugating enzyme) receives an activated ubiquitin from E1 and transfers a ubiquitin to a lysine residue in a target protein with the assistance of an E3 ubiquitin ligase. Repeated cycles via the E1-E2-E3 cascade generate a polyubiquitin chain, namely a death signal, which is subsequently recognized by the regulatory subunit of the 26S proteasome machinery (Fig. 1).

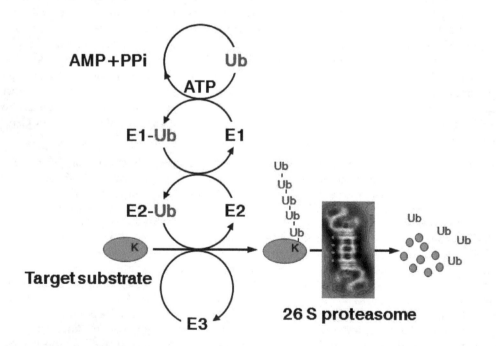

Fig. 1. Overview of the ubiquitination-proteasome pathway. Lysine residue (K) of the substrate is conjugated to ubiquitin (Ub).

2.1 Multiplicity of SCF (Skp-1, Cullins, F-box proteins) complex E3 ubiquitin ligases and their target proteins

The SCF complex E3 ligases or CRLs (Cullin-RING ubiquitin ligases), which are mainly comprised of Skp-1, Cullins, F-box proteins and Rbx/Roc RING finger proteins, are predominate among members of the E3 ubiquitin ligase family that promotes the ubiquitination of target proteins regulating various biological processes, including cell-cycle progression, signal transduction, and differentiation. The substrate specificity of SCF ligase depends on the combination pattern of its components, particularly the F-box binding domain. Numerous regulatory proteins targeted by SCF ligases have just recently been reported, as shown in Table 1. Therefore, deregulation of SCF E3 ligases may reinforce the instability of cellular functions; cell-cycle arrest, apoptosis, tumorigenesis, etc.

2.2 NEDD8, one of the ubiquitin-like proteins (UBLs), conjugation pathway

Several ubiquitin-like proteins (UBLs), including NEDD8, Sentrin/SUMO, ISG15, FAT10, Atg8 and Atg12, have been demonstrated to conjugate to a target molecule in a manner similar to ubiquitin. NEDD8 (neural precursor cell-expressed developmentally downregulated) was originally reported as a novel gene highly enriched in fetal mouse brain (Kumar et al., 1992). NEDD8 encodes a small protein of 81 amino acids, which is 60% identical and 80% homologous to ubiquitin, and equivalently conjugates to substrates (Kamitani et al., 1997). The crystal structure of NEDD8 is quite analogous to that of ubiquitin with the exception of two surface regions which are different (Fig. 2).

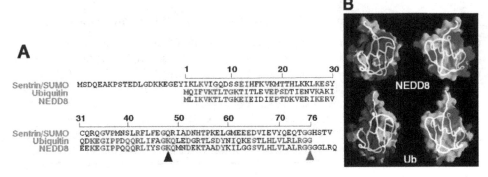

Fig. 2. (A) Alignment of amino acid sequences of human SUMO/Sentrin, Ubiquitin, and NEDD8. Black triangle; site of conjugation with lysine. Red triangle; active cleavage site for glycine. (B). 3D-structures of Ubiquitin and NEDD8.

The NEDD8 conjugation cascade, also known as neddylation, is mediated by E1 NEDD8-activating enzyme (NAE), E2 NEDD8 conjugating enzyme (Ubc12), and E3 NEDD8 ligase, which successively activate and transfer NEDD8 to a target molecule. First, the C-terminal glycine of NEDD8 is adenylated by an E1 NAE, which is composed of APP-BP1 and Uba3 heterodimer, in an ATP-dependent manner and transferred to E1 via a thiolester linkage. Second, activated NEDD8 is consecutively transferred to an E2 NEDD8 conjugation enzyme (Ubc12, Ube2f). Third, an E3 NEDD8 ligase transfers NEDD8 to a substrate lysine residue via an isopeptide bond. On the contrary, covalent neddylation of a substrate is reversibly deconjugated by the action of proteins (e.g. COP9 signalosome, NEDP1/DEN1, USP21) involved in deneddylation (Gong et al., 2000; Lyapina et al., 2001; Rabut & Peter, 2008) or inhibited by Cullin binding to CAND1 (Cullin-associated and neddylation-dissociate 1)(Goldenberg et al., 2004), or negatively down-regulated by NUB1 (NEDD8 ultimate buster 1) linked to the 26S proteasome (Kamitani et al., 2001; Kito et al., 2001) (Fig. 3).

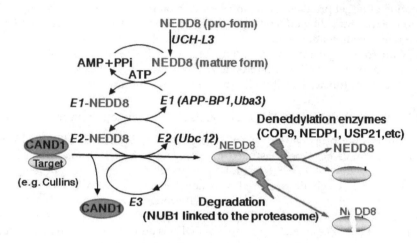

Fig. 3. Overview of the NEDD8 conjugation and deconjugation pathway.

2.2.1 Substrates conjugated by NEDD8; Cullins and other target molecules

Cullins, scaffold proteins assembling other components of an E3 SCF complex, are the substrates usually targeted by NEDD8 (Table 1). To date, seven Cullin family members (Cul-1, -2, -3, -4A, -4B, -5, -7) have been identified. Cul-1-based SCF complexes (CRL1), such as SCF[Skp2], SCF[β-Trcp] and SCF[Fbw7], are the most studied in terms of their cancer-related actions. SCF[Skp2] is involved in the degradation of several cell-cycle regulators (e.g. cyclin D, p27[Kip1], p21[Cip1], p73, p130, etc) (Guardavaccaro & Pagano, 2004). SCF[β-Trcp] promotes degradation of IκBα of the NFκB inhibitor and β-catenin (Skaar et al., 2009). Moreover, SCF[Fbw7] has been reported to promote degradation of cyclin E, c-myc oncoproteins and Notch (Guardavaccaro & Pagano, 2004). A recent study identified more than 350 possible CRL1 substrates by employing global protein stability profiling (Yen & Elledge, 2008). Cul-2 properly generates a CRL2 complex (also known as VBC) with the von Hippel-Lindau gene product (pVHL) through elongin B and elongin C. This complex induces degradation of the hypoxia-inducible factor-1 α subunit (HIF-1α), of which proline residues are hydroxylated by prolyl hydroxylase in an oxygen-dependent manner and then targeted to pVHL for ubiquitination (Kaelin & Ratcliffe, 2008). Bialleic deletion of the VHL gene mainly results in the stability of HIF-1α and thereby ultimately contributes to tumorigenesis of sporadic clear-cell type RCC. The Cul-3-based SCF complex (CRL3), which is produced with Rbx1 and BTB-domain protein, promotes degradation of cyclin E, Mei-1 (a component of mitotic spindle), Dsh (a regulator of Wnt-β-catenin pathway) and NRF2 (a transcriptional factor associated with an anti-oxidant response) (Angers et al., 2006; Furukawa et al., 2003; Furukawa & Xiong, 2005). The CRL4 complex, including Cul-4 (A or B), a damaged DNA binding (DDB1) protein, and a DDB1 and Cul-4-associated factor (DCAF), controls DNA replication and nucleotide excision repair through ubiquitination of CDT1, p21, Histone H2A/H3/H4, XPC, etc (Hu et al., 2004; Jackson & Xiong, 2009; Kapetanaki et al., 2006). Interestingly, knockdown or a specific inhibitor of Cul-4A has attracted research attention as a strategy for treating Cul-4-amplified breast cancer (Chen et al., 1998) and UV-induced skin cancer (Liu et al., 2009). The CRL5 complex, comprised of Cul-5, a suppressor of cytokine signaling (SOCS) family proteins, Elongin B and C, and Rbx1, suppresses JAK-STAT signaling via degradation of JAK family proteins (Hilton, 1999). On the contrary, Cul-5 has been identified as a possible tumor suppressor, overexpression of which induces growth-inhibition of breast cancer cells (Johnson et al., 2007). As regards Cul-7, to date, there have been no reported observations indicating that it is neddylated in the formation of a CRL7 complex.

Scaffold	Adaptor	Receptor	Ring box	Substrates
Cul-1	Skp1	Skp2	Rbx1	p21, p27, p73, p130, Cyclin A/ D
Cul-1	Skp1	β-TrCP	Rbx1	IκBα, β-catenin, Bim EL, Weel, p53
Cul-1	Skp1	Fbxw7	Rbx1	Cyclin E, c-Myc, c-Jun, Notch
Cul-2	Elongin BC	VHL	Rbx1	HIF1α
Cul-3		BTB-domain proteins	Rbx1	Cyclin E, Mei-1, Dsh, NRF2
Cul-4	DDB1	DCAF	Rbx1	CDT1, p21, Histone H2A/H3/H4, XPC
Cul-5	Elongin BC	SOCS	Rbx1	TEL-JAK2, JAK-STAT family proteins
Cul-7	Skp1	Fbxw8	Rbx1	IRS-1, Cyclin D

Table 1. SCF E3 ligases and their substrates.

As to NEDD8-target molecules other than Cullins, p53 is modified with NEDD8 via the function of MDM2, a RING finger E3 ligase, to facilitate its transactivation activity (Xirodimas et al., 2004). MDM2 also neddylates the proapoptotic protein, TAp73, and thereby enhances the localization of NEDD8-conjugated TAp73 in the cytoplasm to suppress its transactivation action (Watson et al., 2006). Moreover, MDM2 itself is also involved in NEDD8 modification, which contributes to its protein stability (Watson et al., 2010; Xirodimas et al., 2004). In addition, breast cancer-associated protein 3 (BCA3), which is highly expressed in breast and prostate cancers, was identified as a NEDD8 substrate (Gao et al., 2006). BCA3 inhibits NFκB-dependent transcription through its ability to bind to NFκB subunit p65 and the cyclin D1 promoter in a neddylation-dependent manner.

3. Focusing on the SCF E3 ligases for anticancer strategy

The SCF ubiquitin E3 ligases have been found to be dysregulated in a wide range of cancers, resulting in unlimited cell-proliferation and carcinogenesis via accumulation of their target-substrates. Consequently, the control of these E3 ligases is attracting attention as a possible strategy for treating cancers. The components (e.g. cullins, Skp-1/2, F-box proteins, Rbx1/2) and the molecules associated with modification by a SCF-activator protein, NEDD8, are potential candidates to be targeted in this approach.

3.1 Potent molecules involved in inhibition of SCF E3 ligases through deneddylation

As mentioned in section **2.2**, neddylation, i.e. conjugation of NEDD8 to target substrates, is catalyzed by certain known enzymes (E1, E2, E3) in a multistep fashion. Recently, MLN4924, a specific inhibitor of E1 NAE, was identified as an adenosine sulfamate derivative based on the results of a high throughput screen (HTS) study designed to identify NAE inhibitors (Soucy et al., 2009). Pharmaceutically, MLN4924 irreversibly forms a covalent adduct with NEDD8 via the NAE involved in the first NEDD8 adenylation step. MLN4924 is a potent ATP-competitive inhibitor that disrupts the thiolester bond between NEDD8 and Uba3, a subunit of NAE. Fundamentally, MLN4924-mediated suppression of cullin neddylation has been shown to increase expression levels of CRL-targeting substrates (Fig. 4). Moreover, MLN4924 was revealed to have antitumor effects against acute myeloid leukemia (AML) cells both in vitro and in xenograft models, simultaneously leading to increases in the amounts of CRL-specific substrates including Iκβα (Milhollen et al., 2010; Swords et al., 2010). Clinical trials using this agent are currently ongoing in AML patients.

Ubc12, an E2 NEDD8-conjugation enzyme, is also a key molecule in the neddylation cascade. Activated NEDD8 is transferred to the active site cystein residue of Ubc12 via a thiolester bond. Finally, Ubc12 conjugates NEDD8 to a single lysine residue of target substrates. Artificial Ubc12-C111S with mutant substitution of Cys-to-Ser in the active site (cys-111) was shown to have a dominant negative effect on the internal function of wild-type Ubc12, attributable to its covalent binding to NEDD8 (Wada et al., 2000) (Fig. 4). This mutant Ubc12-C111S has a forceful anti-proliferative action on cancer cells, concomitant with the instability of cellular morphology due to an actin cytoskeleton irregularity (Leck et al., 2010; Wada et al., 2000).

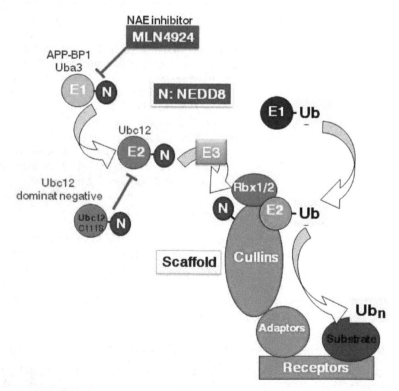

Fig. 4. Targeting the NEDD8 conjugation cascade to obtain antitumor activity.

3.1.1 Potent tumor-suppressor proteins of RCC, NUB1 (NEDD8 ultimate buster 1)/NUB1L

NUB1 is a NEDD8-interacting protein composed of 601 amino acid residues with a calculated molecular mass of 69.1 kDa. It is an interferon (IFN)-inducible protein and predominantly localizes in the nucleus. Moreover, NUB1L, a splicing variant of NUB1, possesses an insertion of 14 amino acids that codes for an additional ubiquitin-associated (UBA) domain, corresponding to a NEDD8-binding site (Fig. 5). Biologically, NUB1/NUB1L recruits NEDD8 and its conjugates to the proteasome for degradation and negatively regulates the NEDD8 conjugation system (Kamitani et al., 2001; Kito et al., 2001; Tanaka et al., 2003).

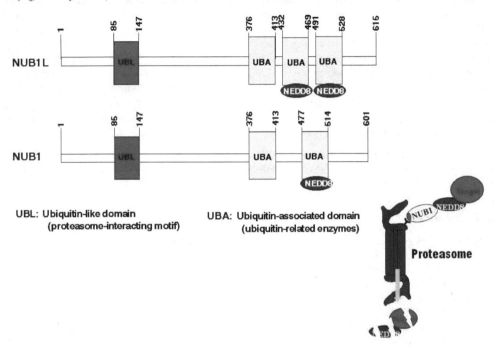

Fig. 5. Functional domains of both NUB1 and NUB1L, which are linked to the proteasome.

Furthermore, NUB1 is expressed in some cancer cell lines, including rectal adenocarcinoma, neuroblastoma, malignant lymphoma, cervical adenocarcinoma and RCC (Kito et al., 2001). Recently, NUB1 was shown to not only correlate with IFNα-induced antimitogenic action, but also exert anticancer effects against RCC cells, concomitant with S-phase transition during the cell cycle and apoptosis via accumulation of p27 and cyclin E (Hosono et al., 2010). Interestingly, overexpression of NUB1 strongly inhibits tumor proliferation in IFNα-resistant RCC cells (Hosono et al., 2010).

In general, tumorigenesis of RCCs, particularly clear cell carcinoma, is mainly attributed to HIF-1α-VEGF-mediated angiogenesis. HIF-1α is stabilized by loss of the function of a CRL2 complex via inactivation of VHL protein and of the hydroxylated oxygen-dependent degradation (ODD) domain of HIF-1α in a state of hypoxia inside RCC cells. For the purpose of developing tumor-specific gene therapy for RCCs, our laboratory constructed a potent delivery plasmid, composed of HIF-1-dependent reporter genes, in which 5 copies of the hypoxia-response element (5HRE) enhanced expression of the ODD domain and target gene under hypoxic conditions. Thus, these novel vectors including 5HRE-ODD-NUB1 or 5HRE-ODD-Ubc12 C111S may be useful for targeting advanced RCCs, even RCCs resistant to IFN, tyrosine kinase inhibitors, or mTOR inhibitors.

4. Conclusion

Potent agents (tyrosine kinase inhibitors, mTOR inhibitors), targeting VEGF and mTOR signal cascades, have recently been used worldwide for the purpose of treating metastatic RCC (mRCC) patients. Although these drugs have produced significant benefits in terms of overall survival and progression-free survival, as compared to traditional immunotherapy with IFN, there is no definitive strategy for the progressive-disease state of mRCC resistant to these target therapies. Alternative molecular targets (e.g. mTORC2, angiopoetin family proteins) complementary to the HIF-VEGF or PI3K-Akt-mTOR signal cascade are anticipated from future research. However, another approach distinct from conventional molecular targeting therapies is needed to prolong the survival of mRCC patients. Targeting neddylation as a procedure for inactivation of SCF E3 ligases was revealed to have a strong potential to suppress cancer cell growth.

Thus, a novel strategy for regulating NEDD8-dependent signal pathways may yield a breakthrough in the field of mRCC treatments, if it meets the criteria of showing high selectivity for cancer cells and being minimally toxic to normal cells.

5. References

Angers, S.; Thorpe, C.J.; Biechele, T.L.; Goldenberg, S.J.; Zheng, N.; MacCoss, M.J. & Moon, R.T. (2006). The KLHL12-Cullin-3 ubiquitin ligase negatively regulates the Wnt-beta-catenin pathway by targeting Dishevelled for degradation. *Nature Cell Biology,* Vol.8, No.4, (April 2006), pp. 348-357, ISSN 1465-7392

Chen, L.C.; Manjeshwar, S.; Lu, Y.; Moore, D.; Ljung, B.M.; Kuo, W.L.; Dairkee, S.H.; Wernick, M.; Collins, C. & Smith, H.S. (1998). The human homologue for the Caenorhabditis elegans cul-4 gene is amplified and overexpressed in primary breast cancers. *Cancer Research,* Vol.58, No.16, (August 1998), pp. 3677-3683, ISSN 0008-5472

Furukawa, M.; He, Y.J.; Borchers, C. & Xiong, Y. (2003). Targeting of protein ubiquitination by BTB-Cullin 3-Roc1 ubiquitin ligases. *Nature Cell Biology,* Vol.5, No.11, (November 2003), pp. 1001-1007, ISSN 1465-7392

Furukawa, M. & Xiong, Y. (2005). BTB protein Keap1 targets antioxidant transcription factor Nrf2 for ubiquitination by the Cullin 3-Roc1 ligase. *Molecular Cell Biology,* Vol.25, No.1, (January 2005), pp. 162-171, ISSN 0270-7306

Gao, F.; Cheng, J.; Shi, T. & Yeh, E.T. (2006). Neddylation of a breast cancer-associated protein recruits a class III histone deacetylase that represses NFkappaB-dependent transcription. *Nature Cell Biology,* Vol.8, No.10, (October 2006), pp. 1171-1177, ISSN 1465-7392

Goldenberg, S.J.; Cascio, T.C.; Shumway, S.D.; Garbutt, K.C.; Liu, J.; Xiong, Y. & Zheng, N. (2004). Structure of the Cand1-Cul1-Roc1 complex reveals regulatory mechanisms for the assembly of the multisubunit cullin-dependent ubiquitin ligases. *Cell,* Vol.119, No.4, (November 2004), pp. 517-528, ISSN 0092-8674

Gong, L.; Kamitani, T.; Millas, S. & Yeh, E.T. (2000). Identification of a novel isopeptidase with dual specificity for ubiquitin- and NEDD8-conjugated proteins. *The Journal Biological Chemistry*, Vol.275, No.19, (November 2000), pp 14212-14216, ISSN 0021-9258

Guardavaccaro, D. & Pagano, M. (2004). Oncogenic aberrations of cullin-dependent ubiquitin ligases. *Oncogene*, Vol.23, No.11, (March 2004), pp. 2037-2049, ISSN 0021-9258

Hershko, A. & Ciechanover, A. (1998). The ubiquitin system. *Annual Review of Biochemistry*, Vol.67, (July 1998), pp. 425-479, ISSN 0066-4154

Hilton, D.J. (1999). Negative regulators of cytokine signal transduction. *Cellular and Molecular Life Science*,Vol.55, No.12, (September 1999), pp. 1568-1577, ISSN 1420-682X

Hosono, T.; Tanaka, T.; Tanji, K.; Nakatani, T. & Kamitani, T. (2010). NUB1, an interferon-inducible protein, mediates anti-proliferative actions and apoptosis in renal cell carcinoma cells through cell-cycle regulation. *British Journal of Cancer*, Vol.102, No.5, (March 2010), pp. 873-882, ISSN 1532-1827

Hu, J.; McCall, C.M.; Ohta, T. & Xiong, Y. (2004). Targeted ubiquitination of CDT1 by the DDB1-CUL4A-ROC1 ligase in response to DNA damage. *Nature Cell Biology*, Vol.6, No.10, (October 2004), pp. 1003-1009, ISSN 1465-7392

Jackson, S. & Xiong, Y. (2009). CRL4s: the CUL4-RING E3 ubiquitin ligases. *Trends in Biochemical Sciences*, Vol.34, No.11, (November 2009), pp. 562-570, ISSN 0968-0004

Johnson, A.E.; Le, I.P.; Buchwalter, A. & Burnatowska-Hledin, M.A. (2007). Estrogen-dependent growth and estrogen receptor (ER)-alpha concentration in T47D breast cancer cells are inhibited by VACM-1, a cul 5 gene. *Molecular and Cellular Biochemistry*, Vol.301, No.1-2, (July 2007), pp. 13-20, ISSN 0300-8177

Kaelin, W.G., Jr.; Ratcliffe, P.J. (2008). Oxygen sensing by metazoans: the central role of the HIF hydroxylase pathway. *Molecular Cell*, Vol.30, No.4, (May 2008), pp. 393-402, ISSN 1097-4164

Kamitani, T.; Kito, K.; Fukuda-Kamitani, T. & Yeh, E.T. (2001). Targeting of NEDD8 and its conjugates for proteasomal degradation by NUB1. *The Journal of Biological Chemistry*, Vol.276, No.49, (December 2001), pp. 46655-46660, ISSN 0021-9258

Kamitani, T.; Kito, K.; Nguyen, H.P. & Yeh, E.T. (1997). Characterization of NEDD8, a developmentally down-regulated ubiquitin-like protein. *The Journal of Biological Chemistry*, Vol.272, No.45, (November 1997), pp. 28557-28562, ISSN 0021-9258

Kapetanaki, M.G.; Guerrero-Santoro, J.; Bisi, D.C.; Hsieh, C.L.; Rapic-Otrin, V. & Levine, A.S. (2006). The DDB1-CUL4ADDB2 ubiquitin ligase is deficient in xeroderma pigmentosum group E and targets histone H2A at UV-damaged DNA sites. *Proceedings of the National Academy of Sciences of the United States of America*, Vol.103, No.8, (February 2006), pp. 2588-2593, ISSN 0027-8424

Kito, K.; Yeh, E.T. & Kamitani, T. (2001). NUB1, a NEDD8-interacting protein, is induced by interferon and down-regulates the NEDD8 expression. *The Journal of Biological Chemistry*, Vol.276, No.23, (March 2001), pp. 20603-20609, ISSN 0021-9258

Kumar, S.; Tomooka, Y. & Noda, M. (1992). Identification of a set of genes with developmentally down-regulated expression in the mouse brain. *Biochemical and Biophysical Research Communications*, Vol.185, No.3, (June 1992), pp. 1155-1161, ISSN 0006-291X

Leck, Y.C.; Choo, Y.Y.; Tan, C.Y.; Smith, P.G. & Hagen, T. (2010). Biochemical and cellular effects of inhibiting Nedd8 conjugation. *Biochemical and Biophysical Research Communications*, Vol.398, No.3, (July 2010), pp. 588-593, ISSN 1090-2104

Liu, L.; Lee, S.; Zhang, J.; Peters, S.B.; Hannah, J.; Zhang, Y.; Yin, Y.; Koff, A.; Ma, L. & Zhou, P. (2009). CUL4A abrogation augments DNA damage response and protection against skin carcinogenesis. *Molecular Cell,* Vol.34, No.4, (May 2009), pp. 451-460, ISSN 1097-4164

Lyapina, S.; Cope, G.; Shevchenko, A.; Serino, G.; Tsuge, T.; Zhou, C.; Wolf, D.A.; Wei, N. & Deshaies, R.J. (2001). Promotion of NEDD-CUL1 conjugate cleavage by COP9 signalosome. *Science,* Vol.292, No.5520, (May 2001), pp. 1382-1385, ISSN 0036-8075

Milhollen, M.A.; Traore, T.; Adams-Duffy, J.; Thomas, M.P.; Berger, A.J.; Dang, L.; Dick, L.R.; Garnsey, J.J.; Koenig, E.; Langston, S.P.; Manfredi, M.; Narayanan, U.; Rolfe, M.; Staudt, L.M.; Soucy, T.A.; Yu, J.; Zhang, J.; Bolen, J.B. & Smith, P.G. (2010). MLN4924, a NEDD8-activating enzyme inhibitor, is active in diffuse large B-cell lymphoma models: rationale for treatment of NF-{kappa}B-dependent lymphoma. *Blood,* Vol.116, No.9, (September 2010), pp. 1515-1523, ISSN 1528-0020

Rabut, G. & Peter, M. (2008). Function and regulation of protein neddylation. 'Protein modifications: beyond the usual suspects' review series. *EMBO Reports,* Vol.9, No.10, (October 2008), pp. 969-976, ISSN 1469-3178

Skaar, J.R.; D'Angiolella, V.; Pagan, J.K. & Pagano, M. (2009). SnapShot: F Box Proteins II. *Cell,* Vol.137, No.7, (June 2009), pp. 1358, 1358 e1, ISSN 1097-4172

Soucy, T.A.; Smith, P.G.; Milhollen, M.A.; Berger, A.J.; Gavin, J.M.; Adhikari, S.; Brownell, J.E.; Burke, K.E.; Cardin, D.P.; Critchley, S.; Cullis, C.A.; Doucette, A.; Garnsey, J.J.; Gaulin, J.L.; Gershman, R.E.; Lublinsky, A.R.; McDonald, A.; Mizutani, H.; Narayanan, U.; Olhava, E.J.; Peluso, S.; Rezaei, M.; Sintchak, M.D.; Talreja, T.; Thomas, M.P.; Traore, T.; Vyskocil, S.; Weatherhead, G.S.; Yu, J.; Zhang, J.; Dick, L.R.; Claiborne, C.F.; Rolfe, M.; Bolen. J.B. & Langston, S.P. (2009). An inhibitor of NEDD8-activating enzyme as a new approach to treat cancer. *Nature,* vol.458, No.7239, (April 2009), pp. 732-736, ISSN 1476-4687

Swords, R.T.; Kelly, K.R.; Smith, P.G.; Garnsey, J.J.; Mahalingam, D.; Medina, E.; Oberheu, K.; Padmanabhan, S.; O'Dwyer, M.; Nawrocki, S.T.; Giles, F.J. & Carew, J.S. (2010). Inhibition of NEDD8-activating enzyme: a novel approach for the treatment of acute myeloid leukemia. *Blood,* Vol.115, No.18, (May 2010), pp. 3796-3800, ISSN 1528-0020

Tanaka, T.; Kawashima, H.; Yeh, E.T. & Kamitani, T. (2003). Regulation of the NEDD8 conjugation system by a splicing variant, NUB1L. *The Journal of Biological Chemistry,* Vol.278, No.35, (August 2003), pp. 32905-32913, ISSN 0021-9258

Wada, H.; Yeh, E.T. & Kamitani, T. (2000). A dominant-negative UBC12 mutant sequesters NEDD8 and inhibits NEDD8 conjugation in vivo. *The Journal of Biological Chemistry,* Vol.275, No.22, (June 2000), pp. 17008-17015, ISSN 0021-9258

Watson, I.R.; Blanch, A.; Lin, D.C.; Ohh, M. & Irwin, M.S. (2006). Mdm2-mediated NEDD8 modification of TAp73 regulates its transactivation function. *The Journal of Biological Chemistry,* Vol.281, No.45, (November 2006), pp. 34096-34103, ISSN 0021-9258

Watson, I.R.; Li, B.K.; Roche, O.; Blanch, A.; Ohh, M. & Irwin, M.S. (2010). Chemotherapy induces NEDP1-mediated destabilization of MDM2. *Oncogene,* Vol.29, No.2, (January 2010), pp. 297-304, ISSN 1476-5594

Xirodimas, D.P.; Saville, M.K.; Bourdon, J.C.; Hay, R.T. & Lane, D.P. (2004). Mdm2-mediated NEDD8 conjugation of p53 inhibits its transcriptional activity. *Cell,* Vol.118, No.1, (July 2004), pp. 83-97, ISSN 0092-8674

Yen, H.C. & Elledge, S.J. (2008). Identification of SCF ubiquitin ligase substrates by global protein stability profiling. *Science,* Vol.322, No.5903, (November 2008), pp. 923-929, ISSN 1095-9203

7

Biological Aspects in Renal Cell Carcinoma

Vanessa Medina Villaamil[1], Guadalupe Aparicio Gallego[1]
and Luis Miguel Antón Aparicio[2,3]
[1]INIBIC, A Coruña University Hospital, A Coruña,
[2]Medical Oncology Service, A Coruña University Hospital, A Coruña,
[3]Medicine Department, University of A Coruña, A Coruña
Spain

1. Introduction

A growing understanding of the underlying molecular biology of renal cell carcinoma (RCC) has identified several pathways pertinent to its pathophysiology. Cellular hypoxia and metabolic stress have been observed in many cancer types. Hypoxia-induced factor (HIF) is considered a central regulator of oxygen homeostasis. The HIF transcription factor complex has been demonstrated to transcriptionally induce the expression of genes involved in angiogenesis, anaerobic glucose metabolism, cell motility and metastasis, growth and survival, apoptosis, and telomere maintenance. Notable genes induced by HIF that are involved in angiogenesis include vascular endothelial growth factor (VEGF) and platelet-derived growth factor (PDGF), as well as other proangiogenic factors, such as angiopoietin-4 (Ang4). These factors promote the proliferation, migration, and maturation of endothelial cells and pericytes supporting the recruitment of vessels or neoangiogenesis necessary to restore blood supply to an ischemic region. In the case of RCC, this process leads to the rampant, disorganised proliferation of vessels in this highly vascular tumour type. Additional factors include proteins involved in promoting the cellular switch to anaerobic glycolysis, such as the glucose transporter Glut1; enzymes of glucose metabolism, such as hexokinase (HK) and lactate dehydrogenase (LDH), the antigen carbonic anhydrase IX (CAIX, also called G250) and the lactate transporter MCT-4. This hypoxic repertoire of gene upregulation likely contributes to the highly glycolytic phenotype of RCC, even in the presence of abundant oxygen with which to perform oxidative phosphorylation for energy generation. Like other processes that integrate endothelial cell vascular network expansion, tumour angiogenesis is dependent on secreted VEGF to promote existing vessel in growth into the tumour and the expansion of vascular networks by neovascularisation. Inappropriate activation of the hypoxia response pathway is a major mechanism of VEGF transcriptional regulation in RCC. A variety of mechanisms account for the increase in VEGF, with activation of the hypoxic response pathway via the transcription factors HIF1-α and HIF2-α as the classic mechanism of induction.

RCC presents a unique clinical setting, in which a tumour type nearly universally usurps a proangiogenic cellular homeostatic mechanism.

Knowledge of the genetic basis of RCC has important implications for diagnosis and management of this disease. Study of the genes for RCC has revealed that kidney cancer is fundamentally a metabolic disorder. The seven RCC genes (*VHL, MET, BHD, TSC1, TSC2, fumarate hydratase (FH)* and *succinate dehydrogenase (SDH)*) represent disorders of energy, nutrient, iron and oxygen sensing.

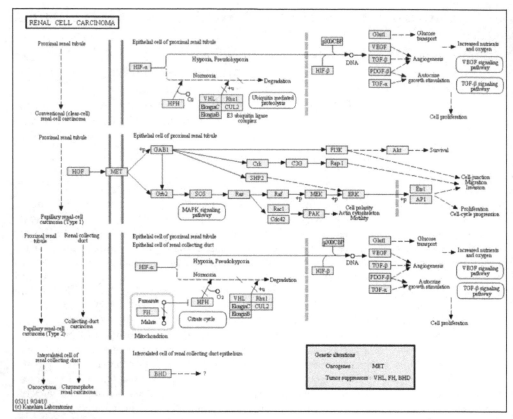

Fig. 1. Renal Cell Carcinoma Pathway (Kanehisa et al., 2010). Renal cell cancer (RCC) accounts for ~3% of human malignancies and its incidence appears to be rising. Although most cases of RCC seem to occur sporadically, an inherited predisposition to renal cancer accounts for 1-4% of cases. RCC is not a single disease, it has several morphological subtypes. Conventional RCC (clear cell RCC) accounts for ~80% of cases, followed by papillary RCC (10-15%), chromophobe RCC (5%), and collecting duct RCC (<1%). Genes potentially involved in sporadic neoplasms of each particular type are VHL, MET, BHD, and FH respectively. In the absence of VHL, hypoxia-inducible factor alpha (HIF- α) accumulates, leading to production of several growth factors, including vascular endothelial growth factor and platelet-derived growth factor. Activated MET mediates a number of biological effects including motility, invasion of extracellular matrix, cellular transformation, prevention of apoptosis and metastasis formation. Loss of functional FH leads to accumulation of fumarate in the cell, triggering inhibition of HPH and preventing targeted pVHL-mediated degradation of HIF- α. BHD mutations cause the Birt-Hogg-Dube syndrome and its associated chromophobe, hybrid oncocytic, and conventional (clear cell) RCC.

Targeting the basic metabolic alterations in RCC has the potential to provide a more durable and effective approach to therapy.

2. Overview of hypoxia-inducible signalling

Over the last decade, major advances have been made in deciphering the molecular mechanisms that allow cells to respond and adapt to low PO2. As key mediators in cellular oxygen homeostasis, hypoxia-inducible factor-1 and -2 (HIF-1 and HIF-2) facilitate both oxygen delivery and adaptation to oxygen deprivation by regulating the expression of gene products that are involved in cellular energy metabolism and glucose transport, angiogenesis, erythropoiesis and iron metabolism, pH regulation, apoptosis, and cell proliferation, as well as cell-cell and cell-matrix interactions (Schofield et al., 2004). Examples of classic HIF target genes are phosphoglycerate kinase-1 (PGK), glucose transporter-1 (GLUT1), vascular endothelial growth factor (VEGF), and erythropoietin (EPO).

HIF-1 and HIF-2 (collectively referred to here as HIF) are members of the Per-ARNT-Sim (PAS) family of heterodimeric basic helix-loop-helix (bHLH) transcription factors and consist of an oxygen-sensitive α-subunit and a constitutively expressed β-unit, also known as the aryl hydrocarbon receptor nuclear translocator (ARNT) or simply HIF-β.

Direct transcriptional regulation occurs through the binding of HIF heterodimers to hypoxia-response elements (HREs), which are present in the regulatory regions of hypoxia-sensitive genes. With regard to their ability to transcriptionally regulate specific hypoxia-responsive genes, HIF-1 and HIF-2 have distinct functions and only partially overlap. For example, glycolytic genes appear to be predominantly regulated by HIF-1 (Hu et al., 2003), whereas HIF-2 has been suggested as the main regulator of hypoxic VEGF and EPO induction in tissues that express both HIF-1 and HIF-2 (Rankin et al., 2005).

In addition to heterodimerisation with HIF-β resulting in the formation of a bHLH transcription factor that mediates the canonical hypoxia response, HIF-α subunits also regulate biological processes through direct protein-protein interaction with other factors. These include, among others, the tumour suppressor protein p53 and the c-Myc proto-oncogene (Koshiji et al., 2004). A more recent example is the ability of HIF-1α to biochemically associate with the intracellular domain of Notch (Notch ICD), thereby increasing Notch signalling through upregulation of Notch target genes such as Hey and Hes (Gustafsson et al., 2005). The observation that HIF-1α modulates Notch signalling through a direct protein-protein interaction underscores the importance of HIF-α as a regulator of important intracellular pathways, independent of its role in HRE-mediated transcription.

HIF activation is dependent on the stabilisation of the oxygen-sensitive α-subunit and its subsequent translocation to the nucleus, where it dimerises with HIF-β and recruits transcriptional cofactors such as CBP and p300 (Schofield et al., 2004). Normally, under conditions of adequate oxygen supply, hydroxylated HIF-α binds to the von Hippel-Lindau tumour suppressor protein (pVHL), which is part of an E3-ubiquitin ligase complex that targets HIF-α for proteasomal degradation. The pVHL/HIF-α interaction is highly conserved between species and requires iron- and oxygen-dependent hydroxylation of specific proline residues within the oxygen-dependent degradation domain (ODD) of HIF-α. Prolyl-hydroxylation by prolyl-4-hydroxylases and binding to pVHL are absolutely required for the execution of HIF proteolysis under normoxia. During hypoxia, prolyl-hydroxylases are inactive, and HIF-α degradation is inhibited. Three major mammalian HIF prolyl-hydroxylases have been identified, all of which are expressed in renal epithelial cells (Soilleux et al., 2005).

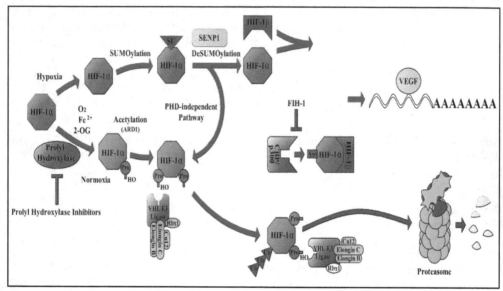

Fig. 2. Regulatory pathway of HIF. HIF-α is hydroxylated in the oxygen dependent destruction domain and at an asparagine residue in the C terminal transactivation domain. Prolyl hydroxylation by PHD is required for binding to the pVHL-E3-ubiquitin ligase complex, whereas asparaginyl hydroxylation prevents the interaction of HIF-α with CBP/p300 transcriptional co-activator. Upon binding to the E3-ligase complex, HIF-α is polyubiquitinated and then degraded by the proteasome. Acetylation of HIF-α by ARD1 enhances binding to pVHL and subsequent ubiquitination. During hypoxia when prolyl-hydroxylases are inactive, HIF-α is stabilized and translocates to the nucleus, where it is SUMOylated by SUMO conjugases. Failure to deSUMOylate HIF-α targets HIF-α for VHL/proteasome-dependent degradation by providing an alternate signal (prolyl hydroxylation-independent) for pVHL binding. DeSUMOylated HIF-α escapes degradation, heterodimerizes with HIF-1β, binds to the hypoxia response elements (consensus binding site), and increases transcription of HIF target genes such as VEGF. Oxygen-dependent asparagine hydroxylation of HIF-α by factor-inhibiting HIF-1 (FIH 1) blocks recruitment of the CBP/p300 co-factor to the HIF transcriptional complex.

A second hypoxic switch operates in the COOH-terminal transactivation domain of HIF-α upon the hydroxylation of a specific asparagine residue. During hypoxia, asparagine hydroxylation is blocked, and CBP/p300 recruitment is facilitated, enabling increased levels of transcription. Factor-inhibiting-HIF (FIH) hydroxylates the asparagine residue. FIH is expressed in renal tubular epithelial cells and glomeruli (Soilleux et al., 2005).

In addition to hypoxic activation, a nonhypoxic increase in HIF transcriptional activity has been shown to be mediated by nitric oxide and TNF-α (Sandau et al., 2001), interleukin 1 (Stiehl et al., 2002), angiotensin II (Richard et al., 2000), and a variety of growth factors, including epidermal growth factor, insulin, and insulin-like growth factors (Jiang et al., 2001; Stiehl et al., 2002; Treins et al., 2002). Nitric oxide, ROS, and certain oncogenes such as v-Src and activated Ras have been shown to inhibit HIF prolyl-hydroxylation (Kaelin 2005). In contrast, HIF activation induced through the phosphoinositide 3-kinase/Akt-1/mammalian target of rapamycin pathway appears to be mediated through increased HIF-α protein translation (Fukuda et al., 2002). Thus, HIF activation is likely to occur in a variety of different renal disease settings even in the absence of significant hypoxia.

Whereas HIF-1α is ubiquitously expressed, HIF-2α expression is more restricted. HIF-2α has been found in hepatocytes, cardiomyocytes, glial cells, type II pneumocytes, and endothelial cells (Wiesener et al., 2003).

The list of HIF-regulated genes (either directly or indirectly regulated by HIF) has grown rapidly. HIF is involved in the regulation of a multitude of biological processes that are relevant to kidney function under physiological and pathological conditions.

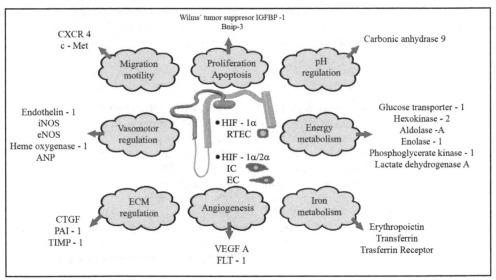

Fig. 3. Overview of selected hypoxia/HIF-regulated biological processes that have been shown or have been proposed to play important roles in the pathogenesis of renal cancer. RTEC (renal tubular epithelial cell), IC (intersticial cell), EC (endothelial cell).

3. Renal injury in cancer patients: Hypoxia and Inflammation

Whereas acutely injured kidneys appear to benefit from the protective effects of HIF-regulated biological processes, chronic hypoxia, mediated in part through HIF-1, can contribute to increased extracellular matrix production and the epithelial-to-mesenchymal transition (EMT), thereby potentially promoting renal fibrosis and the progression of renal disease. HIF may impact the pathogenesis of tubulointerstitial disease through the regulation of inflammatory responses. Microenvironmental changes, such as hypoxia, strongly impact inflammatory cell recruitment (Kong et al., 2004) and function (Cramer et al., 2003). HIF-1 is essential for myeloid cell-mediated inflammation mainly through its effects on cellular ATP generation. Inactivation of HIF-1 results in a profound impairment of myeloid cell aggregation, motility, and invasiveness, whereas forced expression of HIF-1 has the opposite effect (Kong et al., 2004). Alterations in HIF signalling in inflammatory cells may also play a significant role in renal inflammation, subsequent fibrosis and, thus, the progression of chronic renal disease.

Patients with neoplasia are subject to a variety of different types of renal, fluid and electrolyte disorders, either from direct effects such as urinary tract obstruction or infiltration or from indirect effects such as hyperkalaemia. Glomerulonephritis and nephrotic syndrome are due to immunologic reactions associated with neoplasia.

Just as hypoxia can induce inflammation, inflamed lesions often become severely hypoxic. Because of the steep oxygen gradient between the anaerobic intestinal lumen and the metabolically active lamina propria mucosae, intestinal epithelial cells are normally hypoxic (Karhausen et al., 2004).

Contributors to tissue hypoxia during inflammation include an increase in the metabolic demands of cells and a reduction in metabolic substrates caused by thrombosis, trauma, compression (interstitial hypertension), or atelectasis (airway plugging). Moreover, multiplication of intracellular pathogens can deprive infected cells of oxygen (Kempf et al., 2005). In the case of inflamed tissue, hypoxia is not a bystander; rather, it can influence the environment of the tissue, particularly by regulating oxygen-dependent gene expression.

Activation of the prolyl hydroxylase (PHDs)–HIF pathway promotes the resolution of mucosal inflammation in mice (Colgan et al., 2010). Hypoxia-induced changes in gene expression by epithelial cells help to promote mucosal barrier function (e.g., through the activation of intestinal trefoil factor) (Furuta et al., 2001) or to increase the production by the epithelium of anti-inflammatory signalling molecules such as adenosine (Eltzschig 2009). These adaptive responses to hypoxia are activated during mucosal inflammation and promote the resolution of inflammatory bowel disease (Karhausen et al., 2004; Robinson et al., 2008; Eckle et al., 2008) and acute lung injury (Rosenberg et al., 2009; Reutershan et al., 2009; Schingnitz et al., 2010). Several studies have shown that hypoxia enhances the enzymatic conversion of precursor nucleotides, such as ATP, adenosine diphosphate, or AMP, to adenosine (Eltzschig et al., 2003), thereby elevating extracellular levels of adenosine, an anti-inflammatory signalling molecule involved in restraining innate immune responses.

HIF stimulates the production of extracellular adenosine and suppresses both its uptake into the intracellular compartment and its intracellular metabolism (Morote-García et al., 2008). HIF also enhances adenosine receptor signalling by increasing the expression on the cell surface of adenosine receptors (Eckle et al., 2008), an effect that attenuates immune responses, vascular fluid leakage, and neutrophil accumulation in the presence of myocardial, renal, hepatic, or intestinal ischemia or acute lung injury.

Concentrations of oxygen in solid tumors, as compared with those in normal tissues, are frequently lower (Semenza 2003). Solid tumours contain increased levels of HIF-1α and HIF-2α. Hypoxia in a solid tumour stabilises HIF through hypoxia-dependent inhibition of PHDs. Similarly, the activation of oncogenes, or the loss of function of tumour-suppressor genes, results in the stabilisation of HIF, as happens in the case of the VHL tumour-suppressor gene. Hypoxia and inflammation meet at several points in the setting of cancer. In tumour cells oncogenes, inflammatory signals (mediated in part through Toll-like receptors [TLRs]), and hypoxia-activated nuclear factor κB (NF-κB) and hypoxia-inducible factor (HIF) 1α (which activate one another). These factors induce a gene program that recruits and activates leukocytes (through the release of chemokines and cytokines), stimulates angiogenesis and the formation of an abnormal vasculature and endothelium (through release of angiogenic signals), and increases tumour-cell invasion, metastasis, epithelial-to-mesenchymal transition (EMT), survival, proliferation, and metabolic reprogramming. In leukocytes, hypoxia also activates NF-κB and HIF-1α; endogenous ligands, released from necrotic cancer cells, activate TLRs upstream of NF-κB and HIF-1α, and HIF-1α up-regulates TLR expression. The resultant gene-expression profile leads to the production of cytokines and angiogenic signals and skews their polarisation phenotype. Tumour vessels with two PHDs-domain 2 (PHD2) alleles have an abnormal endothelium, are hypo-perfused, and cause tumour hypoxia, which fuels tumour-cell invasiveness and metastasis. In contrast, tumour vessels lacking one PHD2 allele have increased HIF-2α levels, which results in an up-regulation of factors that counteract the development of tumour endothelial abnormalities; this, in turn, results in improved tumour-vessel perfusion and oxygenation and, secondarily, reduced metastasis.

Experimental evidence indicates that inhibition of HIF within the inflamed tumour core attenuates the growth and vascularisation of tumours and enhances the sensitivity of tumours to radiation (Semenza et al., 2010). In contrast, inhibition of PHD2 and stabilisation of HIF within the tumour vasculature may play an important role in tumour therapy, if the means can be found to selectively direct inhibitors of PHD to the tumour vasculature and inhibitors of HIF to the hypoxic core.

4. Hypoxia inducible factor and renal cancer

The most common form of kidney cancer is renal cell cancer of the clear cell type (CC-RCC). A molecular hallmark of sporadic CC-RCC and hereditary CC-RCC associated with the von Hippel-Lindau familial tumour syndrome are mutations in the VHL tumour suppressor pVHL. Loss of pVHL function results in oxygen-independent HIF-α stabilisation, increased HIF transcriptional activity, and constitutive upregulation of HIF target genes. While patients with sporadic CC-RCC are characterised by somatic inactivation of both VHL gene copies in renal epithelial cells, patients with the VHL tumour syndrome transmit germ line mutations of the VHL gene. Although the highly vascular nature of VHL-deficient tumours is easily explained by increased VEGF production as a result of increased HIF transcriptional activity, VHL-associated renal carcinogenesis is more difficult to understand and most likely requires multiple other genetic events beyond the loss of pVHL function. In addition to regulating the degradation of HIF-α-subunits, pVHL has been shown to have additional biological functions, which may or may not be critical for renal tumourigenesis (Haase 2005).

Aside from a regulatory role in tumour angiogenesis, HIF plays a key role in the regulation of factors that are important for the development and invasiveness of CC-RCC. These include, among others, TGF-α, a potent renal epithelial mitogen, cell cycle regulator cyclin D1 (CCND1), and chemokine receptor CXCR4 (Bindra et al., 2002; Raval et al., 2005; Smith et al., 2005; Staller et al., 2003; Wykoff et al., 2004; Zatyka et al., 2002). With regard to the individual contribution of HIF-1 and HIF-2 to renal tumour development, a substantial number of VHL-defective CC-RCC cell lines do not express HIF-1α but do express HIF-2α (Maxwell et al., 1999). This is in contrast to normal, nontransformed renal epithelial cells, in which HIF-2α is not detectable during ischemia (Rosenberger et al., 2002).

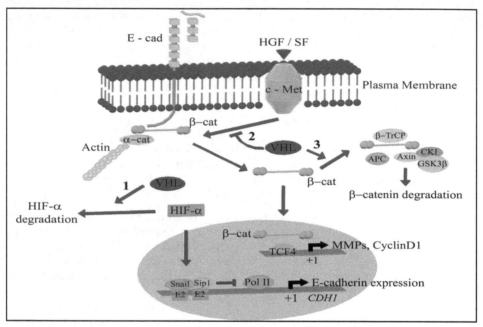

Fig. 4. Role of VHL in the regulation of E-cadherin and β-catenin. Loss of VHL leads to the stabilization of HIFα (1), which promotes the transactivation of E-cadherin-specific repressors, reducing E-caherin expression. Loss of VHL also causes constitutive phosphorylation of c-Met (2) and subsequent release, activation and stabilization of β-catenin (3).

HIF-1 and HIF-2 have diverse functions with regard to VHL renal tumourigenesis. HIF-2 has been proposed to preferentially regulate signalling pathways critical for renal cell growth, such as signalling through the TGF-α/epidermal growth factor receptor pathway and through the cell cycle regulator cyclin D1 (Bindra et al., 2002; Raval et al., 2005; Smith et al., 2005; Staller et al., 2003; Wykoff et al., 2004; Zatyka et al., 2002).

In addition to VHL-associated CC-RCC, HIF-α stabilisation can be found in renal cell cancers that are associated with mutations of the tuberous sclerosis tumour suppressor TSC-2 (Liu et al., 2003) and in rare leiomyomatosis-associated renal cancers. The latter form of renal cancer is characterised by fumarate hydratase deficiency, the inability to convert fumarate to malate, which results in HIF prolyl-hydroxylase inhibition; fumarate acts as a competitive inhibitor of HIF prolyl-hydroxylation (Isaacs et al., 2005). It is unclear whether an increase in HIF-1 and HIF-2 activity in these rare forms of renal cancer has the same biological effects as in VHL-negative CC-RCC, and further investigation is required.

5. Energy disorders in RCC

Tumours are characterised by specific metabolic alterations providing a metabolic signature in malignant transformation at different stages; end stage carcinomas are most dependent on anaerobic glucose degradation (aerobic glycolysis, fermentation) and least dependent on mitochondrial energy supplies. The metabolic endpoint of this transformation is the anaerobic degradation of glucose even in the presence of oxygen (Koppenol et al., 2011).Concomitant with this metabolic switch, high lactate concentrations occur and result in the immune protection of cancer cells, acid-mediated matrix degradation, invasiveness and metastasis (Hutterer et al., 2007).

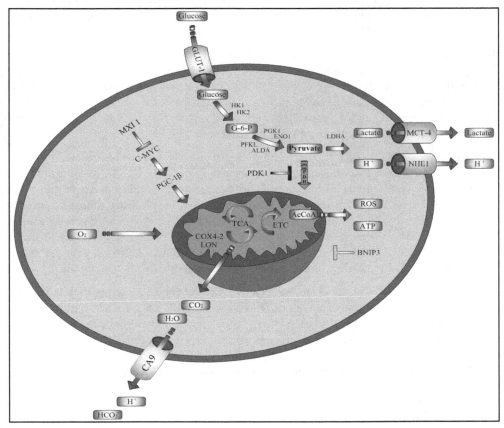

Fig. 5. Regulation of proteins required for glucose uptake and energy metabolism by HIF-1. Metabolic substrates and products are shown in purple and HIF-1-regulated gene products are shown in brown. Red arrows, mitochondrial biogenesis mediated by C-MYC (in renal carcinoma cells). Green blocked arrow, mitochondrial autophagy mediated by BNIP3 (in mouse embryo fibroblasts). AcCoA, acetyl coenzyme A; ALD, aldolase; CA9, carbonic anhydrase; COX, cytochrome c oxidase; ENO, enolase; G-6-P, glucose-6-phosphate; GLUT, glucose transporter; HK, hexokinase; LDH, lactate dehydrogenase; MCT, monocarboxylate transporter; NHE, sodium–hydrogen exchanger; PDH, pyruvate dehydrogenase; PDK, PDH kinase; PFK, phosphofructokinase; PGC, PPAR-γ co-activator; PGK, phosphoglycerate kinase.

Increased total activity of the transketolase-dependent, nonoxidative branch of the pentose phosphate pathway (PPP) in cancer cells is due to the overexpression of the transketolase-like-1 (TKTL1) protein (Hu et al., 2007).

The complex regulation of tumour metabolism switches from mitochondrial oxidative to nonoxidative energy production, which is dependent on the PPP. Both the oxidative and nonoxidative branches of the PPP have been described as activated in carcinogenesis (Ramos-Montoya et al., 2006). It is assumed that the enzymes of the oxidative branch of the PPP [glucose-6-phosphate-dehydrogenase (G6PD) and 6-phosphogluconate dehydrogenase] are triggered by an increased need for NADPH, whereas the enzymes of the nonoxidative branch (TKTL1, transaldolases) are triggered by an increased need for ribose and energy (Ramos-Montoya et al., 2006).

HIF-1 regulates the expression of hundreds of genes in human cells (Manalo et al., 2005; Elvidge et al., 2006) and is essential for embryonic development in mice (Iyer et al., 1998; Ryan et al., 1998). Many of these genes contribute to two essential functions of HIF-1. First, HIF-1 promotes the delivery of oxygen to cells through its control of erythropoiesis and angiogenesis. Second, HIF-1 promotes cell survival under hypoxic conditions by reprogramming cellular glucose and energy metabolism.

Analysis of mRNA expression in mouse embryonic stem cells that were either wild type or homozygous for a knockout allele at the *Hif1a* locus encoding the HIF-1α subunit revealed that expression of the genes encoding glucose transporters 1 and 3 and the glycolytic enzymes hexokinase 1 and 2, glucose phosphate isomerase, phosphofructokinase L, aldolase A and C, triosephosphate isomerase, phosphoglycerate kinase 1, enolase 1, pyruvate kinase M, and lactate dehydrogenase A (LDH-A) was regulated by HIF-1 (Iyer et al., 1998). In human VHL-deficient renal cell carcinoma, upregulation of GLUT1 protein expression has been demonstrated at the earliest stages of tumour formation (Mandriota et al., 2002).

The upregulation of LDH-A results in the increased conversion of pyruvate to lactate at the expense of mitochondrial utilisation of pyruvate as a substrate for pyruvate dehydrogenase (PDH), which converts pyruvate to acetyl CoA. However, recent studies have demonstrated that HIF-1 plays a direct role in actively shunting pyruvate away from the mitochondria through its regulation of the PDK1 gene (encoding PDH kinase 1) in multiple cell types, including VHL deficient renal carcinoma cells (Kim et al., 2006; Papandreou et al., 2006). Phosphorylation of the catalytic subunit of PDH by PDK1 inactivates the enzyme. In mouse embryo fibroblasts cultured from HIF-1α-null embryos, prolonged hypoxic incubation induces ROS production leading to cell death that can be rescued by the forced expression of PDK1 (Kim et al., 2006). HIF-1α-null mouse embryo fibroblasts also manifest increased cell death (relative to wild-type cells) when incubated under hypoxic conditions in the presence of the hypoxic cytotoxin tirapazamine (Papandreou et al., 2006). These results suggest that HIF-1 actively inhibits the oxidative metabolism of glucose under hypoxic conditions.

The decrease in oxygen consumption under moderate hypoxia is likely to be an adaptive mechanism to avoid the development of anoxia. During hypoxia, cells that fail to decrease their oxygen consumption are likely to become anoxic faster than cells that can suppress their rate of oxygen consumption (Denko 2008).

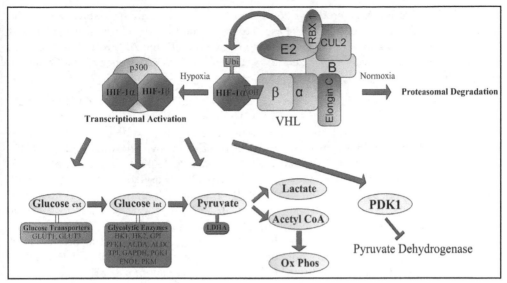

Fig. 6. Regulation of glucose metabolism by HIF-1. Under normoxic conditions, HIF-1α (or HIF-2α) is hydroxylated by PHD2, bound by VHL, ubiquitinated by an E3 ligase complex containing elongin B, elongin C, cullin 2, and Rbx1, and degraded by the proteasome. VHL loss-of-function (in clear cell renal carcinoma) or hypoxic conditions leads to the accumulation of non-hydroxylated, non-ubiquitinated HIF-1α (or HIF-2α), which dimerizes with HIF-1β, recruits the coactivator p300 (or CBP) and activates the transcription of genes encoding glucose transporter (GLUT) 1 and 3, hexokinase (HK) 1 and 2, glucosephosphate isomerase (GPI), phosphofructokinase (PFK) L, aldolase (ALD) A and C, triosephosphate isomerase (TPI), glyceraldephosphate dehydrogenase (GAPDH), phosphoglycerate kinase (PGK) 1, enolase (ENO) 1, pyruvate kinase (PK) M, lactate dehydrogenase (LDH) A, and pyruvate dehydrogenase kinase (PDK) 1.

Mitochondrial respiration in cells is controlled by cellular ATP utilisation. One model suggests that increased cytoplasmic ATP utilisation decreases cytosolic ATP levels and increases cytosolic ADP and Pi levels (Chance et al., 1955). The rise in cytosolic ADP levels leads to a rise in mitochondrial ADP via the increased activity of the adenine nucleotide carrier. The increased mitochondrial ADP concentration stimulates ATP synthase to augment the rate of ATP synthesis. The increased ATP synthesis results in a decrease in the mitochondrial membrane potential, which stimulates the respiratory chain to consume oxygen. Aside from cellular ATP utilisation, the other factors that control mitochondrial respiration are the NADH supply, the respiratory chain, and the degree of proton leak (Jones et al., 1993). The major reason for the decrease in respiration during hypoxia is the decrease in cellular ATP utilisation.

A major ATP consumer that hypoxia inhibits is Na/K-ATPase. The activity of Na/K-ATPase alone can account for 20–70% of the oxygen expenditure of mammalian cells (Milligan et al., 1985). Na/K-ATPase is a transmembrane protein found in higher eukaryotes that transports Na^+ and K^+ across the plasma membrane to maintain ionic gradients (Skou

1957). Na/K-ATPase is a heterodimer composed of α and β subunits (Kaplan 2002). The hypoxia-induced decrease of Na/K-ATPase activity is due to endocytosis of the α subunit from the plasma membrane by PKC zeta. Hypoxia stimulates the AMPK alpha-1 isoform, which directly phosphorylates PKC zeta to promote Na/K-ATPase endocytosis (Gusarova et al., 2009).

The other major ATP consumer that hypoxia inhibits is mRNA translation (Wouters et al., 2005). The mammalian target rapamycin (mTOR) and pancreatic eIF2α kinase(PERK) are the key regulators of translation during hypoxia (Arsham et al., 2003; Koumenis et al., 2002). In growth-promoting conditions, mTOR sustains translation by phosphorylating eIF4E-binding proteins (4EBPs) and ribosomal protein S6 kinases (S6Ks) (Gingras et al., 2001). Hypoxia (1.5% O_2) causes rapid and reversible hypophosphorylation of mTOR and its effectors 4E-BP1 and S6K (Arsham et al., 2003). The rapid inhibition of mTOR is HIF independent and occurs through the activation of AMPK76. Rapid activation of AMPK during hypoxia is dependent on mitochondrial ROS (Emerling et al., 2009). The other major contributor to the decrease in mRNA translation during hypoxia is the activation of PERK73, resulting in eIF2α phosphorylation and the inhibition of mRNA translation initiation. Mitochondrial ROS have been implicated in the activation of PERK.

Mitochondrial respiration is regulated by the availability of oxygen, ADP and reducing equivalents (NADH and $FADH_2$ from the TCA cycle). Oxygen is limiting for respiration under severely hypoxic conditions (<0.5% O_2). Thus, under physiological hypoxia (1–3% O_2), oxygen is not limiting for maximal respiration. The major controller of mitochondrial respiration is ADP availability from cellular ATP utilisation. Hypoxia through mitochondrial ROS also diminishes the activity of Na/K-ATPase and mRNA translation. This results in a decrease in cellular ATP utilisation and a decrease in ADP availability to mitochondria. Hypoxia also stimulates the release of mitochondrial ROS from complex III to activate HIF-1, which induces the transcription of PDK1. PDK1 negatively regulates PDH, an enzyme that converts pyruvate to acetyl-CoA. Thus, an increase in HIF-1 dependent PDK1 expression results in diminished availability of acetyl-CoA. This also contributes to diminished respiration during hypoxia by decreasing TCA cycle activity.

Although HIF-1 and HIF-2 are activated by similar mechanisms by hypoxia, they have both overlapping and distinct gene targets. HIF-1 regulates metabolic genes, whereas HIF-2 regulates EPO and the mitochondrial matrix protein superoxide dismutase 2 (SOD2). Depending on the genetic background, the loss of HIF-2 in adult mice results in profound anaemia (Gruber et al., 2007) or multiple organ pathology due to increased oxidative stress (Scortegagna M., 2003). The role of HIF-2 regulation of oxidative stress is further supported by the observation that SOD2 levels are markedly increased in VHL-null renal cell carcinoma cells (Hervouet et al., 2008). It will be interesting to determine whether activation of HIF-2 prevents oxidative stress-induced injury in other organs, such as brain, lung and heart.

6. Nutrient disorders in RCC

Diets rich in fruits and vegetables have typically been shown to decrease RCC risk, possibly through antioxidant effects, while consumption of fried foods has commonly been shown to increase risk, possibly due to the potential carcinogenic effects of acrylamides (Chow et al., 2008). Recently, epidemiological studies suggest that vitamin D, which is found in food (vitamin D2 and D3) and produced in the body after exposure to ultraviolet (UV) rays from the sun (vitamin D3), may be inversely associated with RCC risk (Karami et al., 2008). Both vitamin D2 and D3 are hydroxylated in the liver and subsequently in the kidney to form active vitamin D (1,25(OH)2D3). Dietary intake of vitamin D accounts for a small (approximately 10%) proportion of vitamin D levels (Holick 2006). However, dietary intake of vitamin D and vitamin D rich foods may play a role in determining RCC risk, given that vitamin D has been associated with anticarcinogenic properties and is primarily metabolised within the kidneys (Holick 2006). Vitamin D and its metabolites are thought to impede carcinogenesis by stimulating cell differentiation, inhibiting cell proliferation, inducing apoptosis, and suppressing invasiveness, angiogenesis, and metastasis (Valdivielso et al., 2006). Vitamin D activation is mediated by binding to vitamin D receptors (VDRs), transcription factors that are part of the nuclear hormone receptor family. Forming a heterodimer complex with the retinoid-X-receptor (RXR) gene, VDR can regulate the transcription of other genes involved in cell regulation, growth, and immunity (Valdivielso et al., 2006; Thibault et al., 2006). Most epidemiological studies have focused on the VDR gene; however, a recent evaluation of 139 single nucleotide polymorphisms (SNPs) across eight genes in the vitamin D pathway found a significant association between RCC risk and certain VDR and RXRA genetic variants (Karami et al., 2009).

The kidney is the most important organ for vitamin D metabolism and activity as well as calcium homeostasis. Within the kidneys, calcium has been shown to influence active vitamin D levels (Holick et al., 2006). Thus, investigations of dietary vitamin D and calcium in RCC aetiology are highly relevant. A Canadian RCC case-control study showed no association for the intake of individual foods rich in vitamin D (i.e., fish and eggs) or calcium (i.e., milk, dairy, and cheese) (Hu et al., 2003). In contrast, calcium supplement intakes were shown to significantly reduce RCC risk as the number of years of intake increased. Different polymorphisms in the VDR gene have been speculated to result in variations of VDR expression and changes to circulating levels of active vitamin D (Ikuyama et al., 2002). For this reason, epidemiological studies suggest that tissue specific expression of vitamin D pathway genes function as the primary mechanism involved in linking vitamin D status with the anticarcinogenic effects of 1,25(OH)2D3. Therefore, a lower renal cancer risk may be associated with higher circulating levels of 25(OH)D, the storage form of vitamin D, by providing substrates for renal tissue-specific synthesis of 1,25(OH)2D3 (McCullough et al., 2008). RXRA, on the other hand, may play a critical role in vitamin D activity, particularly from dietary sources, since this gene has been shown to regulate cholesterol (Hegele et al., 2001), which is abundant in eggs and yogurt, the food groups that were statistically associated with renal cancer risk in this study. RXRA regulated fatty acid and cholesterol metabolism through intestinal cholesterol absorption and bile acid synthesis (Hegele et al., 2001). Cholesterol metabolism has been associated with atherosclerosis, which is associated with hypertension and cardiovascular risk, known risk factors of RCC.

Antioxidant-rich foods have several preventive effects against different diseases, such as cancer, coronary disease, inflammatory disorders, and neurologic degeneration. Honey has been used as a traditional food source since ancient times. It is made when the nectar and sweet deposits from plants are gathered, modified, and stored in the honeycomb by honeybees. The major components of honey are fructose and glucose; honey also contains carbohydrates, proteins, amino acids, vitamins, water, minerals, and enzymes. In general, honey is also rich in antioxidants and has antibacterial properties (Brudzynski 2006). Honey not only promotes growth of new skin tissue by creating a moist environment but also prevents infection by way of its antimicrobial properties. Moreover, honey is harmless; in fact, it enables faster healing of the wounds by forming new tissues. Honey is thought to exhibit a broad spectrum of therapeutic properties, including antibacterial, antifungal, cytostatic, and anti-inflammatory activity (Jeddar et al., 1985). Honey potentiated the antitumour activity of chemotherapeutic drugs, such as 5-fluorouracil and cyclophosphamide, and contains many biologically active compounds, including caffeic acid, caffeic acid phenethyl ester, and flavonoid glycones. These compounds have been shown to have an inhibitory effect on tumour cell proliferation and transformation by the downregulation of many cellular enzymatic pathways, including protein tyrosine kinase, cyclooxygenase, and ornithine decarboxylase pathways (Chinthalapally et al., 1993).

Honey is also a dietary source for flavonoids, which have been demonstrated to have anticarcinogenic and anti-inflammatory activities. Although crude honey was reported by some authors to be a proliferative agent that enhances the proliferation of both normal and malignant cells (Rady 2005), it was also reported to be a promising antitumour agent with pronounced antimetastatic effects (Orsolic et al., 2005). The proliferative effect of honey on tumour cells was suggested to be a nutritional effect rather than a carcinogenic effect, and the antitumour effect was reported to result from many activities, such as the inhibition of DNA synthesis with no signs of cytotoxicity and the downregulation of MMP-2 and MMP-9, which have been implicated in the induction of the angiogenic switch in different model systems (Egeblad et al., 2002). Honey has cytotoxic activity against carcinomic human kidney cells, indicating that honey possesses antitumour and anticarcinogenic activities (Abdel Aziz et al., 2009).

Leptin is an adipocyte-derived hormone/cytokine that links nutritional status with neuroendocrine and immune functions. Leptin was the first adipocyte-derived hormone described, and the amount of leptin produced is directly proportional to the amount of adipose tissue. Leptin activates the anorexigenic axis in the hypothalamus. Leptin is a key intermediary between energy homeostasis and the immune system, and it may play roles in inflammation and obesity-related diseases, including atherosclerosis and cancer. The characterisation of leptin functions and signalling pathways in regulating lipid metabolism, inflammatory mediator production and lipid body biogenesis in macrophages and other cells are important for understanding the roles of leptin in the pathogenesis of inflammatory diseases.

The mTOR kinase pathway is a well-studied and evolutionarily conserved intracellular nutrient-sensing pathway (Lindsley et al., 2004). This pathway integrates nutrient- and growth factor-derived signals to set overall growth rates, and interfaces with the cell cycle machinery to coordinate cell growth and division (Richardson et al., 2004).

New findings are starting to unveil an important role for mTOR in leptin signalling, in the hypothalamic centres as well as in peripheral cells (Cota et al., 2006).

The activation of mTOR complex 1 in the hypothalamus is important for the effects of leptin on the hypothalamic axis, which modulates food intake (Cota et al., 2006). These authors showed that the activation of the mTOR pathway occurs in response to leptin stimulation and that rapamycin inhibits the anorexigenic signal of leptin. Moreover, the amino acid leucine directly activates mTOR in the hypothalamus, functioning as a redundant signal with leptin. Several nutrient sensing mediators that activate mTOR in adipose tissue, including insulin, leucine and UDP-N-acetylglucosamine, also induce leptin synthesis (Lindsley et al., 2004). The role of leptin in regulating lipid accumulation and foam cell formation in macrophages is beginning to be characterised and involves key steps mediated by mTOR-dependent signalling. Typically, increases in the size and numbers of lipid bodies are accompanied by accumulation of triacylglycerides and cholesterol esters in their hydrophobic core. In different cell systems, including adipocytes and macrophages, intracellular lipids are stored and metabolised in hydrophobic organelles called lipid bodies or lipid droplets. Although lipid bodies were long considered inert fat depots, lipid bodies are now viewed as dynamic organelles with roles in integrating lipid metabolism, inflammatory mediator production, membrane trafficking and intracellular signalling (Wang et al., 2007). Accordingly, the regulatory mechanisms of lipid body biogenesis and functions are of major interest for the study of atherosclerosis, obesity, cancer and other inflammatory diseases. In addition, the mTOR inhibitor rapamycin upregulates the expression of genes that promote fatty acid oxidation, while downregulating genes that participate in fatty acid synthesis (Peng et al., 2002). However, it should be noted that depending on the cell type and model system used, leptin might have opposite effects on intracellular lipid storage and metabolism (O'Rourke et al., 2002). In fact, leptin diminishes lipid accumulation in the liver, kidney and adipose tissue (Motomura et al., 2006). These data point to different roles and possibly different signalling pathways for leptin, depending on the tissue.

Numerous studies have established a link between diet and cancer risk or progression; as a result, the World Cancer Research Fund has recently acknowledged that after smoking, diet may be the second most important contributor to the global burden of cancer (http://www.wcrf-uk.org/preventing cancer/index.php.).

7. Iron disorders in RCC

Iron metabolism is crucial in all aspects of energy production in the body (Anderson et al., 2009) and is particularly important for cells that are characterised by high-energy demands, such as tumourous cells. Iron has the ability to shuttle between two oxidative states (ferric and ferrous iron), which makes it an efficient cofactor for several enzymes and the catalyst of numerous biochemical reactions (Anderson et al., 2009). The ferrous form Fe(II) can donate electrons, while the Fe(III) form can accept electrons. Iron plays a crucial role in oxygen transport (as a component of hemoglobin (Hb)), oxygen storage (as a component of myoglobin), and oxidative metabolism (as a component of oxidative enzymes and respiratory chain processes).

Ion is also involved in the synthesis and degradation of lipids, carbohydrates, DNA, and RNA as well as in the metabolism of collagen, tyrosine, and catecholamines.

Therefore, iron deficiency can impair oxidative metabolism, cellular energetics, and cellular immune mechanisms.

Experimental studies in animals have shown that severe iron deficiency can cause diastolic dysfunction and heart failure with pulmonary congestion, left ventricular hypertrophy and dilation, cardiac fibrosis, a reduction in erythropoietin levels and a worsening of the molecular signalling pathways (as measured by cardiac STAT3 phosphorylation), an increase in the inflammatory cytokine TNFα, and proteinuria (Dong et al., 2005). Iron may have anti-inflammatory effects. Compared to haemodialysis patients taking EPO alone, those taking EPO and IV iron had lower proinflammatory TNFα levels and higher anti-inflammatory cytokine IL-4 levels as well as lower levels of total peroxide (a marker of free radical concentration) (Weiss et al., 2003).

The biology of iron and oxygen is closely related, and known regulatory pathways involving HIF and iron-regulatory proteins (IRPs) are responsive to both these stimuli.

In humans, iron is absorbed only in the small intestine, stored in the liver and the reticuloendothelial (RE) system, and is mainly used in bone marrow. Intestinal absorption of iron depends on four types of proteins of iron metabolism: duodenal cytochrome b (Dcytb), divalent metal transporter 1 (DMT1), ferroportin 1 (FP1) and hephaestin (Hp).

Many proteins of iron metabolism show a high degree of expression in tumour cells, indicating that iron plays an important role in tumourigenesis and development. However, regulatory factors of iron metabolism and their mechanisms remain to be studied. New treatment strategies may be developed by combining imaging agents or targeted drugs with proteins related to iron metabolism. Recently, magnetic nanoparticles carrying chemotherapeutic drugs provide a new thinking for solid tumour targeted therapy. For example, the combination of the magnetic nanoparticle Fe_3O_4 with cisplatin (DDP) is used to reverse DDP resistance in the human ovarian cancer cell line SKOV3/DDP through increasing intracellular drug concentrations and promoting cell apoptosis by reducing mRNA expression of the antiapoptosis genes *bcl2* and *survivin* (Jiang et al., 2009).

8. Oxygen sensing and RCC

Tumours are characterised by specific metabolic alterations providing a metabolic signature in malignant transformation at different stages; end stage carcinomas are most dependent on anaerobic glucose degradation (aerobic glycolysis, fermentation) and least dependent on mitochondrial energy supplies (Ramanathan et al., 2005). The metabolic endpoint of this transformation, the anaerobic degradation of glucose even in the presence of oxygen, was first described by Nobel laureate Otto Warburg (Warburg et al., 1924). Concomitant with this metabolic switch, high lactate concentrations occur and result in immune protection of cancer cells, acid-mediated matrix degradation, invasiveness and metastasis. Furthermore, transformation to a more malignant phenotype is associated with resistance to chemo- and radiation-therapy (Cao et al., 2007).

Increased total activity of the transketolase-dependent, nonoxidative branch of the pentose phosphate pathway (PPP) in cancer cells is due to the overexpression of the transketolase-like-1 (TKTL1) protein (Hu et al., 2007).

The complex regulation of tumour metabolism switches from mitochondrial oxidative to nonoxidative energy production, which is dependent on the PPP. Both the oxidative and nonoxidative branches of the PPP have been described as activated in carcinogenesis. It is assumed that the enzymes of the oxidative branch of the PPP [glucose-6-phosphate-dehydrogenase (G6PD) and 6-phosphogluconate dehydrogenase] are triggered by an increased need for NADPH, whereas the enzymes of the nonoxidative branch (TKTL1, transaldolases) are triggered by an increased need for ribose and energy (Ramos-Montoya et al., 2006).

During malignant transformation of cancer cells, a metabolic switch from mitochondrially based, oxygen-dependent ATP production (oxidative phosphorylation) to anaerobic glucose degradation (aerobic glycolysis, fermentation) leading to oxygen- and mitochondria-independent ATP generation takes place, even in the presence of oxygen (Ramanathan et al., 2005).

Activation of HIF-1, a key transcription factor that upregulates genes involved in glycolytic energy metabolism, is a common feature of RCC and has been linked to malignant transformation, metastasis and treatment resistance. In the absence of a functional von Hippel-Lindau tumour suppressor protein (70% of sporadic RCCs), irrespective of oxygen concentration, HIF-1α is not degraded and translocates to the nucleus where it dimerises with HIF-1β to form transcriptionally active HIF. HIF-1α is increased by hypoxia, insulin, insulin-like growth factor, epidermal growth factor and angiotensin II. The glycolysis-activated accumulation of HIF-1 protein once again stresses the crucial role of aerobic glycolysis in carcinogenesis and has been demonstrated to be a potent target in anticancer therapy (Oh et al., 2008).

Increased lactic-acid production and excretion by fermenting tumour cells results in suppression of cytokine production, T-cell inactivation, acid-mediated matrix degradation and apoptosis of surrounding healthy cells, leading to invasion and metastasis. Thus, high lactate production results in an exceptional growth advantage for tumour cells. The correlation between mitochondrial dysfunction and increased aerobic glycolysis in carcinogenesis has been investigated, but the competitive advantage for tumour cells is still under discussion (Ramanathan et al., 2005; Brandon et al., 2006). Mitochondrial energy production is correlated with release of reactive oxygen species (ROS) that damage proteins and macromolecules such as DNA. During proliferation, DNA is exposed to ROS that leads to severe DNA damage and mutations. Fermentative cancer cells do not produce mitochondrial ROS, thus preventing ROS-induced DNA alterations.

Anaerobic glucose metabolism is believed to have a poorer energy output in relation to the energy stored in the glucose molecule. Therefore, the elevated demand for glucose is compensated by the upregulation of glucose transporters and the onset of aerobic glycolysis in a PI-3K-dependent manner, resulting in high lactate concentrations (Walenta et al., 2004). The switch to anaerobic energy production by the TKTL1-dependent, nonoxidative branch of the PPP supports the enormous demand for (ROS-free) energy and anabolic substrates, such as ribose, NADPH and acetyl-CoA. The modified, TKTL1-dependent PPP seems a general biochemical program suitable for safe and enhanced energy release, and the anabolic substrate production necessary for rapid cell proliferation.

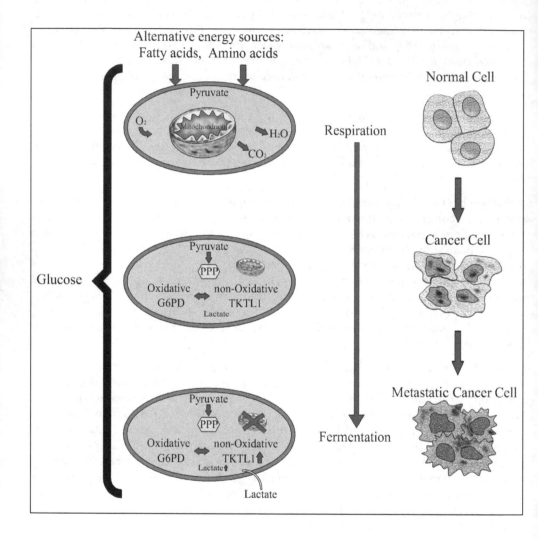

Fig. 7. Malignant transformation of cancer cells: renal tumors are present with an altered glucose metabolism. Enhanced glycolysis leads to increased activity of the enzymes in the oxidative (G6PD) and nonoxidative branches (TKTL1) of the PPP. Progressing tumors are characterized by specific upregulation of the nonoxidative branch of the PPP, ensuring ribose and energy, and supporting acidification of the tumor microenvironment. Acidification is a major step in invasive tumor growth, metastasis and immune escape. Additionally, upregulation of the anaerobic energy supply without ROS production, and G6PD activity for increased reducing equivalents, protects cancer cells from oxidative stress.

9. Conclusions

The oxygen-dependent regulation of HIF activity involves very complex pathways that involve prolyl hydroxylases and the VHL tumour suppressor protein, both of which are highly modulated by environmental and physiologic cues. The exact roles of the different HIF-α isoforms in these processes are still under intense investigation.

In the past decade, studying the regulation of HIFs has led to an appreciation that mitochondrial metabolism and ROS are essential regulators of HIFs. Conversely, HIFs have also been shown to regulate mitochondrial metabolism and ROS levels. Because mitochondria are the major consumers of oxygen, it is not surprising that HIFs and mitochondria are inter-connected.

The evidence accumulated from ecologic and case control studies show that diet has an important role in the development of RCC. Energy intake and several dietary factors should be considered as potentially involved in the development of renal cell cancer at different stages of tumourigenesis.

In this chapter, we have summarised the most recent findings in HIF signalling and have attempted to provide a perspective on how recent advances in HIF biology may affect our understanding of renal cancer.

10. References

Abdel Aziz A, Rady H, Amer MA, and Kiwan HS. (2009) Effect of Some Honey Bee Extracts on the Proliferation, Proteolytic and Gelatinolytic Activities of the Hepatocellular Carcinoma Hepg2 Cell Line. *Aus J Basic App Sci* 3, 2754–69

Anderson GJ and Vulpe CD (2009) Mammalian iron transport. *Cellular and Molecular Life Sciences* 66, 3241–3261

Arsham AM, Howell JJ, and Simon MC. (2003) A novel hypoxia-inducible factor-independent hypoxic response regulating mammalian target of rapamycin and its targets. *J Biol Chem* 278, 29655–29660

Bindra RS, Vasselli JR, Stearman R, Linehan WM, and Klausner RD. (2002) VHL-mediated hypoxia regulation of cyclin D1 in renal carcinoma cells. *Cancer Res* 62, 3014–3019

Brandon M, Baldi P, and Wallace DC. (2006) Mitochondrial mutations in cancer. *Oncogene* 25, 4647–62

Brudzynski K. (2006) Effect of hydrogen peroxide on antibacterial activities of Canadian honeys. *Can J Microbiol.* 52, 1228–37

Cao X, Fang L, Gibbs S, Huang Y, Dai Z, Wen P, Zheng X, Sadee W, and Sun D. (2007) Glucose uptake inhibitor sensitizes cancer cells to daunorubicin and overcomes drug resistance in hypoxia. *Cancer Chemother Pharmacol* 59:495–505

Chance B and Williams GR. (1955) Respiratory enzymes in oxidative phosphorylation. I. Kinetics of oxygen utilization. *J Biol Chem* 217, 383–393

Chinthalapally V, Dhimant D, Barbara S, Nalini K, Shantu A, and Bandaru R. (1993) Inhibitory effect of caffeic acid esters on azoxymethane-induced biochemical changes and aberrant crypt foci formation in rat colon. *Cancer Res* 53, 4182–8

Chow WH and Devesa SS. (2008) Contemporary epidemiology of renal cell cancer *Cancer Journal* 14, 288–301

Colgan SP, and Taylor CT. (2010) Hypoxia: an alarm signal during intestinal inflammation. *Nat Rev Gastroenterol Hepatol* 7, 281-7

Cota D, Proulx K, Smith KA, Kozma SC, Thomas G, Woods SC, and Seeley RJ.(2006) Hypothalamic mTOR signaling regulates food intake. *Science* 312, 927-30

Cramer T, Yamanishi Y, Clausen BE, Forster I, Pawlinski R, Mackman N, Haase VH, Jaenisch R, Corr M, Nizet V, Firestein GS, Gerber HP, Ferrara N, and Johnson RS.(2003) HIF-1α is essential for myeloid cell-mediated inflammation. *Cell* 112, 645–657

Denko NC. (2008) Hypoxia, HIF1 and glucose metabolism in the solid tumour. *Nat Rev Cancer* 8, 705–713

Dong F, Zhang X, Culver B, Chew HG, Kelley RO, and Ren J (2005) Dietary iron deficiency induces ventricular dilation, mitochondrial ultrastructural aberrations and cytochrome c release: involvement of nitric oxide synthase and protein tyrosine nitration. *Clinical Science* 109, 277–286

Eckle T, Grenz A, Laucher S, and Eltzschig HK. A2B adenosine receptor signaling attenuates acute lung injury by enhancing alveolar fluid clearance in mice. *J Clin Invest* 118, 3301-15

Eckle T, Köler D, Lehmann R, El Kasmi KC, and Eltzschig HK. (2008) Hypoxia-inducible factor-1 is central to cardioprotection: a new paradigm for ischemic preconditioning. *Circulation* 118, 166-75

Egeblad M, and Werb Z. (2002) New functions for the matrix metalloproteinases in cancer progression. *Nat Rev Cancer* 2, 161–74

Eltzschig HK, Ibla JC, Furuta GT, Leonard MO, Jacobson KA, Enjyoji K, Robson SC, and Colgan SP. (2003) Coordinated adenine nucleotide phosphohydrolysis and nucleoside signaling in posthypoxic endothelium: role of ectonucleotidases and adenosine A2B receptors. *J Exp Med* 198, 783-96

Eltzschig HK. (2009) Adenosine: an old drug newly discovered. *Anesthesiology* 111, 904-15

Elvidge GP, Glenny L, Appelhoff RJ, Ratcliffe PJ, Ragoussis J, and Gleadle JM (2006) Concordant regulation of gene expression by hypoxia and 2-oxoglutarate-dependent dioxygenase inhibition: the role of HIF-1alpha, HIF-2alpha, and other pathways. *J Biol Chem* 281, 15215–15226

Emerling BM, Weinberg F, Snyder C, Burgess Z, Mutlu GM, Viollet B, Budinger GR, and Chandel NS. (2009) Hypoxic activation of AMPK is dependent on mitochondrial ROS but independent of an increase in AMP/ATP ratio. *Free Radic Biol Med* 46, 1386–1391

Fukuda R, Hirota K, Fan F, Jung YD, Ellis LM, and Semenza GL. (2002) Insulin-like growth factor 1 induces hypoxia-inducible factor 1-mediated vascular endothelial growth factor expression, which is dependent on MAP kinase and phosphatidylinositol 3-kinase signaling in colon cancer cells. *J Biol Chem* 277, 38205–38211

Furuta GT, Turner JR, Taylor CT, Hershberg RM, Comerford K, Narravula S, Podolsky DK, and Colgan SP. (2001) Hypoxia-inducible factor 1-dependent induction of intestinal trefoil factor protects barrier function during hypoxia. *J Exp Med* 193, 1027-34

Gingras AC, Raught B, Gygi SP, Niedzwiecka A, Miron M, Burley SK, Polakiewicz RD, Wyslouch-Cieszynska A, Aebersold R, and Sonenberg N. (2001) Hierarchical phosphorylation of the translation inhibitor 4EBP1.*Genes Dev* 15, 2852–2864

Gruber M, Hu CJ, Johnson RS, Brown EJ, Keith B, and Simon MC. (2007) Acute postnatal ablation of Hif-2alpha results in anemia. *Proc Natl Acad Sci U S A*. 104, 2301–2306

Gusarova GA, Dada LA, Kelly AM, Brodie C, Witters LA, Chandel NS, and Sznajder JI. (2009) Alpha1-AMP-activated protein kinase regulates hypoxia-induced Na,K-ATPase endocytosis via direct phosphorylation of protein kinase C zeta. *Mol Cell Biol* 29, 3455–3464

Gustafsson MV, Zheng X, Pereira T, Gradin K, Jin S, Lundkvist J, Ruas JL, Poellinger L, Lendahl U, and Bondesson M. (2005) Hypoxia requires notch signaling to maintain the undifferentiated cell state. *Dev Cell* 9, 617–628

Haase VH. (2005) The VHL tumor suppressor in development and disease: functional studies in mice by conditional gene targeting. *Semin Cell Dev Biol* 16, 564–574

Hegele RA and Cao H. (2001) Single nucleotide polymorphisms of RXRA encoding retinoid X receptor alpha. *Journal of Human Genetics* 46, 423–425

Hervouet E, Cízková A, Demont J, Vojtísková A, Pecina P, Franssen-van Hal NL, Keijer J, Simonnet H, Ivánek R, Kmoch S, Godinot C, and Houstek J. (2008) HIF and reactive oxygen species regulate oxidative phosphorylation in cancer. Carcinogenesis 29, 1528–1537

Holick MF (2006) Vitamin D: its role in cancer prevention and treatment *Progress in Biophysics and Molecular Biology* 92, 49–59

Hu CJ, Wang LY, Chodosh LA, Keith B, and Simon MC. (2003) Differential roles of hypoxia-inducible factor 1α (HIF-1α) and HIF-2α in hypoxic gene regulation. *Mol Cell Biol* 23, 9361–9374

Hu J, Mao Y, and White K. (2003) Diet and vitamin or mineral supplements and risk of renal cell carcinoma in Canada. *Cancer Causes Control* 14, 705–714

Hu LH, Yang JH, Zhang DT, Zhang S, Wang L, Cai PC, Zheng JF, and Huang JS. (2007) The TKTL1 gene influences total transketolase activity and cell proliferation in human colon cancer LoVo cells. *Anticancer Drugs* 18, 427–33

Hu LH, Yang JH, Zhang DT, Zhang S, Wang L, Cai PC, Zheng JF, and Huang JS. (2007) The TKTL1 gene influences total transketolase activity and cell proliferation in human colon cancer LoVo cells. *Anticancer Drugs* 18, 427–33

Hutterer GC, Patard JJ, Perrotte P, Ionescu C, de La Taille A, Salomon L, Verhoest G, Tostain J, Cindolo L, Ficarra V, Artibani W, Schips L, Zigeuner R, Mulders PF, Valeri A, Chautard D, Descotes JL, Rambeaud JJ, Mejean A, and Karakiewicz PI. (2007) Patients with renal cell carcinoma nodal metastases can be accurately identified: external validation of a new nomogram. *Int J Cancer* 121, 2556–61

Ikuyama T, Hamasaki T, Inatomi H, Katoh T, Muratani T, and Matsumoto T. (2002) Association of vitamin D receptor gene polymorphism with renal cell carcinoma in Japanese *Endocrine Journal* 49, 433–438

Isaacs JS, Jung YJ, Mole DR, Lee S, Torres-Cabala C, Chung YL, Merino M, Trepel J, Zbar B, Toro J, Ratcliffe PJ, Linehan WM, and Neckers L. (2005) HIF overexpression correlates with biallelic loss of fumarate hydratase in renal cancer: novel role of fumarate in regulation of HIF stability. *Cancer Cell* 8, 143–153

Iyer NV, Kotch LE, Agani F, Leung SW, Laughner E, Wenger RH, Gassmann M, Gearhart JD, Lawler AM, Yu AY, and Semenza GL (1998) Cellular and developmental control of O2 homeostasis by hypoxia-inducible factor 1 alpha. *Genes Dev* 12, 149–162

Jeddar A, Khassany A, Ramsaroop VG, Bhamjei IE, Moosa A. (1985) The antibacterial action of honey: an in vitro study. *S Afr Med J* 67, 257–9

Jiang BH, Jiang G, Zheng JZ, Lu Z, Hunter T, and Vogt PK. (2001) Phosphatidylinositol 3-kinase signaling controls levels of hypoxia-inducible factor 1. *Cell Growth Differ* 12, 363–369

Jiang Z, Chen BA, Wu Q, Xia GH, Zhang Y, Gao F, Hong TY, Xu CR, Cheng J, Li GH, Chen WJ, Liu LJ, Li XM, and Wang XM. (2009) Reversal effect of Fe3O4-magnetic nanoparticles on multi-drug resistance of ovarian carcinoma cells and its correlation with apoptosis-associated genes *J Chin J Cancer* 28, 1158-1162

Jones DP, Shan X and Park Y. (1993) Coordinated multisite regulation of cellular energy metabolism. *Annu Rev Nutr* 12, 327–343

Kaelin WG. Proline hydroxylation and gene expression. (2005) *Annu Rev Biochem* 74, 115–128

Kanehisa M, Goto S, Furumichi M, Tanabe M, and Hirakawa M. (2010) KEGG for representation and analysis of molecular networks involving diseases and drugs. *Nucleic Acids Res.* 38, D355-D360

Kaplan JH. (2002) Biochemistry of Na,K-ATPase. *Annu Rev Biochem* 71, 511–535

Karami S, Brennan P, Hung RJ, Boffetta P, Toro J, Wilson RT, Zaridze D, Navratilova M, Chatterjee N, Mates D, Janout V, Kollarova H, Bencko V, Szeszenia-Dabrowska N, Holcatova I, Moukeria A, Welch R, Chanock S, Rothman N, Chow WH, and Moore LE. (2008)Vitamin D receptor polymorphisms and renal cancer risk in Central and Eastern Europe *Journal of Toxicology and Environmental Health A* 6, 367–372

Karami S, Brennan P, Rosenberg PS, Navratilova M, Mates D, Zaridze D, Janout V, Kollarova H, Bencko V, Matveev V, Szeszenia-Dabrowska N, Holcatova I, Yeager M, Chanock S, Menashe I, Rothman N, Chow WH, Boffetta P, and Moore LE. (2009) Analysis of SNPs and haplotypes in vitamin D pathway genes and renal cancer risk. PLoS ONE 4, e7013

Karhausen J, Furuta GT, Tomaszewski JE, Johnson RS, Colgan SP, Haase VH. (2004) Epithelial hypoxia-inducible factor-1 is protective in murine experimental colitis. *J Clin Invest* 114, 1098-106

Kempf VA, Lebiedziejewski M, Alitalo K, Wälzlein JH, Ehehalt U, Fiebig J, Huber S, Schütt B, Sander CA, Müller S, Grassl G, Yazdi AS, Brehm B, and Autenrieth IB. (2005) Activation of hypoxia-inducible factor-1 in bacillary angiomatosis: evidence for a role of hypoxia-inducible factor- 1 in bacterial infections. *Circulation* 111, 1054-62

Kim J-W, Tchernyshyov I, Semenza GL, and Dang CV (2006) HIF-1-mediated expression of pyruvate dehydrogenase kinase: a metabolic switch required for cellular adaptation to hypoxia. *Cell Metab* 3, 177–185

Kong T, Eltzschig HK, Karhausen J, Colgan SP, and Shelley CS. (2004) Leukocyte adhesion during hypoxia is mediated by HIF-1-dependent induction of β2 integrin gene expression. *Proc Natl Acad Sci USA* 101, 10440–10445

Koppenol WH, Bounds PL, and Dang CV. (2011) Otto Warburg's contributions to current concepts of cancer metabolism. *Nat Rev Cancer* 11, 325-37

Koshiji M, Kageyama Y, Pete EA, Horikawa I, Barrett JC, and Huang LE. (2004) HIF-1α induces cell cycle arrest by functionally counteracting Myc. *EMBO J* 23, 1949–1956

Koumenis C, Naczki C, Koritzinsky M, Rastani S, Diehl A, Sonenberg N, Koromilas A, and Wouters BG. (2002) Regulation of protein synthesis by hypoxia via activation of the endoplasmic reticulum kinase PERK and phosphorylation of the translation initiation factor eIF2alpha. *Mol Cell Biol* 22, 7405–7416

Lindsley JE, and Rutter J. (2004) Nutrient sensing and metabolic decisions. *Comp Biochem Physiol B Biochem Mol Biol* 139, 543-59

Liu MY, Poellinger L, and Walker CL. (2003) Up-regulation of hypoxiainducible factor 2α in renal cell carcinoma associated with loss of Tsc-2 tumor suppressor gene. *Cancer Res* 63, 2675–2680

Manalo DJ, Rowan A, Lavoie T, Natarajan L, Kelly BD, Ye SQ, Garcia JG, and Semenza GL (2005) Transcriptional regulation of vascular endothelial cell responses to hypoxia by HIF-1. *Blood* 105, 659–669

Mandriota SJ, Turner KJ, Davies DR, Murray PG, Morgan NV, Sowter HM, Wykoff CC, Maher ER, Harris AL, Ratcliffe PJ, and Maxwell PH (2002) HIF activation identifies early lesions in VHL kidneys: evidence for site-specific tumor suppressor function in the nephron. *Cancer Cell* 1, 459–468

McCullough ML, Bandera EV, Moore DF, and Kushi LH. (2008) Vitamin D and calcium intake in relation to risk of endometrial cancer: a systematic review of the literature. *Prev Med* 46, 298-302

Morote-Garcia JC, Rosenberger P, Kuhlicke J, and Eltzschig HK. (2008) HIF-1-dependent repression of adenosine kinase attenuates hypoxia-induced vascular leak. *Blood* 111, 5571-80

Motomura W, Inoue M, Ohtake T, Takahashi N, Nagamine M, Tanno S, Kohgo Y, and Okumura T. (2006) Upregulation of ADRP in fatty liver in human and liver steatosis in mice fed with high fat diet. *Biochem Biophys Res Commun* 340, 1111-8

Multiple organ pathology, metabolic abnormalities and impaired homeostasis of reactive oxygen species in Epas1-/- mice. (2003) Multiple organ pathology, metabolic abnormalities and impaired homeostasis of reactive oxygen species in Epas1−/− mice. *Nat Genet* 35, 331–340

O'Rourke L, Gronning LM, Yeaman SJ, and Shepherd PR. (2002) Glucose-dependent regulation of cholesterol ester metabolism in macrophages by insulin and leptin. *J Biol Chem* 277, 42557-62

Oh SH, Woo JK, Jin Q, Kang HJ, Jeong JW, Kim KW, Hong WK, and Lee HY. (2008) Identification of novel antiangiogenic anticancer activities of deguelin targeting hypoxia-inducible factor-1a. *Int J Cancer* 122, 5–14

Orsolic N, Terzic S, Sver L, and Basic I. (2005) Honey-bee products in prevention and/or therapy of murine transplantable tumours. *J Sci Food Agri* 85, 363–70

Papandreou I, Cairns RA, Fontana L, Lim AL, and Denko NC (2006) HIF-1 mediates adaptation to hypoxia by actively downregulating mitochondrial oxygen consumption. *Cell Metab* 3, 187-197

Peng T, Golub TR, and Sabatini DM. (2002) The immunosuppressant rapamycin mimics a starvation-like signal distinct from amino acid and glucose deprivation. *Mol Cell Biol* 22, 5575-84

Rady H. (2005) Faculty of Science. Cairo University; Phytochemical and biological study of an antitumor agent of plant origin mixed withhoney on malignant human cells in vitro.

Ramanathan A, Wang C, and Schreiber SL. (2005) Perturbational profiling of a cell-line model of tumorigenesis by using metabolic measurements. *Proc Natl Acad Sci USA* 102, 5992-7

Ramos-Montoya A, Lee WN, Bassilian S, Lim S, Trebukhina RV, Kazhyna MV, Ciudad CJ, Noe V, Centelles JJ, and Cascante M. (2006) Pentose phosphate cycle oxidative and nonoxidative balance: a new vulnerable target for overcoming drug resistance in cancer. *Int J Cancer* 119, 2733-41

Ramos-Montoya A, Lee WN, Bassilian S, Lim S, Trebukhina RV, Kazhyna MV, Ciudad CJ, Noe V, Centelles JJ, and Cascante M. (2006) Pentose phosphate cycle oxidative and nonoxidative balance: a new vulnerable target for overcoming drug resistance in cancer. *Int J Cancer* 119, 2733-41

Rankin EB, Higgins DF, Walisser JA, Johnson RS, Bradfield CA, and Haase VH. (2005) Inactivation of the arylhydrocarbon receptor nuclear translocator (Arnt) suppresses von Hippel-Lindau disease-associated vascular tumors in mice. *Mol Cell Biol* 25, 3163-3172

- Raval RR, Lau KW, Tran MG, Sowter HM, Mandriota SJ, Li JL, Pugh CW, Maxwell PH, Harris AL, and Ratcliffe PJ. (2005) Contrasting properties of hypoxia-inducible factor 1 (HIF-1) and HIF-2 in von Hippel-Lindau-associated renal cell carcinoma. *Mol Cell Biol* 25, 5675-5686

Reutershan J, Vollmer I, Stark S, Wagner R, Ngamsri KC, and Eltzschig HK. (2009) Adenosine and inflammation: CD39 and CD73 are critical mediators in LPS-induced PMN trafficking into the lungs. *FASEB J* 23, 473-82

Richard DE, Berra E, and Pouyssegur J. (2000) Nonhypoxic pathway mediates the induction of hypoxia-inducible factor 1α in vascular smooth muscle cells. *J Biol Chem* 275, 26765-26771

Richardson CJ, Schalm SS, and Blenis J. (2004) PI3-kinase and TOR: PIKTORing cell growth. *Semin Cell Dev Biol* 15, 147-59

Robinson A, Keely S, Karhausen J, Gerich ME, Furuta GT, and Colgan SP. (2008) Mucosal protection by hypoxia-inducible factor prolyl hydroxylase inhibition. *Gastroenterology* 134, 145-55

Rosenberger C, Mandriota S, Jurgensen JS, Wiesener MS, Horstrup JH, Frei U, Ratcliffe PJ, Maxwell PH, Bachmann S, and Eckardt KU. (2002) Expression of hypoxia-inducible factor-1α and -2α in hypoxic and ischemic rat kidneys. *J Am Soc Nephrol* 13, 1721-1732

Rosenberger P, Schwab JM, Mirakaj V, Masekowsky E, Mager A, Morote-Garcia JC, Unertl K, and Eltzschig HK. (2009) Hypoxia-inducible factor-dependent induction of netrin-1 dampens inflammation caused by hypoxia. *Nat Immunol* 10, 195-202

Ryan HE, Lo J, and Johnson RS (1998) HIF-1 alpha is required for solid tumor formation and embryonic vascularization. *EMBO J* 17, 3005-3015

Sandau KB, Zhou J, Kietzmann T, and Brune B. (2001) Regulation of the hypoxia-inducible factor 1α by the inflammatory mediators nitric oxide and tumor necrosis factor-α in contrast to desferroxamine and phenylarsine oxide. *J Biol Chem* 276, 39805-39811

Schingnitz U, Hartmann K, Macmanus CF, Eckle T, Zug S, Colgan SP, Eltzschig HK. (2010) Signaling through the A2B adenosine receptor dampens endotoxininduced acute lung injury. *J Immunol* 184, 5271-9

Schofield CJ and Ratcliffe PJ. (2004) Oxygen sensing by HIF hydroxylases. *Nat Rev Mol Cell Biol* 5, 343-354

Semenza GL. (2003) Targeting HIF-1 for cancer therapy. *Nat Rev Cancer* 3, 721-32

Skou JC. (1957) The influence of some cations on an adenosine triphosphatase from peripheral nerves. *Biochim Biophys Acta* 23, 394-401

Smith K, Gunaratnam L, Morley M, Franovic A, Mekhail K, and Lee S. (2005) Silencing of epidermal growth factor receptor suppresses hypoxiainducible factor-2-driven VHL-/- renal cancer. *Cancer Res* 65: 5221-5230

Soilleux EJ, Turley H, Tian YM, Pugh CW, Gatter KC, and Harris AL. (2005) Use of novel monoclonal antibodies to determine the expression and distribution of the hypoxia regulatory factors PHD-1, PHD-2, PHD-3 and FIH in normal and neoplastic human tissues. *Histopathology* 47, 602-610

Staller P, Sulitkova J, Lisztwan J, Moch H, Oakeley EJ, and Krek W. (2003) Chemokine receptor CXCR4 downregulated by von Hippel-Lindau tumour suppressor pVHL. *Nature* 425, 307-311

The Word Cancer Resarch Fund, June 2009, http://www.wcrf-uk.org/preventing cancer/index.php.

Thibault F, Cancel-Tassin G, and Cussenot O. (2006) Low penetrance genetic susceptibility to kidney cancer *BJU International* 98, 735-738

Treins C, Giorgetti-Peraldi S, Murdaca J, Semenza GL, and Van Obberghen E. (2002) Insulin stimulates hypoxia-inducible factor 1 through a phosphatidylinositol 3-kinase/target of rapamycin-dependent signalling pathway. *J Biol Chem* 277: 27975-27981

Valdivielso JM and Fernandez E. (2006) Vitamin D receptor polymorphisms and diseases *Clinica Chimica Acta* 371, 1-12

Walenta S, and Mueller-Klieser WF. (2004) Lactate: mirror and motor of tumor malignancy. *Semin Radiat Oncol* 14, 267-74

Warburg O, Posener K, and Negelein E. (1924) Über den Stoffwechsel der Carcinomcelle. *Biochem* 152, 309-44

Weiss G, Meusburger E, Radacher G, Garimorth K, Neyer U, and Mayer G. (2003) Effect of iron treatment on circulating cytokine levels in ESRD patients receiving recombinant human erythropoietin. *Kidney International* 64, 572-578

Wouters BG, van den Beucken T, Magagnin MG, Koritzinsky M, Fels D, and Koumenis C.
    (2005) Control of the hypoxic response through regulation of mRNA translation.
    Semin Cell Dev Biol 16, 487–501

Wykoff CC, Sotiriou C, Cockman ME, Ratcliffe PJ, Maxwell P, Liu E, and Harris AL. (2004)
    Gene array of VHL mutation and hypoxia shows novel hypoxia-induced genes and
    that cyclin D1 is a VHL target gene. *Br J Cancer* 90, 1235–1243

Zatyka M, da Silva NF, Clifford SC, Morris MR, Wiesener MS, Eckardt KU, Houlston RS,
    Richards FM, Latif F, and Maher ER. (2002) Identification of cyclin D1 and other
    novel targets for the von Hippel-Lindau tumor suppressor gene by expression
    array analysis and investigation of cyclin D1 genotype as a modifier in von Hippel-
    Lindau disease. *Cancer Res* 62, 3803–3811

8

Immunotherapy of Renal Cell Carcinoma – From Antigen Identification to Patient Treatment

Heiko Schuster[1], Mathias Walzer[1,2] and Stefan Stevanović[1]
[1]Department of Immunology, Institute for Cell Biology, University of Tübingen
[2]Applied Bioinformatics Group, Center for Bioinformatics, University of Tübingen
Germany

1. Introduction

Renal cell carcinoma (RCC) ist the 3rd most common urologic cancer leading to an estimated 271 000 new cancer cases worldwide each year (Ferlay *et al.* 2010). RCC is generally associated with poor prognosis because of late diagnosis and bad responsiveness to classical radio- and chemotherapy. For a long period of time immunotherapy with IL-2 or Interferon alpha (IFNα) have been the only therapeutic options to treat advanced stage RCCs. In recent years targeted therapy with tyrosine kinase inhibitors (TKIs; Sunitinib, Sorafenib) or mTor inhibitors (Everolimus, Temsirolimus) has replaced cytokine based immunotherapy as a first line treatment in the management of metastatic RCCs (mRCC). IFNα is nevertheless still playing an important role in the treatment of mRCC not as a monotherapy, but rather in combination with the antibody Bevacizumab which is directed against proangiogenic vascular endothelial growth factor (VEGF).

Despite these recent improvements resistance to this new class of drugs frequently occurs and curative treatment of RCC is still only possible by surgical resection of the tumor mass at an early non-metastatic stage (Rini & Atkins 2009). A lot of effort has therefore been put into the development of a targeted immunotherapeutic approach that aims at the *in vivo* induction or reinforcement of an anti tumor immune response.

2. Cancer immunotherapy In the course of history

The underlying idea that the immune system is able to recognise and kill transformed cells is actually not new (Parish 2003). As early as the 19th century William Coley and others noticed that cancer patients suffering from a bacterial infection sometimes experienced tumor regression. William Coley was also the first to translate this observation into clinical practice by treating cancer patients with a bacterial preparation of Streptococcus pyogenes known as Coley's toxin (Coley 1893). In 1909 Paul Ehrlich evaluated the role of the immune system in tumor control and suggested that without the immune system cancers would occur in much higher frequency (Ehrlich 1909). Unfortunately it took more than half a century before Ehrlich's idea regained attention. First experimental evidence during the 1950s could show that syngenic animals could be immunized against transplantable tumors. In the early 1960s Lewis Thomas argued that long-lived organisms must have developed mechanisms that resemble homograft rejection in order to counter neoplastic diseases

(Lawrence 1959). Based on Thomas' views Frank M. Burnet formulated in 1967 his revolutionary „Immunosurveillance Theory" in which he stated that immune cells were constantly surveying host tissues for the presence of transformed cells that could be recognized by neo-antigens acquired during the transformation process (Burnet 1967). However Burnet's idea remained controversial simply because many people could not believe that the immune system could properly differentiate between healthy tissue and transformed cancer cells. Experiments with athymic nude mice also argued against Burnets idea (Stutman 1979). Despite their supposed lack of mature T cells (which was later shown to be not completely true (Maleckar & Sherman 1987)) these mice had no higher incidence in tumor development as originally predicted by Ehrlich. Since the late 80s, more and more evidence accumulated that revived the immunosurveillance theory. The discovery of tumor associated antigens (TAA) in mice and humans as well as the observation that truly immunodeficient knockout mice (*e.g.* RAG2$^{-/-}$, STAT1$^{-/-}$) really showed a higher incidence in cancer development finally proved Burnets idea.

3. Immunotherapeutical studies in RCC

RCC, along with melanoma, are considered to be the most immunogenic tumor in humans. This is based on the occurence of spontaneous regressions even in metastatic disease (Lokich 1997), the high amount of lymphocytic infiltrates found in tumor tissue (Van den Hove *et al.* 1997) and the comparably good response to nonspecific immunotherapy with cytokines like IL-2 or IFNα, at least in some part of the patients (10-20%) (Negrier *et al.* 1998). First clinical trials using a specific immunotherapy for RCC were therefore conducted during the mid - 90s already. Table 1 provides a comprehensive summary of published results regarding anti-tumor vaccination approaches from that time until today. Many different strategies involving lysate from autologous tumor tissue, allogenic tumor cell lines, whole tumor cell RNA as well as defined antigens (*e.g.* peptides derived from TAAs CAIX or MUC1) have been used. In most cases these antigens were applied in combination with an adjuvant (*e.g.* GM-CSF, BCG or incomplete Freunds adjuvant) or after loading onto dendritic cells (DCs) usually from the same patient. Dendritic cells are professional antigen presenting cells that have the capacity to take up tumor derived products spontaneously (in some trials also inforced by electrofusion with tumor cells) and to present antigen derived peptides *via* HLA class I and II molecules to cytotoxic- and also T helper cells. In most trials dendritic cells were generated from autologous peripheral blood derived monocytes or CD34$^+$ bone marrow cells that can both develop *ex vivo* into immature dendritic cells (iDCs). More recent studies almost uniformly apply a cytokine maturation step to generate mature dendritic cells (mDCs) as iDCs have been shown to posess tolerogenic rather than immune stimulatory functionality (Figdor *et al.* 2004). Keyhole limpet hemocyanin has been also applied in many trials as an immunostimulant because it was previously shown to improve dendritic cell based vaccinations by inducing a potent CD4$^+$ T helper cell response at least in mouse models (Shimizu *et al.* 2001). Other approaches to enhance the immunogenicity of the vaccine have been tried by virally transducing autologous tumor cells and allogenic cell lines with cytokines (GM-CSF, IL2) or T-cell costimulatory molecule CD80 (B7.1).

Vaccination with all these different approaches has proven to be well tolerated and side effects have been rare and were usually limited to allergic reactions at the site of injection as well as induration or erythema. In trials in which additional cytokine treatment (IL-2, IFNα) was employed, further side effects like fatigue, fever, vomiting and hypotension could be observed.

In some cases systemic application of high dose cytokines can however also lead to serious and life-threatening side effects. These symptoms have been known for a long time to also occur under cytokine monotherapy and are therefore not directly associated with the vaccine.

Inactivated tumor cells and gene modified tumor vaccines:

Author	Setting	Antigen	Adjuvant	N*	Results
(Galligioni et al. 1996)	Adjuvant after nephrectomy	Autol. Irradiated tumor cells	BCG	60 (60)	5-year DFS 63% vs. control 72%; 5-year OS 69% vs. control 78%
(Simons & Mikhak 1998)	mRCC	Autol. Irradiated tumor cells transduced with GM-CSF	None	16	1 PR
(Schwaab et al. 2000)	metastatic RCC	Autol. Irradiated tumor cells	BCG IFNg+ IFNa	14	3 MR, 5 SD, 1 PD
Dillman(Dillman et al. 2004)	8 primary RCC, 17 mRCC	Autol. Irradiated tumor cells	BCG, GM-CSF, IFNa, IFNg, IL2, CP	25	median PFS 2.4 months, median OS 10,2 months
(Jocham et al. 2004)	Adjuvant after nephrectomy	Autol. tumor lysate vaccine (Reniale)	None	177 (202)	5 year PFS 77.4% vs control 67.8%
(Dudek et al. 2008)	stage IV RCC	Autol. large multivalent immunogen vaccine	none, CP, IL-2 + CP	31	median PFS 12.2, 1 PR, 12 SD
(May et al. 2009)	Adjuvant after nephrectomy	Autol. tumor lysate vaccine (Reniale)	None	495 (495)	5-year OS 80.6% vs. control 79,2%, 10-year OS 79,2% vs. control 62,1%
(Antonia et al. 2002)	mRCC	Autol. Irradiated tumor cells transduced with B7-1	IL-2	15	2 PR, 2SD
(Tani et al. 2004)	stage IV RCC	Autol. Irradiated tumor cells transduced with GM-CSF	none, low dose IL-2	4	1 SD, 1MR
(Pizza et al. 2004)	mRCC	Autol. fixed tumor cells + allog. ACHN cell line transduced with IL-2	None	30 (131)	1 CR, 4 PR, 9 SD
(Moiseyenko et al. 2005)	mRCC after cytoreductive surgery	Autol. Irradiated tumor cells transfected with tag7/PGRP-S	None	4	1 SD
(Fishman et al. 2008)	stage IV RCC	Autol. Irradiated tumor cells transduced with B7-1	IL-2	39	1 CR, 24 SD
(Buchner et al. 2010)	mRCC	Allog.RCC-26 tumor cell line transduced with CD80 and IL 2	None	15	median PFS 5.3 months, median OS 15.6 months

Peptide based vaccines

Authors	Setting	Antigen	Adjuvant	N*	Results
(Uemura et al. 2006)	mRCC, HLA-A*24 pos.	CA9 derived peptides (p219-227, p288-296, p323-331)	IFA	23	3 PR, 6SD, median OS 21 months
(Iiyama et al. 2007)	mRCC, HLA-A*24 pos.	WT1 anchor modified peptide	IFA	3	2 SD
(Suekane et al. 2007)	mRCC, HLA-A*24 pos or HLA-A*2 pos.	Personalized cocktail of 4 peptides based on presence of Anti Peptide IgG or CTLs	IFA	10	6 SD
(Wood et al. 2008)	Adjuvant after nephrectomy	Autol. tumor derived heat-shock protein-peptide complex (Vitespen)	None	367 (361)	No difference in RFS
(Jonasch et al. 2008)	mRCC	Autol. tumor derived heat-shock protein-peptide complex (Vitespen)	None, IL2	60	2 CR, 2PR, 7SD
(Reinhardt et al. 2010)	mRCC, HLA-A*02 pos.	IMA901, 9 HLA-A*02 + 1 panDR restricted peptides	GMCSF, single dose CP before vaccination	64	OS after 18 months 63% and 80% with CP pretreament

Dendritic cell based vaccines					
Authors	Setting	DC + Antigen	Adjuvant/ Additional Treatment	N*	Results
(Oosterwijk-Wakka et al. 2002)	mRCC	Autol. iDCs loaded with autol. tumor cell lysate	IL-2;/ DC pulsed with KLH,none	12	8 SD
(Marten et al. 2002)	mRCC	Autol. mDCs loaded with autol. tumor cell lysate	none;/ DC pulsed with KLH, none	15	1 PR, 7 SD
(Holtl et al. 2002)	mRCC	Autol. mDCs loaded with autol. tumor cell lysate or allog. A498 cell line lysate	none / DC pulsed with KLH	35	2 CR, 1 PR, 7 SD
(Azuma et al. 2002)	mRCC	Autol. iDCs loaded with autol. tumor cell lysate	none / DC pulsed with KLH	3	1 SD
(Marten et al. 2003)	mRCC	Allog. mDCs fused with autol. tumor cells	None	12	4 SD
(Marten et al. 2006)	mRCC, HLA matched	Autol. mDCs loaded with a telomerase derived peptide	none; DC pulsed with KLH	10	1 MR, 1 SD
(Gitlitz et al. 2003)	mRCC	Autol. iDCs loaded with autol. tumor cell lysate	None	12	1 PR, 3 SD
(Barbuto et al. 2004)	mRCC	Allog. mDCs fused with autol. tumor derived cells	None	19	3 OR, 14 SD
(Avigan et al. 2007)	stage IV RCC	Allog. mDCs fused with autol. tumor derived cells	None	20	2 PR, 8 SD
(Avigan et al. 2004)	mRCC	Allog. iDCs fused with autol. tumor derived cells	DC pulsed with KLH	13	5 SD
(Pandha et al. 2004)	mRCC	Autol. iDCs loaded with allog. lysate of tumor cell line JM-RCC	KLH	5	2 SD
(Arroyo et al. 2004)	mRCC	Autol. mDCs loaded with autol. tumor cell lysate	DC pulsed with KLH	5	3 SD
(Dannull et al. 2005)	mRCC	Autol. mDCs transfected with whole tumor RNA	Pretreatment with ONTAK (Treg depletion)	11	not evaluated
(Holtl et al. 2005)	mRCC	Allog. mDCs laded with autol. tumor cell lysate	none/ Cyclophosphamide; DC pulsed with KLH	20	2 MR, 3 SD
(Wierecky et al. 2006)	mRCC HLA-A*02	Autol. mDCs loaded with two HLA-A*02 MUC1 peptides	pan DR-peptide PADRE, IL-2 (post vaccination period)	20	1 CR, 2 PR, 2 MR, 5 SD
(Bleumer et al. 2007)	metastatic ccRCC HLA-A*02	Autol. mDCs loaded with an HLA-A*02 and HLA-DR restricted CA9 derived peptide	DC pulsed with KLH	6	all PD
(Wei et al. 2007)	mRCC	Autol. mDCs fused with autol. tumor derived cells (Dendritomas)	IL-2	10	1 PR, 3 SD
(Matsumoto et al. 2007)	mRCC	Autol. mDCs loaded with autol. Primary tumor derived cell lysate	DC pulsed with KLH	3	1 SD
(Kim et al. 2007)	mRCC	Autol. mDCs loaded with autol. Primary tumor derived cell lysate	DC pulsed with KLH	9	1 PR, 5 SD
(Berntsen et al. 2008)	mRCC, HLA-A*02 pos or neg	Autol. mDCs loaded with allog. cell line lysate (A*02 neg) or a mix of 9 different hTERT and 11 Survivin derived peptides (A*02 pos)	IL-2, pan DR-peptide PADRE, DC pulsed with KLH (only A*02 neg)	27	13 SD
(Tatsugami et al. 2008)	mRCC	Autol. mDCs loaded with autol. Primary tumor derived cell lysate	IFNa	7	5 SD
(Schwaab et al. 2009)	mRCC	Autol. mDCs loaded with autol. Primary tumor derived cell lysate	IL-2 and IFNa	18	3 CR, 6 PR, 6 SD

*Number of patients treated versus number of patients in control group in brackets. mRCC: metastatic renal cell carcinoma, ccRCC: clear cell renal cell carcinoma, autol.: autologous, allog.: allogenic, mDC: mature dendritic cells, iDC: immature dendritic cells, BCG: Bacille Calmette Guerin, IFA: Incomplete Freunds adjuvant CP: Cyclophosphamide, CR: complete response, PR: partial response, MR: mixed response, OR: objective response, SD: stable disease, PD: progressive disease, OS.: overall survival RFS.: regression free survival, PFS: progression free survival, DFS: disease free survival.

Table 1. Immunotherapeutical studies in RCC

Apart from the tumor vaccination studies mentioned above other approaches involving the transfer of leukocytes such as adoptive T-cell transfer and even stem cell transplantation have been applied in some cases. Allogenic stem cell transplantation has been used succesfully for several decades in hematological cancers. Lymphocytes, in particular T-cells of HLA identical donors, are thought to exert a graft-vs-leukaemia effect mainly by recognition of minor histocompatibility antigens on recipient tissues (Bleakley & Riddell 2004) but probably also tumor cell specific antigens (Tykodi *et al.* 2004). The curative or graft-vs-leukaemia effect (GvL) therefore often directly correlates with the appearance of graft vs host disease (GvHD). The use of stem cell transplantation in solid tumors has been shown to provide a similiar graft-vs-tumor (GvT) effect in renal cell carcinoma, but also in ovarian (Bay *et al.* 2002) and breast cancer patients (Bishop *et al.* 2004). In the context of solid tumors non-myeloablative regimens have been preferred to avoid the substantial side effects of myeloablation with high dose chemotherapy and irradiation. Engraftment thus does not lead to complete substitution of the host's immune system but rather to a chimeric state incorperationg both the recipient's and the donor's hematological system. First studies of non-myeloablative allogenic stem cell transplantation (NST) in 17 mRCC patients showed quite promising results (Childs *et al.* 2000) with partial regression in over 50% including three patients with prolonged complete response. Further studies have been conducted (for a comprehensive overview see (Demirer *et al.* 2008)) with small patient numbers and varying response rates ranging from 0% (Rini *et al.* 2006) to more than 50% (Bregni *et al.* 2002) . However, NST is also facing several other difficulties. Besides the need for an HLA matched donor, severe and sometimes fatal complications from transplantation and subsequent GvHD can occur. Furthermore the time from treatment to response can take several months and in order to avoid graft rejection, patients have to be kept in an immunosuppressive state which allows for and might even accelerate rapid disease progression.

Adoptive T cell transfer in RCC has played a rather minor role compared to trials in other immunogenic tumors, especially in melanoma. Initial studies with isolated and *ex vivo* expanded tumor infiltrating lymphocytes (TILs) that have been reinfused into the patient usually in combination with IL-2, showed only modest response (Topalian *et al.* 1988; Kradin *et al.* 1989). In a larger phase III trial involving 160 patients with metastatic RCC, treatment with *ex vivo* expanded TILs and IL-2 showed no benefit compared to IL-2 alone (Figlin *et al.* 1999). Because of these disappointing results and because of the lack of tumor specific T-cell epitopes further use of (antigen specific) adoptive T-cell transfer has been limited although recently the usage of gammadelta T cells in RCC patients has moved into the focus of ongoing research (Bennouna *et al.* 2008; Kobayashi *et al.* 2010). In order to complete the picture of current immunotherapeutic approaches, WX-G250 (Girentuximab) has to be mentioned. This is an antibody developed by Wilex that is specifically intended for adjuvant use in non-metastatic RCC patients and is currently undergoing Phase III clinical trials (Reichert 2011). The chimeric IgG1 antibody is directed against Carbonic anhydrase 9, which is a tumor associated antigen expressed by more than 90% of clear cell renal cell carcinoma. Data from a recent Phase I/II trial of Girentuximab in combination with IFNα for metastatic RCC patients have shown good tolerability, safety and also clinical benefit (Siebels *et al.* 2011).

Considering the diversity of different immunotherapeutic approaches, especially in tumor vaccination, the question remains why many of these studies failed or showed rather limited clinical success, with only a few trials progressing to clinical phase III. In order to answer this question we will first look at the main problem of all immunotherapeutic approaches, namely the ability of a tumor to escape a directed immune response by inducing an immunosuppresive environment. In this context we will also discuss methodological deficiencies and contradictions that have contributed to clinical failure and describe more promising directions for future immunotherapy.

4. Immunosuppression and tumor escape

As mentioned above, renal cell carcinomas, like other tumors, are highly infiltrated by leukocytes and especially T cells (> 60%) mainly of the CD8+ rather than the CD4+ phenotype. Natural killer cells have also been found to be enriched within the TIL population in some studies at least whereas B cells make up only a minor subset. (Van den Hove, Van Gool et al. 1997). Infiltrating T cells are predominantly of the antigen experienced effector memory type (T_{EM}), and CD8+ cells also encompass highly differentiated T_{EMRA} effector cells (Attig *et al.* 2009). Expression of several lymphocyte activation markers such as CD69 or HLA-DR on TILs has been confirmed and oligoclonal expansion of certain TCR-Vβ regions indicates that a selection of potentially tumor specific T cells has taken place (Angevin *et al.* 1997). Furthermore, after isolation and ex vivo culture T cells are able to express cytokines and show normal cytotoxic activity. However if these TILs show functionality *ex vivo* then why are they not reactive within the tumor microenvironment? Indeed, freshly isolated uncultured TILs often show a reduced capacity of their cytotoxic function (Van den Hove, Van Gool et al. 1997) and also an impaired cytokine production or altered cytokine profile, demonstrating that some kind of immunosuppressive milieu must be present within the tumor microenvironment (Gouttefangeas *et al.* 2007). Defects in T-cell signalling and downregulation of the CD3 ζ-chain, which is necessary for TCR signal transduction into the cell, can be frequently found in T cells isolated from RCC patients (Frey & Monu 2008). Several mechanisms responsible for this locoregional immunosuppression have been discovered within the last decades and only the most important findings will be described here. Some of these mechanisms, such as the activation of T regulatory cells (T_{regs}), have been intentionally developed by evolution to counteract deleterious long term activation of an immune response in order to avoid autoimmune diseases. Others, such as the generation of inhibitory signals have been developed or rather selected within the heterogeneity of tumor cells to escape an existing immune response and thereby provide a selection advantage. Among the latter are immunosuppressive cytokines IL-10 or TGF-β, which are known to inhibit T-cell activation as well as proliferation and can also lead to downregulation of MHC class I molecules (Khong & Restifo 2002; Li *et al.* 2006). In renal cell carcinoma, proangiogenic vascular endothelial growth factor (VEGF), which acts also immunosuppressively by inhibiting DC maturation (Ohm & Carbone 2001) plays a major role because it is usually found highly overexpressed in clear cell RCCs (Rini 2005). Apart from the expression of immunosuppressive factors, tumor cells can also downregulate costimulatory molecules from their surface. Despite the fact that tumor cells are not professional APCs and therefore not supposed to prime T cells, the complete lack of costimulatory molecules such as CD80 (B7.1) or CD86 (B7.2) can lead to a decreased T-cell activation or even induction of T-cell anergy (Jung *et al.* 1999; Lang *et al.* 2000). In this context another B7 family member should be mentioned which, in contrast to the aforementioned, is often found highly upregulated in different types of cancer. B7-H1

(PDL1) is usually expressed on macrophages and provides costimulatiory function for T cells. However, due to its high abundance on tumor cells it has a predominantly negative regulatory activity. After binding to its receptor PD1 on activated T cells B7-H1 can downmodulate T cell activation and even induce apoptosis (Dong et al. 2002). B7-H1, and more recently another associate of the B7 family with a similiar function, B7-H4, have been shown to be expressed in RCC patients and their expression correlated with adverse clinical prognosis (Thompson et al. 2005).

In order to escape an already existing specific immune response, cancer cells can either escape by downregulating the antigen or even parts of the HLA presentation machinery. Indeed downregulation of HLA expression can be observed in several cancer types preferentially in late metastasized stages (Marincola et al. 2000; Campoli et al. 2002). Different mechanisms underlying this process of downregulation or even complete loss of HLA expression have been elucidated from several tumor cell lines and seem to affect nearly all parts of the antigen processing machinery (Seliger et al. 2002). To which extent HLA downregulation or loss plays a role in RCC is still controversial. Whereas some publications suggest that HLA downregulation is a frequent event (Romero et al. 2006) other more recent data could clearly show that HLA-expression is not diminished but rather upregulated in comparison to benign kidney tissue (Saenz-Lopez et al. 2010; Stickel et al. 2011).

Tumor cells can also indirectly inhibit an immune response by depriving proliferating immune cells of essential nutrients. Indoleamine-2,3-dioxygenase (IDO) is an enzyme that catalyzes the first and also rate-limiting step in the degradation of the essential amino acid tryptophane. IDO has been found to be nearly ubiquitously expressed in human tumors (Uyttenhove et al. 2003). By locally depleting tryptophane, IDO can inhibit the proliferation of TILs and also induce or recruit T_{regs} (Prendergast et al. 2009).

CD4+ CD25high FoxP3+ regulatory T cells have become a major field of investigation in immunotherapy because of their potential to induce tolerance by suppressing (tumor) antigen specific priming of T cells and also T cell effector functions (Zou 2006). T_{regs} are known to accumulate within the microenvironment of different tumors (Woo et al. 2001) and higher levels of T_{regs} in the peripheral blood of cancer patients have been detected. In RCC patients a higher frequency of T_{regs} within the tumor and periphery have been described and correlate with an adverse clinical outcome (Liotta et al. 2011). A plethora of different mechanisms have been described on how T_{regs} exert their immunosuppressive functions that range from the expression of immunosuppressive cytokines (IL 10, TGFβ)(Taylor et al. 2006), induction of IDO and B7-H4 in APCs (Fallarino et al. 2003; Sica et al. 2003), and consumption of IL-2 (von Boehmer 2005) to direct cell mediated cytotoxicity (Grossman et al. 2004). Antigen specific T_{regs} have been described (Wang et al. 2004) but after activation, the suppressive activity of CD4+ T_{regs} seems to be antigen non-specific affecting T cells of varying specificity (Thornton & Shevach 2000). Another type of immunosuppresive cells are the myeloid derived suppressor cells (MDSCs) which have recently acquired increasing attention (Kusmartsev & Vieweg 2009). MDSCs are a heterogeneous population of progenitor cells of the myeloid lineage. Under healthy conditions these cells rapidly differentiate into mature granulocytes, macrophages and also dendritic cells. However, in patients suffering from different types of cancer that include RCC (Rodriguez et al. 2009), these immature cells have been shown to strongly accumulate in peripheral blood and also

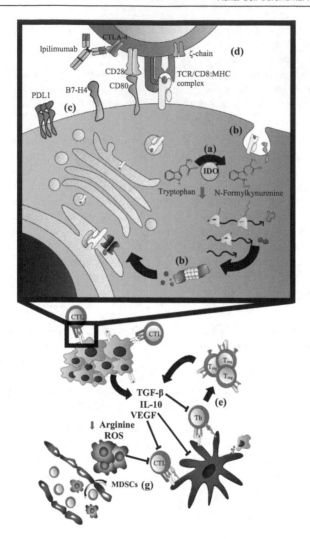

Fig. 1. Immunosuppressive Mechanisms: (a) Overexpression of Indoleamin-2.3-
dioxyngenase (IDO) leads to reduced extracellular tryptophan levels thereby inhibiting T
cell proliferation. (b) Defects in antigen presentation machinery or downregulation of MHC
molecules prevent recognition by cytotoxic lymphocytes (CTLs). (c) Aberrant expression of
PDL1 or upregulation of coinhibitory molecules B7-H4 decrease costimulation. (d)
Downregulation of T-cell receptor (TCR) ζ-chain inhibits intracellular signalling. (e)
Secretion of immunosuppressive cytokines by tumor cells or regulatory T cells (Tregs)
inhibits activation of T cells (IL-10, TGF-β) and dendritic cells (VEGF). In addition induction
of Tregs (f) from the CD4+ T helper cell (Th) population is inceased. (g) Infiltration of
myeloid derived suppressor cells (MDSCs) from the blood lead to production of reactive
oxygen species (ROS)) and enhanced arginine catabolism through arginase and iNOS
thereby further hampering T cell proliferation.

within the tumor microenvironment (Young *et al.* 1997; Nagaraj & Gabrilovich 2010) where they exert potent immunosuppressive effects. Myeloid suppressor cells seem to highly express two enzymes involved in the arginine metabolism: Arginase and inducible nitric oxid synthase (iNOS). These enzymes drive the enhanced catabolism of arginine which subsequently leads to an arginine depletion from the tumor microenvironment thereby strongly inhibiting T-cell proliferation (Ochoa *et al.* 2007; Gabrilovich & Nagaraj 2009). Higher arginase activity in PBMCs from RCC patients could indeed be demonstrated (Zea *et al.* 2005). Other mechanisms of MDSC mediated immunosuppression, such as the production of reactive oxygen species (ROS) *e.g.* peroxynitrite (Kusmartsev *et al.* 2004), the secretion of immunosuppressive cytokine TGF-β (Filipazzi *et al.* 2007) and the induction of other immune suppressive cells such as T_{regs} (Serafini *et al.* 2008) could also be observed.

Despite all these different immunosuppressive cells and the mechanisms discussed (see Figure 1), the infiltration of cancer tissue by leukocytes still remains a reliable marker for patient outcome and correlates positively with clinical prognosis in RCC patients (Pages *et al.* 2010). Galon et. al have shown that the presence and composition of the immunological infiltrate is highly predictive for clinical outcome in colon cancer patients and can even be superior to classical TNM staging (Galon *et al.* 2006).

5. Counteracting immunosuppression

In view of all these sophisticated immunosuppresive mechanisms there are doubts that we will ever be able to overcome immunosuppression and tumor escape. In order to generate a long lasting immune response which keeps the immune system up and running, tumor associated antigens ant T-cell epitopes represent only a part of the whole picture. Adjuvants are therefore urgently needed to specifically address this difficult task. Adjuvants or „Immunologist's dirty little secrets" as Janeway termed them (Janeway 1989) are an active component of most protective vaccines against infectious diseases particularly intended to enhance or modulate a specific immune response. Most of the adjuvants approved for human treatment (Alumn, MPL) were actually developed for passive vaccination of healthy patients against infectious diseases - a setting in which an enormously high safety profile of the adjuvant is clearly necessary. However, considering the highly immunosuppressive environment of late stage tumors in particular, the need for stronger immunostimulatory adjuvants has emerged even if they reduce safety and bear the risk of provoking autoimmunity. In the majority of trials involving RCC patients (Table 1) cytokines such as GM-CSF, IL-2 or IFNα have been used to ensure effective priming of T cells and enhance the immune response. Regardless of toxicity problems considering the systemic application of IL-2 and Interferon α, new studies could show that IL-2 also leads to the induction and stimulation of regulatory T cells (Brandenburg *et al.* 2008). Similarly GM-CSF has been shown to stimulate the recruitment of myeloid derived suppressor cells (Serafini *et al.* 2004) and its beneficial effect in cancer vaccination has been challenged by two randomized vaccination trials in melanoma in which patients that additionally received GM-CSF had an inferior immunologic and patient outcome (Faries *et al.* 2009; Slingluff *et al.* 2009). The use of incomplete Freund's adjuvant and BCG as adjuvants in cancer immunotherapy appears rather outdated. Nevertheless, BCG is still approved for the treatment of superficial bladder cancer. Metabolizable squalene based emulsions (MF59, AF03) and saponins (Quil-A, ISCOM, QS-2) have replaced mineral oil based formulations like Freunds adjuvant. The use of live-attenuated bacteria like BCG has been discontinued in favor of molecularly defined

TLR agonists. The discovery that toll like receptors (TLRs) constitute part of the innate immune system and can act as pattern recognition receptors (PRRs) for different pathogen associated molecular patterns (PAMPs) has boosted the search for agonistic TLR ligands. Synthetic TLR ligands can, as their natural counterparts, bind to TLRs on different cell types and subsequently lead to the activation of the cell (*e.g.* maturation, release of proinflammatory cytokines, enhanced antigen presentation or effector function). In theory a combination of different TLR agonists can be used to tailor an immune response to fit individual needs (Adams 2009). For example, TLRs 3, 7/8 and 9 have been shown to lead to the preferential activation of a Th1 response which has been known for a long time to be a prognostic factor in cancer immunotherapy correlating with favourable outcome. Several of these synthetic TLR agonists such as PolyI:C (TLR3 agonist), Resimiquimod (TLR7/8 agonist) and CpG (TLR9 agonist) are currently being evaluated in clinical trials (Adams *et al.* 2008; Cheever 2008).

Only very few studies in RCC patients have attempted to address the specific requirements needed to overcome immune escape. Some groups have used cyclophosphamide prior to or during vaccination because it is known that low doses of this chemotherapeutic drug lead to improved immune responses potentially by depleting T_{regs}. (Ghiringhelli *et al.* 2004; Lutsiak *et al.* 2005). Denileukin (Diftitox, Ontak), a recombinant fusion protein of IL-2 and diphtheria toxin has been also used successfully for the same purpose (Atchison *et al.* 2010). However some studies have described severe side effects in conjunction with Denileukin like vision loss and vascular leak syndrome (Park *et al.* 2007; Avarbock *et al.* 2008), treatment failure has also been reported (Welters *et al.* 2009). Recent studies are suggesting that pretreatment with less toxic Sunitinib might have a similar effect on regulatory T cells (Finke *et al.* 2008).

The most promising agents that are currently being developed to overcome tumor induced immunosuppression are immune modulating antibodies that inhibit immune checkpoint controls (Fife & Bluestone 2008). The first antibody with this mode of action (Ipilimumab) has just recently been approved by regulatory authorities in the US and Europe as a monotherapy for the treatment of late stage melanoma. Ipilimumab is directed against cytotoxic T-lymphocyte antigen 4 (CTLA-4), a negative immunoregulatory receptor expressed by activated T cells, in particular T_{regs}. CTLA-4 binds to costimulatory molecules (*e.g.* CD80, CD86) on APCs or tumor cells and thereby directly competes with T cell coactivating molecule CD28. However whereas signalling through CD28 is leads to T cell activation CTLA-4 signalling is rather inhibitory and promotes T cell tolerization and anergy. Blocking of CTLA-4 by Ipilimumab consequently leads to an increase in T-cell activating signals resulting in a greatly sustained activation of an immune repsonse. Considering its unspecific mechanism of action it is not surprising that among the different side effects experienced after treatment with Ipilimumab, the induction of autoimmune phenomena was also quite frequent. Nevertheless, in most cases the treatment with corticosteroids was effective and did not interfere with clinical benefit.

Based on this very recent breakthrough, several trials are currently evaluating combinations of Ipilimumab with targeted immunotherapeutic approaches in order to highlight the direction to activated T cells. Another immunomodulating antibody directed against PD1 (MDX-1106) is currently being applied in late phase clinical trials. Interaction of PD1 with its ligand B7-H1, which is broadly overexpressed on tumor cells has already been discussed as an established tumor escape mechanism.

The advent of new immunotherapies has also clearly revealed another problem regarding the kinetics and study endpoints of clinical immunotherapeutic trials (Hoos *et al.* 2010). Evaluation of clinical benefit is usually based on world health organization (WHO) (World Health Organization. 1979) or response evaluation criteria in solid tumors (RECIST) (Therasse *et al.* 2000; Eisenhauer *et al.* 2009). These are criteria that were originally developed for treatment with cytotoxic agents. However, patterns of clinical response may greatly differ in immunotherapeutic trials. Compared to chemotherapeutics, the manifestation of clinical response is often delayed in immunotherapeutic trials and develops after an initial phase of stable disease or even tumor progression. This effect is frequently observed in immunotherapeutic trials and is expressed by a delayed separation of Kaplan-Meyer survival curves (Hoos *et al.* 2010). Furthermore, a well-known discrepancy of many immunotherapies that fail to achieve clinical benefit in progression-free survival but do show an objective effect on overall survival can be explained by this effect. In order to accommodate these observations, new immune related response criteria (irRC) have been proposed and are currently being tested for their significance and applicability in immunotherapeutical trials (Wolchok *et al.* 2009).

Another question that remains in this context is the appropriate general setting of an immunotherapeutic approach. Nearly all trials mentioned in Table 1 focus on late stage patients with metastatic RCC that have often not responded to previous therapies and have acquired a resistance to cytokine treatment and targeted therapy. Some authors have suggested that this might be a rather unfavourable setting for testing the efficiency of an immunotherapeutic approach because the immune system has probably lost the battle against the cancer at a much earlier stge and immune suppressive mechanisms may have progressed to an irreversible state. The use of immunotherapies should therefore be tested preferentially in an adjuvant or minimal residual disease setting (Morse *et al.* 2005; Hoos *et al.* 2007).

6. Tumor associated antigens: the good, the bad, and the ugly

The lack of defined tumor specific antigens in RCC can already be deduced from the list of studies undertaken so far. Only few invoke defined antigens, most make use of autologous tumor tissue alone, in combination with adjuvant or after loading on dendritic cells. The use of non-defined antigens has several inherent problems however. First, the quality of the vaccine is critically dependent on the purity of the antigen and tissue material received from surgery is undoubtedly of varying quality. Furthermore, some studies have shown that only apoptotic and not necrotic cell vaccines can induce a regular immune response (Scheffer *et al.* 2003). Second, a mixture of different unknown antigens always has the potential of partially or preferentially inducing tolerogenic T cells or, even worse, inducing autoimmunity against self-antigens. Last but not least, immunomonitoring of patients, which has become a powerful tool in recent immunotherapeutic studies, can only be carried out accurately if the antigen is known in advance. Compared with full length proteins, antigenic peptides have the advantage of simple chemically defined production in GMP quality. This allows for the combination of different antigenic peptides to a multi-epitope vaccine. Thereby the individuality of a patient's immune response is taken into account, indicating that not every patient will develop an equally strong immune response against one and the same antigen. The major disadvantage of defined T-cell epitopes is that they are usually restricted to for one HLA allotype requiring the patient to match to a certain HLA in order to benefit from the treatment. This further underlines the need for the identification of additional tumor-associated antigen-derived peptides for less common HLA alleles (Klug *et al.* 2009).

How can we now decide whether an identified antigen is also a good vaccination candidate and what are the hallmarks of these antigens? The most important but often carelessly neglected requirement of any good vaccination candidate is the presence of the antigen on the tumor cell. In terms of an immunotherapy this means that the antigen needs to be accessible in order to be recognized by immune cells, preferentially T cells. At first glance this sounds trivial but in fact most studies have made use of antigens that have actually never been found to be presented by MHC molecules and instead emanated from *in vitro* tested or *in silico* predicted T cell epitopes of previously known tumor associated antigens that were shown to be overexpressed within tumor tissue at the mRNA or protein level. In doing so basic principles of immunology are ignored since T cells are not given insight into tumor cells but have to rely on a showcase of peptide antigens presented by MHC molecules. Indeed it could be shown that the gene expression level of a certain protein and presentation of corresponding protein-derived peptides only reveal a very faint correlation (Weinzierl *et al.* 2007).

The second most important requirement is the immunogenicity of the antigen. This is indeed a crucial point, since many of the tumor antigens are derived from self proteins and hence show only weak immunogenicity if at all because of central or peripheral T-cell tolerance. One great exception are unique antigens that arise from gene mutations or fusion proteins which accumulate during the course of tumor development. These neo-antigens are therefore not affected by tolerance mechanisms, either in the thymus during lymphocyte maturation by clonal deletion or in the periphery by anergy induction. Because of the large set of distinct mutations acquired within each tumor not only within different genes, but also at a multitude of locations within the gene, the application of mutated antigens in tumor vaccination will be restricted to a patient individualized approach.

Other frequently examined antigens including cancer testis or differentiation antigens show a rather restricted expression pattern that can in some cases also be considered to be tumor specific. During the course of tumorigenesis cancer cells often acquire epigenetic alterations that lead to the expression of genes (MAGE, NY-ESO-1) which are usually only transcribed during embryonic development and hence remain silenced within adult tissue. Some of these cancer testis antigens (CTA) have, however, also been found to be expressed in thymic epithelium so that central tolerance by deletion of CTA-specific T cells cannot be excluded (Gotter *et al.* 2004). Differentiation antigens are commonly expressed in malignant and normal cells of the same lineage *e.g.* Melan-A, gp100 and TRP1 in melanoma tumor tissue and benign melanocytes. In cases in which the benign tissue expressing the differentiation antigen is dispensable as, for instance, in prostate cancer patients after prostatectomy, differentiation antigens like PSA become highly specific for the tumor. The great majority of potential vaccination antigens is, however, derived from tumor antigens that are rather ubiquitously expressed but show a (high) overexpression on cancer tissue (CA9, Her2/neu, MUC1) (Kessler & Melief 2007). Differentiation and overexpressed antigens are usually subject to central and peripheral tolerance mechanisms. Self tolerance for many antigens, however is not always complete. The prior testing of T-cell immunogenicity for theses antigens is therefore absolutely essential.

Another aspect that should be considered before choosing a vaccination antigen is its impact on tumor oncogenicity. Preferentially, antigens should be targeted that are involved in the oncogenic process and hence indispensable for tumor growth and maintenance of the neoplastic state.

Based on similar but not identical criteria, a ranking of potentially suitable tumor associated antigens for clinical use has been published in an initiative from the National Cancer Institute involving different working groups in the US (Cheever *et al.* 2009). They used an analytical hiearchy process generated ranking which further included objective criteria like therapeutic functionality, the expression of the antigen within stem cells, number of patients expressing the antigen, the number of known antigen derived T-cell epitopes and also the cellular localisation of the antigen.

7. Identification of new tumor associated antigens

Having described the hallmarks of optimal tumor associated and specific antigens in the context of an anti-tumor vaccine we would now like to present state-of-the-art technology for the identification of respective antigens with a clear focus on tumor associated HLA ligands. There are several strategies which can be divided into two basic sets: Top-down approaches carried out - by directly analysing the tumor antigens present within or presented by tumor cells, and bottom-up. The latter represent a reverse approach usually starting from the gene level *via* the protein level and subsequently to the HLA ligand level.

7.1 Bottom-up

One of the first approaches developed for the large scale identification of tumor associated antigens is the serological identification of antigens by recombinant expression cloning SEREX (Sahin *et al.* 1995). The method is based on cDNA expression libraries created from tumor cell lines or tissues which are subsequently packaged into lambda-phage vectors that can be used to infect *E. coli* bacteria. During the lytic phase the production of recombinant proteins is induced and clones can be screened for the presence of tumor reactive antibodies using cancer patient sera. Selection, cloning and sequencing of antibody reacting clones allows for the straightforward molecular description of the antigen, as the recombinant proteins are located in the same *E.coli* clone plaque as the respective cDNA (Tureci *et al.* 2005). The major advantage of cDNA expression libraries is that only genes that are actually expressed within the cell/tissue of origin are incorporated and that they can be generated from various sources that include patient derived autologous tumor tissue. SEREX is still a valued, commonly used tool for antigen identification (Wang *et al.* 2009; Kiyamova *et al.* 2010). Several modifications have been incoporated to overcome restrictions for instance regarding the prokaryotic expression system, which does not allow for posttranslational modifications (Kim *et al.* 2007). With the advent of the „omics" era a comparatively high throughput analysis of differences in the gene expression level could be done with relative ease. Now large databases summarizing these data are publicly available (Edgar *et al.* 2002). New approaches aim at gaining a deeper understanding of the tumor and its genetic basis by sequencing the complete tumor genome. The whole genome approach has profited from the rapid progress in next-generation sequencing techniques over the last few years which is fortunately accompanied by decreasing costs (Wong *et al.* 2011). The complete and differential sequencing of tumor tissue and corresponding normal tissue shows alterations directly on genomic level that the tumor has acquired during its development (see Fig. 2 blue section). The subset of potential tumor antigens can be assessed by the selection of non-silent mutational events. Further reconciliation with databases of known sequence polymorphisms (dbSNP, (Smigielski *et al.* 2000)) or known mutations in cancer (COSMIC, (Bamford *et al.* 2004)) can help to distinguish tumor driver from passenger mutations.

The bottom-up approach yields proteins without any post-translational modifications. A prerequisite for successful peptide vaccination therapy is the presentation on the tumor cell surface by MHC molecules. *In silico* digestion and HLA binding prediction (Feldhahn *et al.* 2009) of the respective parts can shed light on which of these are putative tumor antigens suitable for further evaluation of immunogenicity in T-cell arrays.

A major determinant for peptide:HLA binding is the steric configuration defined by the MHC molecule and the amino acid sequence of the peptide (Bjorkman *et al.* 1987). The HLA molecule forms a peptide binding groove with prominent binding pockets for individual amino acid side chains. The polymorphism of the HLA alleles results in different polypeptides and therefore different binding pocket properties. This yields characteristic peptide sequence motifs for ligands to bind the HLA molecule. The most conserved positions in these motifs form the anchor residues, whose side chains fit best in the binding pockets for strong interaction.

With sufficient ligandome analysis that takes sequence statistics for the given peptide:HLA molecule pairs into consideration one can generate Position Specific Scoring Matrices (PSSMs). Each position holds higher scores for more frequently occurring amino acids. Summing up the scores for each position, these matrices can be used to estimate the binding capability with an HLA molecule for any given peptide sequence. The SYFPEITHI method uses PSSMs generated from naturally processed HLA ligands from the SYFPEITHI database (Rammensee *et al.* 1999) in an expert system fashion also accounting for given chemical conditions. The assumption of independent contribution of each amino acid to the overall binding affinity is one drawback of PSSM approaches. Non-linear fashion machine learning methods can create prediction models that address this issue with different techniques (support vector machine (SVM) based SVMHC (Dönnes & Kohlbacher 2006), artificial neural network (ANN) training method based NetMHC (Buus *et al.* 2003). Prediction quality for all approaches is heavily dependent on the sampling coverage for an an allele-specific HLA ligandome available (discussion of efficiency is out of scope).

There also exist prediction methods for the steps preceding peptide presentation, the proteasomal cleavage of proteins (PAProC (Nussbaum *et al.* 2001), NetChop, (Kesmir *et al.* 2002)) and the TAP transport (TAPPred, (Bhasin & Raghava 2004)). As these steps are very complex and depend on a huge variety of parameters, the results may not adequately reflect the naturally occurring process. The framework for T-cell epitope detection FRED provides easy accession to most prediction methods for MHC binding as well as creating a general infrastructure for the handling of antigen sequence data. It includes the possibility for integrated analysis of protein polymorphisms influences and simultaneous accession of different prediction methods. Analysis pipelines intended for high throughput capability profit immensely from such frameworks. They integrate different algorithms with differing input and output types and therefore provide a flexible means to implement of accelerating the analysis process.

7.2 Top-down

Until now straightforward proteomics approaches have mainly focused on the identification of serum cancer biomarkers rather than target antigens for cancer therapy (Seliger *et al.* 2003). One exception is serological proteome analysis, SERPA, a modified SEREX approach translated to the protein level. In contrast to SEREX, screening with autologous patient sera is not carried out against cDNA expression libraries but against protein lysates separated by two dimensional polyacrylamide gel electrophoresis (2D-PAGE) or directly against protein arrays (Desmetz *et al.* 2009). The comparative full proteome analysis of tumor and benign tissue usually requires the pre-separation of proteins, for example by 2D-PAGE or multidimensional liquid chromatography, due to the overall complexity of the protein lysate. This approach has in the past suffered from low sensitivity and weak reproducibility (Baggerman *et al.* 2005). Identification of tumor associated target antigens has remained rare since standard proteomics approaches often fail to detect low abundant proteins (Joshi *et al.* 2011). Nevertheless proteomics is a rapidly developing field. Taking the steadily increasing mass spectrometric sensitivity (Yates *et al.* 2009), the use of *in vitro* (*e.g.* chemical modification) or *in vivo* (*e.g.* SILAC) differential labeling approaches for quantification (Schulze & Usadel 2010) and also MALDI imaging technology (Fournier *et al.* 2008) into account, proteomics will clearly contribute to a greater extent to TAA identification in the future.

In contrast to standard proteomics, HLA ligandomics is a well established, straightforward approach and perfectly suited for the identification of tumor associated HLA ligands (Schirle *et al.* 2000). HLA molecules can be directly isolated from dissected tumors and autologous normal tissue. The method of choice is immunoaffinity chromatography using antibodies specific for different HLA molecules (see table 2) immobilised on a sepharose matrix. Application of a crude tissue lysate leads to the binding of respective HLA molecules which can be subsequently eluted by acid treatment. At the same time, pH shift also leads to the release of bound peptides from the HLA binding grooves. Due to the narrow mass range of these peptide ligands, they can be easily separated from higher molecular weight substances (>10 kDa) by ultra-filtration. Lyophilisation of the filtrate yields a mixture of different HLA derived peptides ready for concomitant separation and analysis using liquid-chromatography coupled mass spectrometry (LC-MS, see Fig. 2a).

Clone	∝HLA	Reference
W6/32	A,B,C	(Barnstable *et al.* 1978)
B1.23.2	B,C	(Rebai & Malissen 1983)
BB7.2	A2	(Parham & Brodsky 1981)
GAP-A3	A3	(Berger *et al.* 1982)
Spv-L3	DQ	(Spits *et al.* 1983)
Tü-39	DR, DQ, DP	(Maeda & Hirata 1984)
L243	DR	(Lampson & Levy 1980)
IVD-12	DQ	(Kolstad *et al.* 1987)

Table 2. HLA directed antibodies

The greates benefit is that the described procedure yields natural ligands, so that neither the proteasomal cleavage nor intracellular transport and loading onto HLA molecules has to be determined for the respective peptide. The challenge is the molecular characterisation of the heterogenous mixture of isolated peptides.

Peptide and protein sequencing can be accomplished via tandem mass spectrometry. This is an advanced technique of proteomics analysis and offers a versatile, high-throughput procedure for investigation of protein samples, including sequence identification. The measurement is conducted by recording the mass-to-charge ratio (m/z) of peptide ions with high sensitivity down to the sub-femtomole level. For better identification a second mass analyzer can be added in tandem, where molecules of selected masses are further fragmented (Roepstorff & Fohlman 1984; Johnson *et al.* 1987) and the resulting mass-to-charge ratios measured (see Table 3). Fragmentation of peptides occurs most prominently at the backbone structure, *i.e.* the peptide bonds concatenating the amino acids. The result of a tandem mass spectrometric analysis is a spectrum of fragment m/z values. The fragments containing the N-terminus of the peptide are called „b-ions" whereas those containing the C-terminus are called „y-ions", each enumerated by the number of retained amino acids. *Via* the masses of the fragments the spectra can be annotated with the peptide's sequence.

	b-ions	Mass	y-ions	Mass	
1	(S)	-	YFPEITHI	1019.5197	8
2	SY	251.1026	FPEITHI	856.4563	7
3	SYF	398.1710	PEITHI	709.3879	6
4	SYFP	495.2238	EITHI	612.3352	5
5	SYFPE	624.2664	ITHI	483.2926	4
6	SYFPEI	737.3505	THI	370.2085	3
7	SYFPEIT	838.3981	HI	269.1608	2
8	SYFPEITH	975.4571	I	132.1019	1

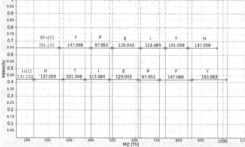

Table 3. Theoretical fragmentation spectrum of SYFPEITHI peptide.

Missing peaks make the spectrum annotation a complex problem. These are due to: technical detection thresholds, complex or incomplete fragmentation, contamination and measurement noise. This can be addressed by computational methods for mass spectrometry proteomics. Spectra can be identified by either algorithmic comparison to a database of known spectra (Eng *et al.* 1994), directly by de novo methods (Bertsch *et al.* 2009) that do not depend on databases or by comparison with a sequence database (Perkins *et al.* 1999).

The latter and in most cases very robust method infers theoretical spectra from a set of compatible sequences and matches the experimentally determined masses with those calculated. The method is robust because it is possible to infer a statistical significance evaluation, *i.e.* a score, from the size of the database as well as the number and quality of matches. Another technique to introduce robustness to the results is the use of a false discovery cut off. The introduction of a decoy database (most commonly the inverse input database) allows for calculation of a false discovery rate, defined as the number of false discoveries (from the decoy) over the number of false and correct discoveries (from both databases) given a score. A false discovery rate of 5% discerns a score within one experiment which guarantees that scores equal or better will be false discoveries only by the chance of p=0.05 (i.e. 5%).

Sophisticated methods for high throughput identification of natural HLA ligands are beginning to emerge. Established proteomics methods are specifically suited for this task. OpenMS (Sturm *et al.* 2008) is an open and flexible framework for proteomics data analysis. As explained, integrated analysis is a major advantage for high throughput oriented analysis. In the case of individualized cancer therapy, different disciplines with diverse methods come together which does not permit a comprehensive framework. One solution for maintaining high throughput capability is a tailored workflow development that integrates analysis tools of different trades. OpenMS/TOPP also comes with tools for workflow development (Kohlbacher *et al.* 2007) for virtually seamless integration of other computational aspects of immunology, such as the *in silico* prediction of HLA presented peptides or database connection and reconciliation containing very different types of data.

7.3 Validation and selection of peptide candidates

The final verification step of identified HLA ligands includes the chemical synthesis of peptides. The tandem mass spectrometric measurement of the synthesized peptide represents a crucial aspect of reliability. As fragmentation patterns define the sequence and are preserved throughout the measurements, the corresponding spectra as well as the retention time of the synthetic and identified peptide will be nearly identical. A putative T-cell epitope needs to be further validated in T-cell priming experiments. For this reason a plethora of protocols has been established to prime naive T cells usually from healthy donors with either natural (*e.g.* dendritic cells) or artificial APCs presenting the synthetic peptide. Proliferation and priming efficiency can subsequently be assayed by a variety of functional tests, *e.g.* enzyme linked immunospot technique (ELISPOT), intracellular cytokine staining (ICS) or tetramer staining.

In order to work reasonably well in a preferably diverse target group, the design of a vaccine also poses the challenge of combining several vaccination candidate peptides to a multi-epitope vaccine. Recently, Toussaint et al. (Toussaint & Kohlbacher 2009) proposed a mathematical framework for the selection of an optimal set of peptides for vaccination. Given a set of candidate epitopes, a target population, information on the respective T-cell reactivities to the peptides (or HLA binding affinities), along with other user-defined information to be incorporated in the selection process, the framework efficiently determines an optimal epitope set.

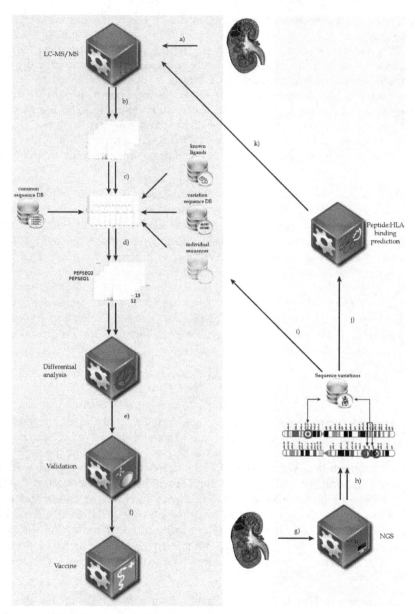

Fig. 2. The workflow for standard HLA ligandome analysis (red) and with mounted bottom-up approach methods (blue) for patient individualisation. a) sample preparation, b) MS analysis, c) peptide identification, d) FDR filter, e) differential analys f) HLA ligand validation, g) vaccine design and application, h) genome sequencing, i) variation detection, j) peptide:HLA binding prediction, k) identification of peptides with sequence variation, l) targeted search. Chromosome figures are modified from a screenshot at http://genome.ucsc.edu (Kent et al. 2002).

8. Outlook

The therapeutic situation in advanced stage renal cell carcinoma leaves much rome for improvement with frequent resistance development to TKIs and still no cure in sight. Despite the lack of convincing clinical succes, targeted immunotherapy remains a promising approach. We are only just beginning to understand the complex relationship between the tumor and the surrounding microenvironment. The sophisticated mechanisms of immune evasion that hamper an active immune response are still a major hindrance on the road to success. First steps to overcoming this are by specifically addressing immunosuppression presented through the advent of immune modulatory antibodies such as Ipilimumab. However improvement of targeted immunotherapy is also clearly dependent on the identification of new tumor associated and also specific antigens as well as HLA ligands (Stevanovic 2002). This stresses the need for concise epitope libraries comprising ligands from different tumor entities and benign tissue for various HLA alleles (Krüger et al. 2005).

8.1 Targeting the individual patient

The greatest leap forward in the struggle for a successful immunotherapy, at least from the authors' point of view are expected from a patient individualised approach. Tremendous progress in DNA sequencing during the last few years has enabled us to look at the genetic basis of each individual cancer. Comparison of somatic mutations within different tumors has shown that distinct mutational patterns are not only present between different tumor types but also between tumors of the same entity clearly underlining the need for an individualized approach (Ocana & Pandiella 2010).

Combination of whole genome sequencing with HLA ligandome analysis will in future lead to the identification of mutated tumor specific HLA ligands presented on tumor cells. The advanced utilisation of computer-aided high throughput methods enables fast and accurate identification of vaccine candidates. This demonstrates that individualised anti-tumor therapy is also feasible within a certain time frame (first vaccination estimated 5-7 weeks post surgery see Table 4).

Step	Approx. Duration	Section in Figure 2
Genome sequencing	> 2 Weeks	Blue
Ligandome analysis	1-2 weeks	Red
GMP grade peptide synthesis	>2 Weeks	Red

$$\sum \sim 6 \text{ Weeks}$$

Table 4. Current time limitations until vaccine availability

The use of mutated HLA ligands should also eliminate the need for time consuming *in vitro* T-cell immunogenicity testing since these antigens are tumor specific neoantigens and thus foreign to the immune system. Differences in the strength of an immune response towards a certain mutated peptide antigen can, however, not be excluded. Nevertheless, the probability of response failure can be greatly reduced by a combination of several mutated peptides to a multi-epitope vaccine.

Compared to other treatment strategies, immunotherapy aimed at mutated antigens does not necessarily need to target tumor driver mutations, which are usually key to oncogenic properties. Instead, any mutation specific for a certain tumor which is found to be expressed and presented by HLA molecules can be used. Thereby the amount of possible vaccination candidate peptides is greatly increased. The importance of this fact is obvious given that only 2-5 driver mutations among the 1000-10000 somatic mutations found can be unambiguously identified within each tumor (Stratton 2011).

8.2 Targeting the tumor microenvironment

Failure to eradicate cancer by targeting tumor cells exclusively has extended the focus in anticancer therapy during the last few years to include the tumor microenvironment (Kenny et al. 2007). Evidence is accumulating to confirm intense crosstalk between tumor cells and their surroundings. Tumor cells not just passively profit from nutritional factors but actively shape their own environment towards their specific needs in a process of coevolution (Polyak et al. 2009). Clear cell renal cell carcinoma are a prime example of this since they are usually hypervascularized. This is nearly always the result of a genetic defect in the hypoxia inducible factor 1 signalling cascade leading to secretion of large amounts of proangiogenic VEGF (Sufan et al. 2004). Other well established mechanisms of tumor-stroma interaction are the remodelling of the extracellular matrix by tumor-associated macrophages(Mantovani et al. 2006), the expression of stimulatory growth factors by tumor asociated fibroblasts (Bhowmick et al. 2004) and of course the attraction of immune suppressive cells (Baglole et al. 2006). The idea of targeting the cancer's „safe haven" might therefore not only deprive the tumor from its nutritional basis but hopefully also, at least in part reverse immunosuppression. Targeting the tumor stroma in RCC is already being done: tyrosine kinase inhibitors, which currently represent first line treatment for metastatic RCC, are thought to act primarily on endothelial cells, thereby inhibiting angiogenesis.

Combination therapy of TKIs together with cytokine treatment (Miller & Larkin 2009) as well as TKIs with targeted immunotherapy (Rini et al. 2011) are already being tested in clinical trials. But what about targeting the stroma directly with a specific immunotherapy? Stroma cells within tumor cells seem to differ in various aspects from their normal counterparts. Endothelial cells within the tumor show a highly fenestrated chaotic organization and often lack supportive smooth muscle cells as well as a regular basement membrane (Aird 2009). Cancer associated fibroblasts have an activated phenotype with high proliferative capacity, less growth requirements and show a high capacity to recruit endothelial progenitor cells (Orimo & Weinberg 2006; Li et al. 2007). Differences between normal and tumor stroma can also be observed on the level of gene expression (Ma et al. 2009) and are probably based on different epigenetic alterations (Hu et al. 2005). Some groups have reported that tumor associated stroma cells are also subject to clonally selected somatic mutations in tumor suppressor genes (TP53) (Kurose et al. 2002) and oncogenes (EGFR) (Weber et al. 2005) and further show a high degree of genomic instability (loss of chromosomal heterozygosity) (Moinfar et al. 2000). However these results are still controversial and might also be due to technical issues (Polyak, Haviv et al. 2009).

Nevertheless, considering the overall changes within tumor associated stroma might render these cells susceptible to an attack by different immune cells. In order to include the targeting of tumor stroma cells into an immunotherapeutic approach, immunological accessible antigens, especially HLA ligands which are exclusively expressed on tumor stroma need to be identified.

8.3 Targeting cancer stem cells

Another upcoming field in cancer therapy is based on the observation that tumor cells within some cancer types at least show a hierarchical organization which is closely resembling that of normal benign tissue. According to the cancer stem cell hypothesis only a rare population of tumor cells termed cancer stem cells (CSC) or tumor initiating cells (TIC) are ultimately responsible for initiating and driving tumor growth. CSCs share some characteristics with normal tissue stem cells including the potential of self renewal, indefinite division, slow replication rate, greatly increased DNA repair capacity and finally the ability to divide asymmetrically, thereby giving rise to new cancer stem cells and rapidly dividing more differentiated tumor cells that make up the bulk of the tumor (Wang & Dick 2005). Evidence for the existence of a tumor initiating cell population was first provided in acute myeloid leukaemia by John Dick and colleagues in the mid 90s (Lapidot *et al.* 1994; Bonnet & Dick 1997). They demonstrated that tumorigenicity of leukaemia cells was much higher in a subpopulation of CD34+CD38- tumor cells. Less than 500 cells exhibiting this particular phenotype were sufficient to engraft immunodeficient mice, whereas even a 100-fold higher number of CD34+CD38+ tumor cells, which constitute the gross of leukaemic cells, could not initiate engraftment. Even more important engraftment of isolated CD34+CD38- cells repeated the composition of the original tumor in that CD34+CD38- cells also gave rise to the major leukaemic cell population of CD34+CD38+ cells.

Several years later, the presence of a cancer stem cell population in solid tumors was shown for breast cancer (Al-Hajj *et al.* 2003). Since then, the existence of a CSC-population has been shown for many different types of cancer including brain, prostate, liver, colon and lung (for a review see (Visvader & Lindeman 2008)). In renal cell carcinoma, the existence of a CD105+ cancer stem cell population has also been postulated but final proof regarding its existence is still missing (Bussolati *et al.* 2008). The attraction of the cancer stem cell model is in part based on its ability to explain long known but still poorly understood clinical phenomena, the relapse of cancer patients after a period of tumor regression and even absence of detectable lesions. CSC are known to be highly resistant to chemo- and radiotherapy. They can remain quiescent for a prolonged period of time and then restart tumor growth at a distant site leading to metastasis. This bears a fundamental clinical impact for the treatment of cancer patients. As long as CSCs are not effectively killed by a treatment we won't be able to completely eradicate a certain tumor (Clevers 2011). Considering the resistance mechanisms to standard therapeutic approaches, immunotherapy may indeed be the only therapeutic option to directly target these cells. Therefore cancer stem cell specific antigens urgently need to be discovered and their potential for a targeted immunotherapy evaluated.

There is ample evidence that specific immunotherapy will play a very important role in the future not only in RCC but rather for the treatment of different cancer types. The first targeted immunotherapy Provenge (Sipuleucel-T) manufactured by Dendreon has just recently been approved by the FDA for the treatment of advanced prostate cancer. Provenge consists of an autologous dendritic cell vaccine loaded with a fusion protein of GM-CSF with the prostate specific antigen prostatic acid phosphatase (PAP). Although it is far too early to speak of a triumphal course of this new category of cancer treatment at least a start has been made.

9. Acknowledgements

We specially thank Lynne Yakes for expert proofreading.

10. References

Adams, S. (2009). Toll-like receptor agonists in cancer therapy. *Immunotherapy*, 1, 6, (Nov, 2009) pp. 949-964

Adams, S., et al. (2008). Immunization of malignant melanoma patients with full-length NY-ESO-1 protein using TLR7 agonist imiquimod as vaccine adjuvant. *J Immunol*, 181, 1, (Jul 1, 2008) pp. 776-784

Aird, W. C. (2009). Molecular heterogeneity of tumor endothelium. *Cell Tissue Res*, 335, 1, (Jan, 2009) pp. 271-281

Al-Hajj, M., et al. (2003). Prospective identification of tumorigenic breast cancer cells. *Proc Natl Acad Sci U S A*, 100, 7, (Apr 1, 2003) pp. 3983-3988

Angevin, E., et al. (1997). Analysis of T-cell immune response in renal cell carcinoma: polarization to type 1-like differentiation pattern, clonal T-cell expansion and tumor-specific cytotoxicity. *Int J Cancer*, 72, 3, (Jul 29, 1997) pp. 431-440

Antonia, S. J., et al. (2002). Phase I trial of a B7-1 (CD80) gene modified autologous tumor cell vaccine in combination with systemic interleukin-2 in patients with metastatic renal cell carcinoma. *J Urol*, 167, 5, (May, 2002) pp. 1995-2000

Arroyo, J. C., et al. (2004). Immune response induced in vitro by CD16- and CD16+ monocyte-derived dendritic cells in patients with metastatic renal cell carcinoma treated with dendritic cell vaccines. *J Clin Immunol*, 24, 1, (Jan, 2004) pp. 86-96

Atchison, E., et al. (2010). A pilot study of denileukin diftitox (DD) in combination with high-dose interleukin-2 (IL-2) for patients with metastatic renal cell carcinoma (RCC). *J Immunother*, 33, 7, (Sep, 2010) pp. 716-722

Attig, S., et al. (2009). Simultaneous infiltration of polyfunctional effector and suppressor T cells into renal cell carcinomas. *Cancer Res*, 69, 21, (Nov 1, 2009) pp. 8412-8419

Avarbock, A. B., et al. (2008). Lethal vascular leak syndrome after denileukin diftitox administration to a patient with cutaneous gamma/delta T-cell lymphoma and occult cirrhosis. *Am J Hematol*, 83, 7, (Jul, 2008) pp. 593-595

Avigan, D., et al. (2004). Fusion cell vaccination of patients with metastatic breast and renal cancer induces immunological and clinical responses. *Clin Cancer Res*, 10, 14, (Jul 15, 2004) pp. 4699-4708

Avigan, D. E., et al. (2007). Phase I/II study of vaccination with electrofused allogeneic dendritic cells/autologous tumor-derived cells in patients with stage IV renal cell carcinoma. *J Immunother*, 30, 7, (Oct, 2007) pp. 749-761

Azuma, T., et al. (2002). Dendritic cell immunotherapy for patients with metastatic renal cell carcinoma: University of Tokyo experience. *Int J Urol*, 9, 6, (Jun, 2002) pp. 340-346

Baggerman, G., et al. (2005). Gel-based versus gel-free proteomics: a review. *Comb Chem High Throughput Screen*, 8, 8, (Dec, 2005) pp. 669-677

Baglole, C. J., et al. (2006). More than structural cells, fibroblasts create and orchestrate the tumor microenvironment. *Immunol Invest*, 35, pp. 297-325

Bamford, S., et al. (2004). The COSMIC (Catalogue of Somatic Mutations in Cancer) database and website. *Br J Cancer*, 91, 2, (Jul, 2004) pp. 355--358

Barbuto, J. A., et al. (2004). Dendritic cell-tumor cell hybrid vaccination for metastatic cancer. *Cancer Immunol Immunother*, 53, 12, (Dec, 2004) pp. 1111-1118

Barnstable, C. J., et al. (1978). Production of monoclonal antibodies to group A erythrocytes, HLA and other human cell surface antigens-new tools for genetic analysis. *Cell*, 14, 1, (May, 1978) pp. 9-20

Bay, J. O., et al. (2002). Allogeneic hematopoietic stem cell transplantation in ovarian carcinoma: results of five patients. *Bone Marrow Transplant*, 30, 2, (Jul, 2002) pp. 95-102

Bennouna, J., et al. (2008). Phase-I study of Innacell gammadelta, an autologous cell-therapy product highly enriched in gamma9delta2 T lymphocytes, in combination with IL-2, in patients with metastatic renal cell carcinoma. *Cancer Immunol Immunother*, 57, 11, (Nov, 2008) pp. 1599-1609

Berger, A. E., et al. (1982). Monoclonal antibody to HLA-A3. *Hybridoma*, pp. 87-90

Berntsen, A., et al. (2008). Therapeutic dendritic cell vaccination of patients with metastatic renal cell carcinoma: a clinical phase 1/2 trial. *J Immunother*, 31, 8, (Oct, 2008) pp. 771-780

Bertsch, A., et al. (2009). De novo peptide sequencing by tandem MS using complementary CID and electron transfer dissociation. *Electrophoresis*, 30, 21, (Nov, 2009) pp. 3736--3747

Bhasin, M. & G. P. S. Raghava (2004). Analysis and prediction of affinity of TAP binding peptides using cascade SVM. *Protein Sci*, 13, 3, (Mar, 2004) pp. 596--607

Bhowmick, N. A., et al. (2004). Stromal fibroblasts in cancer initiation and progression. *Nature*, 432, 7015, (Nov 18, 2004) pp. 332-337

Bishop, M. R., et al. (2004). Allogeneic lymphocytes induce tumor regression of advanced metastatic breast cancer. *J Clin Oncol*, 22, 19, (Oct 1, 2004) pp. 3886-3892

Bjorkman, P. J., et al. (1987). Structure of the human class I histocompatibility antigen, HLA-A2. *Nature*, 329, 6139, (Oct, 1987) pp. 506-512

Bleakley, M. & S. R. Riddell (2004). Molecules and mechanisms of the graft-versus-leukaemia effect. *Nat Rev Cancer*, 4, 5, (May, 2004) pp. 371-380

Bleumer, I., et al. (2007). Preliminary analysis of patients with progressive renal cell carcinoma vaccinated with CA9-peptide-pulsed mature dendritic cells. *J Immunother*, 30, 1, (Jan, 2007) pp. 116-122

Bonnet, D. & J. E. Dick (1997). Human acute myeloid leukemia is organized as a hierarchy that originates from a primitive hematopoietic cell. *Nat Med*, 3, 7, (Jul, 1997) pp. 730-737

Brandenburg, S., et al. (2008). IL-2 induces in vivo suppression by CD4(+)CD25(+)Foxp3(+) regulatory T cells. *Eur J Immunol*, 38, 6, (Jun, 2008) pp. 1643-1653

Bregni, M., *et al.* (2002). Nonmyeloablative conditioning followed by hematopoietic cell allografting and donor lymphocyte infusions for patients with metastatic renal and breast cancer. *Blood*, 99, 11, (Jun 1, 2002) pp. 4234-4236

Buchner, A., *et al.* (2010). Phase 1 trial of allogeneic gene-modified tumor cell vaccine RCC-26/CD80/IL-2 in patients with metastatic renal cell carcinoma. *Hum Gene Ther*, 21, 3, (Mar, 2010) pp. 285-297

Burnet, F. M. (1967). Immunological aspects of malignant disease. *Lancet*, 1, 7501, (Jun 3, 1967) pp. 1171-1174

Bussolati, B., *et al.* (2008). Identification of a tumor-initiating stem cell population in human renal carcinomas. *FASEB J*, 22, 10, (Oct, 2008) pp. 3696-3705

Buus, S., *et al.* (2003). Sensitive quantitative predictions of peptide-MHC binding by a 'Query by Committee' artificial neural network approach. *Tissue Antigens*, 62, 5, (Nov, 2003) pp. 378--384

Campoli, M., *et al.* (2002). HLA class I antigen loss, tumor immune escape and immune selection. *Vaccine*, 20 Suppl 4, (Dec 19, 2002) pp. A40-45

Cheever, M. A. (2008). Twelve immunotherapy drugs that could cure cancers. *Immunol Rev*, 222, (Apr, 2008) pp. 357-368

Cheever, M. A., *et al.* (2009). The prioritization of cancer antigens: a national cancer institute pilot project for the acceleration of translational research. *Clin Cancer Res*, 15, 17, (Sep 1, 2009) pp. 5323-5337

Childs, R., *et al.* (2000). Regression of metastatic renal-cell carcinoma after nonmyeloablative allogeneic peripheral-blood stem-cell transplantation. *N Engl J Med*, 343, 11, (Sep 14, 2000) pp. 750-758

Clevers, H. (2011). The cancer stem cell: premises, promises and challenges. *Nat Med*, 17, 3, (Mar, 2011) pp. 313-319

Coley, W. B. (1893). The treatment of malignant tumors by repeated inoculations of erysipelas. With a report of ten original cases. *Am. J. Med. Sci.*, 105, (Jan, 1893) pp. 487-511

Dannull, J., *et al.* (2005). Enhancement of vaccine-mediated antitumor immunity in cancer patients after depletion of regulatory T cells. *J Clin Invest*, 115, 12, (Dec, 2005) pp. 3623-3633

Demirer, T., *et al.* (2008). Transplantation of allogeneic hematopoietic stem cells: an emerging treatment modality for solid tumors. *Nat Clin Pract Oncol*, 5, 5, (May, 2008) pp. 256-267

Desmetz, C., *et al.* (2009). Humoral response to cancer as a tool for biomarker discovery. *J Proteomics*, 72, 6, (Aug 20, 2009) pp. 982-988

Dillman, R., *et al.* (2004). Autologous tumor cell line-derived vaccine for patient-specific treatment of advanced renal cell carcinoma. *Cancer Biother Radiopharm*, 19, 5, (Oct, 2004) pp. 570-580

Dong, H., *et al.* (2002). Tumor-associated B7-H1 promotes T-cell apoptosis: a potential mechanism of immune evasion. *Nat Med*, 8, 8, (Aug, 2002) pp. 793-800

Dönnes, P. & O. Kohlbacher (2006). SVMHC: a server for prediction of MHC-binding peptides. *Nucleic Acids Res*, 34, Web Server issue, (Jul, 2006) pp. 194-197

Dudek, A. Z., *et al.* (2008). Autologous large multivalent immunogen vaccine in patients with metastatic melanoma and renal cell carcinoma. *Am J Clin Oncol*, 31, 2, (Apr, 2008) pp. 173-181

Edgar, R., *et al.* (2002). Gene Expression Omnibus: NCBI gene expression and hybridization array data repository. *Nucleic Acids Res*, 30, 1, (Jan 1, 2002) pp. 207-210

Ehrlich, P. (1909). Über den jetzigen Stand der Karzinomforschung. *Ned. Tijdschr. Geneeskd.*, 5, pp. 273-290

Eisenhauer, E. A., *et al.* (2009). New response evaluation criteria in solid tumours: revised RECIST guideline (version 1.1). *Eur J Cancer*, 45, 2, (Jan, 2009) pp. 228-247

Eng, J. K., *et al.* (1994). An approach to correlate tandem mass spectral data of peptides with amino acid sequences in a protein database. *Journal of the American Society for Mass Spectrometry*, 5, 11, (November, 1994) pp. 976--989

Fallarino, F., *et al.* (2003). Modulation of tryptophan catabolism by regulatory T cells. *Nat Immunol*, 4, 12, (Dec, 2003) pp. 1206-1212

Faries, M. B., *et al.* (2009). Effect of granulocyte/macrophage colony-stimulating factor on vaccination with an allogeneic whole-cell melanoma vaccine. *Clin Cancer Res*, 15, 22, (Nov 15, 2009) pp. 7029-7035

Feldhahn, M., *et al.* (2009). FRED--a framework for T-cell epitope detection. *Bioinformatics*, 25, 20, (Oct, 2009) pp. 2758--2759

Ferlay, J., *et al.* (2010). Estimates of worldwide burden of cancer in 2008: GLOBOCAN 2008. *Int J Cancer*, 127, 12, (Dec 15, 2010) pp. 2893-2917

Fife, B. T. & J. A. Bluestone (2008). Control of peripheral T-cell tolerance and autoimmunity via the CTLA-4 and PD-1 pathways. *Immunol Rev*, 224, (Aug, 2008) pp. 166-182

Figdor, C. G., *et al.* (2004). Dendritic cell immunotherapy: mapping the way. *Nat Med*, 10, 5, (May, 2004) pp. 475-480

Figlin, R. A., *et al.* (1999). Multicenter, randomized, phase III trial of CD8(+) tumor-infiltrating lymphocytes in combination with recombinant interleukin-2 in metastatic renal cell carcinoma. *J Clin Oncol*, 17, 8, (Aug, 1999) pp. 2521-2529

Filipazzi, P., *et al.* (2007). Identification of a new subset of myeloid suppressor cells in peripheral blood of melanoma patients with modulation by a granulocyte-macrophage colony-stimulation factor-based antitumor vaccine. *J Clin Oncol*, 25, 18, (Jun 20, 2007) pp. 2546-2553

Finke, J. H., *et al.* (2008). Sunitinib reverses type-1 immune suppression and decreases T-regulatory cells in renal cell carcinoma patients. *Clin Cancer Res*, 14, 20, (Oct 15, 2008) pp. 6674-6682

Fishman, M., *et al.* (2008). Phase II trial of B7-1 (CD-86) transduced, cultured autologous tumor cell vaccine plus subcutaneous interleukin-2 for treatment of stage IV renal cell carcinoma. *J Immunother*, 31, 1, (Jan, 2008) pp. 72-80

Fournier, I., *et al.* (2008). Tissue imaging using MALDI-MS: a new frontier of histopathology proteomics. *Expert Rev Proteomics*, 5, 3, (Jun, 2008) pp. 413-424

Frey, A. B. & N. Monu (2008). Signaling defects in anti-tumor T cells. *Immunol Rev*, 222, (Apr, 2008) pp. 192-205

Gabrilovich, D. I. & S. Nagaraj (2009). Myeloid-derived suppressor cells as regulators of the immune system. *Nat Rev Immunol*, 9, 3, (Mar, 2009) pp. 162-174

Galligioni, E., *et al.* (1996). Adjuvant immunotherapy treatment of renal carcinoma patients with autologous tumor cells and bacillus Calmette-Guerin: five-year results of a prospective randomized study. *Cancer*, 77, 12, (Jun 15, 1996) pp. 2560-2566

Galon, J., *et al.* (2006). Type, density, and location of immune cells within human colorectal tumors predict clinical outcome. *Science*, 313, 5795, (Sep 29, 2006) pp. 1960-1964

Ghiringhelli, F., *et al.* (2004). CD4+CD25+ regulatory T cells suppress tumor immunity but are sensitive to cyclophosphamide which allows immunotherapy of established tumors to be curative. *Eur J Immunol*, 34, 2, (Feb, 2004) pp. 336-344

Gitlitz, B. J., *et al.* (2003). A pilot trial of tumor lysate-loaded dendritic cells for the treatment of metastatic renal cell carcinoma. *J Immunother*, 26, 5, (Sep-Oct, 2003) pp. 412-419

Gotter, J., *et al.* (2004). Medullary epithelial cells of the human thymus express a highly diverse selection of tissue-specific genes colocalized in chromosomal clusters. *J Exp Med*, 199, 2, (Jan 19, 2004) pp. 155-166

Gouttefangeas, C., *et al.* (2007). Immunotherapy of renal cell carcinoma. *Cancer Immunol Immunother*, 56, 1, (Jan, 2007) pp. 117-128

Grossman, W. J., *et al.* (2004). Human T regulatory cells can use the perforin pathway to cause autologous target cell death. *Immunity*, 21, 4, (Oct, 2004) pp. 589-601

Holtl, L., *et al.* (2005). Allogeneic dendritic cell vaccination against metastatic renal cell carcinoma with or without cyclophosphamide. *Cancer Immunol Immunother*, 54, 7, (Jul, 2005) pp. 663-670

Holtl, L., *et al.* (2002). Immunotherapy of metastatic renal cell carcinoma with tumor lysate-pulsed autologous dendritic cells. *Clin Cancer Res*, 8, 11, (Nov, 2002) pp. 3369-3376

Hoos, A., *et al.* (2010). Improved endpoints for cancer immunotherapy trials. *J Natl Cancer Inst*, 102, 18, (Sep 22, 2010) pp. 1388-1397

Hoos, A., *et al.* (2010). Development of ipilimumab: contribution to a new paradigm for cancer immunotherapy. *Semin Oncol*, 37, 5, (Oct, 2010) pp. 533-546

Hoos, A., *et al.* (2007). A clinical development paradigm for cancer vaccines and related biologics. *J Immunother*, 30, 1, (Jan, 2007) pp. 1-15

Hu, M., *et al.* (2005). Distinct epigenetic changes in the stromal cells of breast cancers. *Nat Genet*, 37, 8, (Aug, 2005) pp. 899-905

Iiyama, T., *et al.* (2007). WT1 (Wilms' tumor 1) peptide immunotherapy for renal cell carcinoma. *Microbiol Immunol*, 51, 5, pp. 519-530

Janeway, C. A., Jr. (1989). Approaching the asymptote? Evolution and revolution in immunology. *Cold Spring Harb Symp Quant Biol*, 54 Pt 1, 1989) pp. 1-13

Jocham, D., *et al.* (2004). Adjuvant autologous renal tumour cell vaccine and risk of tumour progression in patients with renal-cell carcinoma after radical nephrectomy: phase III, randomised controlled trial. *Lancet*, 363, 9409, (Feb 21, 2004) pp. 594-599

Johnson, R. S., *et al.* (1987). Novel fragmentation process of peptides by collision-induced decomposition in a tandem mass spectrometer: differentiation of leucine and isoleucine. *Anal Chem*, 59, 21, (Nov, 1987) pp. 2621--2625

Jonasch, E., *et al.* (2008). Vaccination of metastatic renal cell carcinoma patients with autologous tumour-derived vitespen vaccine: clinical findings. *Br J Cancer*, 98, 8, (Apr 22, 2008) pp. 1336-1341

Joshi, S., *et al.* (2011). Oncoproteomics. *Clin Chim Acta*, 412, 3-4, (Jan 30, 2011) pp. 217-226

Jung, D., *et al.* (1999). Gene transfer of the Co-stimulatory molecules B7-1 and B7-2 enhances the immunogenicity of human renal cell carcinoma to a different extent. *Scand J Immunol,* 50, 3, (Sep, 1999) pp. 242-249

Kenny, P. A., *et al.* (2007). Targeting the tumor microenvironment. *Front Biosci,* 12, 2007) pp. 3468-3474

Kent, W. J., *et al.* (2002). The human genome browser at UCSC. *Genome Res,* 12, 6, (Jun, 2002) pp. 996--1006

Kesmir, C., *et al.* (2002). Prediction of proteasome cleavage motifs by neural networks. *Protein Eng,* 15, 4, (Apr, 2002) pp. 287-296

Kessler, J. H. & C. J. Melief (2007). Identification of T-cell epitopes for cancer immunotherapy. *Leukemia,* 21, 9, (Sep, 2007) pp. 1859-1874

Khong, H. T. & N. P. Restifo (2002). Natural selection of tumor variants in the generation of "tumor escape" phenotypes. *Nat Immunol,* 3, 11, (Nov, 2002) pp. 999-1005

Kim, J. H., *et al.* (2007). Phase I/II study of immunotherapy using autologous tumor lysate-pulsed dendritic cells in patients with metastatic renal cell carcinoma. *Clin Immunol,* 125, 3, (Dec, 2007) pp. 257-267

Kim, M. S., *et al.* (2007). Optimized serological isolation of lung-cancer-associated antigens from a yeast surface-expressed cDNA library. *J Microbiol Biotechnol,* 17, 6, (Jun, 2007) pp. 993-1001

Kiyamova, R., *et al.* (2010). Identification of tumor-associated antigens from medullary breast carcinoma by a modified SEREX approach. *Mol Biotechnol,* 46, 2, (Oct, 2010) pp. 105-112

Klug, F., *et al.* (2009). Characterization of MHC ligands for peptide based tumor vaccination. *Curr Pharm Des,* 15, 28, 2009) pp. 3221-3236

Kobayashi, H., *et al.* (2010). Complete remission of lung metastasis following adoptive immunotherapy using activated autologous gammadelta T-cells in a patient with renal cell carcinoma. *Anticancer Res,* 30, 2, (Feb, 2010) pp. 575-579

Kohlbacher, O., *et al.* (2007). TOPP--the OpenMS proteomics pipeline. *Bioinformatics,* 23, 2, (Jan, 2007) pp. e191--e197

Kolstad, A., *et al.* (1987). A human-human hybridoma antibody (TrB12) defining subgroups of HLA-DQw1 and -DQw3. *Hum Immunol,* 20, 3, (Nov, 1987) pp. 219-231

Kradin, R. L., *et al.* (1989). Tumour-infiltrating lymphocytes and interleukin-2 in treatment of advanced cancer. *Lancet,* 1, 8638, (Mar 18, 1989) pp. 577-580

Krüger, T., *et al.* (2005). Lessons to be learned from primary renal cell carcinomas: novel tumor antigens and HLA ligands for immunotherapy. *Cancer Immunol Immunother,* 54, 9, (Sep, 2005) pp. 826-836

Kurose, K., *et al.* (2002). Frequent somatic mutations in PTEN and TP53 are mutually exclusive in the stroma of breast carcinomas. *Nat Genet,* 32, 3, (Nov, 2002) pp. 355-357

Kusmartsev, S., *et al.* (2004). Antigen-specific inhibition of CD8+ T cell response by immature myeloid cells in cancer is mediated by reactive oxygen species. *J Immunol,* 172, 2, (Jan 15, 2004) pp. 989-999

Kusmartsev, S. & J. Vieweg (2009). Enhancing the efficacy of cancer vaccines in urologic oncology: new directions. *Nat Rev Urol,* 6, 10, (Oct, 2009) pp. 540-549

Lampson, L. A. & R. Levy (1980). Two populations of Ia-like molecules on a human B cell line. *J Immunol*, 125, 1, (Jul, 1980) pp. 293-299

Lang, S., *et al.* (2000). B7.1 on human carcinomas: costimulation of T cells and enhanced tumor-induced T-cell death. *Cell Immunol*, 201, 2, (May 1, 2000) pp. 132-143

Lapidot, T., *et al.* (1994). A cell initiating human acute myeloid leukaemia after transplantation into SCID mice. *Nature*, 367, 6464, (Feb 17, 1994) pp. 645-648

Lawrence, H. S., (1959). *Cellular and humoral aspects of the hypersensitive states*, P.B. Hoeber, ISBN, New York, USA

Li, H., *et al.* (2007). Tumor microenvironment: the role of the tumor stroma in cancer. *J Cell Biochem*, 101, 4, (Jul 1, 2007) pp. 805-815

Li, M. O., *et al.* (2006). Transforming growth factor-beta regulation of immune responses. *Annu Rev Immunol*, 24, pp. 99-146

Liotta, F., *et al.* (2011). Frequency of regulatory T cells in peripheral blood and in tumour-infiltrating lymphocytes correlates with poor prognosis in renal cell carcinoma. *BJU Int*, 107, 9, (May, 2011) pp. 1500-1506

Lokich, J. (1997). Spontaneous regression of metastatic renal cancer. Case report and literature review. *Am J Clin Oncol*, 20, 4, (Aug, 1997) pp. 416-418

Lutsiak, M. E., *et al.* (2005). Inhibition of CD4(+)25+ T regulatory cell function implicated in enhanced immune response by low-dose cyclophosphamide. *Blood*, 105, 7, (Apr 1, 2005) pp. 2862-2868

Ma, X. J., *et al.* (2009). Gene expression profiling of the tumor microenvironment during breast cancer progression. *Breast Cancer Res*, 11, 1, 2009) pp. R7

Maeda, H. & R. Hirata (1984). Separation of four class II molecules from DR2 and DRw6 homozygous B lymphoid cell lines. *Immunogenetics*, 20, 6, pp. 639-647

Maleckar, J. R. & L. A. Sherman (1987). The composition of the T cell receptor repertoire in nude mice. *J Immunol*, 138, 11, (Jun 1, 1987) pp. 3873-3876

Mantovani, A., *et al.* (2006). Role of tumor-associated macrophages in tumor progression and invasion. *Cancer Metastasis Rev*, 25, 3, (Sep, 2006) pp. 315-322

Marincola, F. M., *et al.* (2000). Escape of human solid tumors from T-cell recognition: molecular mechanisms and functional significance. *Adv Immunol*, 74, 2000) pp. 181-273

Marten, A., *et al.* (2002). Therapeutic vaccination against metastatic renal cell carcinoma by autologous dendritic cells: preclinical results and outcome of a first clinical phase I/II trial. *Cancer Immunol Immunother*, 51, 11-12, (Dec, 2002) pp. 637-644

Marten, A., *et al.* (2003). Allogeneic dendritic cells fused with tumor cells: preclinical results and outcome of a clinical phase I/II trial in patients with metastatic renal cell carcinoma. *Hum Gene Ther*, 14, 5, (Mar 20, 2003) pp. 483-494

Marten, A., *et al.* (2006). Telomerase-pulsed dendritic cells: preclinical results and outcome of a clinical phase I/II trial in patients with metastatic renal cell carcinoma. *Ger Med Sci*, 4, 2006) pp. Doc02

Matsumoto, A., *et al.* (2007). Immunotherapy against metastatic renal cell carcinoma with mature dendritic cells. *Int J Urol*, 14, 4, (Apr, 2007) pp. 277-283

May, M., *et al.* (2009). [Adjuvant autologous tumour cell vaccination in patients with renal cell carcinoma. Overall survival analysis with a follow-up period in excess of more than 10 years]. *Urologe A*, 48, 9, (Sep, 2009) pp. 1075-1083

Miller, R. E. & J. M. Larkin (2009). Combination systemic therapy for advanced renal cell carcinoma. *Oncologist*, 14, 12, (Dec, 2009) pp. 1218-1224

Moinfar, F., *et al.* (2000). Concurrent and independent genetic alterations in the stromal and epithelial cells of mammary carcinoma: implications for tumorigenesis. *Cancer Res*, 60, 9, (May 1, 2000) pp. 2562-2566

Moiseyenko, V. M., *et al.* (2005). Phase I/II trial of gene therapy with autologous tumor cells modified with tag7/PGRP-S gene in patients with disseminated solid tumors: miscellaneous tumors. *Ann Oncol*, 16, 1, (Jan, 2005) pp. 162-168

Morse, M. A., *et al.* (2005). Recent developments in therapeutic cancer vaccines. *Nat Clin Pract Oncol*, 2, 2, (Feb, 2005) pp. 108-113

Nagaraj, S. & D. I. Gabrilovich (2010). Myeloid-derived suppressor cells in human cancer. *Cancer J*, 16, 4, (Jul-Aug, 2010) pp. 348-353

Negrier, S., *et al.* (1998). Recombinant human interleukin-2, recombinant human interferon alfa-2a, or both in metastatic renal-cell carcinoma. Groupe Francais d'Immunotherapie. *N Engl J Med*, 338, 18, (Apr 30, 1998) pp. 1272-1278

Nussbaum, A. K., *et al.* (2001). PAProC: a prediction algorithm for proteasomal cleavages available on the WWW. *Immunogenetics*, 53, 2, (Mar, 2001) pp. 87-94

Ocana, A. & A. Pandiella (2010). Personalized therapies in the cancer "omics" era. *Mol Cancer*, 9, 2010) pp. 202

Ochoa, A. C., *et al.* (2007). Arginase, prostaglandins, and myeloid-derived suppressor cells in renal cell carcinoma. *Clin Cancer Res*, 13, 2 Pt 2, (Jan 15, 2007) pp. 721s-726s

Ohm, J. E. & D. P. Carbone (2001). VEGF as a mediator of tumor-associated immunodeficiency. *Immunol Res*, 23, 2-3, 2001) pp. 263-272

Oosterwijk-Wakka, J. C., *et al.* (2002). Vaccination of patients with metastatic renal cell carcinoma with autologous dendritic cells pulsed with autologous tumor antigens in combination with interleukin-2: a phase 1 study. *J Immunother*, 25, 6, (Nov-Dec, 2002) pp. 500-508

Orimo, A. & R. A. Weinberg (2006). Stromal fibroblasts in cancer: a novel tumor-promoting cell type. *Cell Cycle*, 5, 15, (Aug, 2006) pp. 1597-1601

Pages, F., *et al.* (2010). Immune infiltration in human tumors: a prognostic factor that should not be ignored. *Oncogene*, 29, 8, (Feb 25, 2010) pp. 1093-1102

Pandha, H. S., *et al.* (2004). Dendritic cell immunotherapy for urological cancers using cryopreserved allogeneic tumour lysate-pulsed cells: a phase I/II study. *BJU Int*, 94, 3, (Aug, 2004) pp. 412-418

Parham, P. & F. M. Brodsky (1981). Partial purification and some properties of BB7.2. A cytotoxic monoclonal antibody with specificity for HLA-A2 and a variant of HLA-A28. *Hum Immunol*, 3, 4, (Dec, 1981) pp. 277-299

Parish, C. R. (2003). Cancer immunotherapy: the past, the present and the future. *Immunol Cell Biol*, 81, 2, (Apr, 2003) pp. 106-113

Park, M., *et al.* (2007). Vision loss following denileukin diftitox treatment: a case report of possible posterior ischemic optic neuropathy. *Leuk Lymphoma*, 48, 4, (Apr, 2007) pp. 808-811

Perkins, D. N., *et al.* (1999). Probability-based protein identification by searching sequence databases using mass spectrometry data. *Electrophoresis*, 20, 18, (Dec, 1999) pp. 3551--3567

Pizza, G., *et al.* (2004). Allogeneic gene-modified tumour cells in metastatic kidney cancer. Report II. *Folia Biol (Praha)*, 50, 6, pp. 175-183

Polyak, K., *et al.* (2009). Co-evolution of tumor cells and their microenvironment. *Trends Genet*, 25, 1, (Jan, 2009) pp. 30-38

Prendergast, G. C., *et al.* (2009). IDO recruits Tregs in melanoma. *Cell Cycle*, 8, 12, (Jun 15, 2009) pp. 1818-1819

Rammensee, H., *et al.* (1999). SYFPEITHI: database for MHC ligands and peptide motifs. *Immunogenetics*, 50, 3-4, (Nov, 1999) pp. 213-219

Rebai, N. & B. Malissen (1983). Structural and genetic analyses of HLA class I molecules using monoclonal xenoantibodies. *Tissue Antigens*, 22, 2, (Aug, 1983) pp. 107-117

Reichert, J. M. (2011). Antibody-based therapeutics to watch in 2011. *MAbs*, 3, 1, (Jan-Feb, 2011) pp. 76-99

Reinhardt, C., *et al.* (2010). Results of a randomized Phase 2 study investigating multi-peptide vaccination with IMA901 in advanced renal cell carcinoma (RCC). *Proceedings of the American Society of Clinical Oncology (ASCO)*, Chicago, IL, USA, June 2010

Rini, B. I. (2005). VEGF-targeted therapy in metastatic renal cell carcinoma. *Oncologist*, 10, 3, (Mar, 2005) pp. 191-197

Rini, B. I. & M. B. Atkins (2009). Resistance to targeted therapy in renal-cell carcinoma. *Lancet Oncol*, 10, 10, (Oct, 2009) pp. 992-1000

Rini, B. I., *et al.* (2006). Adoptive immunotherapy by allogeneic stem cell transplantation for metastatic renal cell carcinoma: a CALGB intergroup phase II study. *Biol Blood Marrow Transplant*, 12, 7, (Jul, 2006) pp. 778-785

Rini, B. I., *et al.* (2011). IMA901 multi-peptide vaccine randomized INTernational phase III trial (IMPRINT): A randomized, controlled Phase III study investigating IMA901 multipeptide cancer vaccine in patients receiving sunitinib as first-line therapy for advanced/metastatic RCC, Retrieved 12 Jul 2011, Available from http://www.immatics.com/

Rodriguez, P. C., *et al.* (2009). Arginase I-producing myeloid-derived suppressor cells in renal cell carcinoma are a subpopulation of activated granulocytes. *Cancer Res*, 69, 4, (Feb 15, 2009) pp. 1553-1560

Roepstorff, P. & J. Fohlman (1984). Letter to the editors. *Biological Mass Spectrometry*, 11, 11, 1984) pp. 601--601

Romero, J. M., *et al.* (2006). Analysis of the expression of HLA class I, proinflammatory cytokines and chemokines in primary tumors from patients with localized and metastatic renal cell carcinoma. *Tissue Antigens*, 68, 4, (Oct, 2006) pp. 303-310

Saenz-Lopez, P., *et al.* (2010). Higher HLA class I expression in renal cell carcinoma than in autologous normal tissue. *Tissue Antigens*, 75, 2, (Feb, 2010) pp. 110-118

Sahin, U., *et al.* (1995). Human neoplasms elicit multiple specific immune responses in the autologous host. *Proc Natl Acad Sci U S A*, 92, 25, (Dec, 1995) pp. 11810--11813

Scheffer, S. R., *et al.* (2003). Apoptotic, but not necrotic, tumor cell vaccines induce a potent immune response in vivo. *Int J Cancer*, 103, 2, (Jan 10, 2003) pp. 205-211

Schirle, M., *et al.* (2000). Identification of tumor-associated MHC class I ligands by a novel T cell-independent approach. *Eur J Immunol*, 30, 8, (Aug, 2000) pp. 2216-2225

Schulze, W. X. & B. Usadel (2010). Quantitation in mass-spectrometry-based proteomics. *Annu Rev Plant Biol*, 61, 2010) pp. 491-516

Schwaab, T., *et al.* (2000). A randomized phase II trial comparing two different sequence combinations of autologous vaccine and human recombinant interferon gamma and human recombinant interferon alpha2B therapy in patients with metastatic renal cell carcinoma: clinical outcome and analysis of immunological parameters. *J Urol*, 163, 4, (Apr, 2000) pp. 1322-1327

Schwaab, T., *et al.* (2009). Clinical and immunologic effects of intranodal autologous tumor lysate-dendritic cell vaccine with Aldesleukin (Interleukin 2) and IFN-{alpha}2a therapy in metastatic renal cell carcinoma patients. *Clin Cancer Res*, 15, 15, (Aug 1, 2009) pp. 4986-4992

Seliger, B., *et al.* (2002). HLA class I antigen abnormalities and immune escape by malignant cells. *Semin Cancer Biol*, 12, 1, (Feb, 2002) pp. 3-13

Seliger, B., *et al.* (2003). Detection of renal cell carcinoma-associated markers via proteome- and other 'ome'-based analyses. *Brief Funct Genomic Proteomic*, 2, 3, (Oct, 2003) pp. 194-212

Serafini, P., *et al.* (2004). High-dose granulocyte-macrophage colony-stimulating factor-producing vaccines impair the immune response through the recruitment of myeloid suppressor cells. *Cancer Res*, 64, 17, (Sep 1, 2004) pp. 6337-6343

Serafini, P., *et al.* (2008). Myeloid derived suppressor cells promote cross-tolerance in B-cell lymphoma by expanding regulatory T cells. *Cancer Res*, 68, 13, (Jul 1, 2008) pp. 5439-5449

Shimizu, K., *et al.* (2001). Enhancement of tumor lysate- and peptide-pulsed dendritic cell-based vaccines by the addition of foreign helper protein. *Cancer Res*, 61, 6, (Mar 15, 2001) pp. 2618-2624

Sica, G. L., *et al.* (2003). B7-H4, a molecule of the B7 family, negatively regulates T cell immunity. *Immunity*, 18, 6, (Jun, 2003) pp. 849-861

Siebels, M., *et al.* (2011). A clinical phase I/II trial with the monoclonal antibody cG250 (RENCAREX(R)) and interferon-alpha-2a in metastatic renal cell carcinoma patients. *World J Urol*, 29, 1, (Feb, 2011) pp. 121-126

Simons, J. W. & B. Mikhak (1998). Ex-vivo gene therapy using cytokine-transduced tumor vaccines: molecular and clinical pharmacology. *Semin Oncol*, 25, 6, (Dec, 1998) pp. 661-676

Slingluff, C. L., Jr., *et al.* (2009). Effect of granulocyte/macrophage colony-stimulating factor on circulating CD8+ and CD4+ T-cell responses to a multipeptide melanoma vaccine: outcome of a multicenter randomized trial. *Clin Cancer Res*, 15, 22, (Nov 15, 2009) pp. 7036-7044

Smigielski, E. M., *et al.* (2000). dbSNP: a database of single nucleotide polymorphisms. *Nucleic Acids Res*, 28, 1, (Jan, 2000) pp. 352--355

Spits, H., *et al.* (1983). Characterization of monoclonal antibodies against cell surface molecules associated with cytotoxic activity of natural and activated killer cells and cloned CTL lines. *Hybridoma*, 2, 4, 1983) pp. 423-437

Stevanovic, S. (2002). Identification of tumour-associated T-cell epitopes for vaccine development. *Nat Rev Cancer*, 2, 7, (Jul, 2002) pp. 514-520

Stickel, J. S., *et al.* (2011). Quantification of HLA class I molecules on renal cell carcinoma using Edman degradation. *BMC Urol*, 11, pp. 1

Stratton, M. R. (2011). Exploring the genomes of cancer cells: progress and promise. *Science*, 331, 6024, (Mar 25, 2011) pp. 1553-1558

Sturm, M., *et al.* (2008). OpenMS - an open-source software framework for mass spectrometry. *BMC Bioinformatics*, 9, 2008) pp. 163

Stutman, O. (1979). Spontaneous tumors in nude mice: effect of the viable yellow gene. *Exp Cell Biol*, 47, 2, 1979) pp. 129-135

Suekane, S., *et al.* (2007). Phase I trial of personalized peptide vaccination for cytokine-refractory metastatic renal cell carcinoma patients. *Cancer Sci*, 98, 12, (Dec, 2007) pp. 1965-1968

Sufan, R. I., *et al.* (2004). The role of von Hippel-Lindau tumor suppressor protein and hypoxia in renal clear cell carcinoma. *Am J Physiol Renal Physiol*, 287, 1, (Jul, 2004) pp. F1-6

Tani, K., *et al.* (2004). Phase I study of autologous tumor vaccines transduced with the GM-CSF gene in four patients with stage IV renal cell cancer in Japan: clinical and immunological findings. *Mol Ther*, 10, 4, (Oct, 2004) pp. 799-816

Tatsugami, K., *et al.* (2008). Dendritic cell therapy in combination with interferon-alpha for the treatment of metastatic renal cell carcinoma. *Int J Urol*, 15, 8, (Aug, 2008) pp. 694-698

Taylor, A., *et al.* (2006). Mechanisms of immune suppression by interleukin-10 and transforming growth factor-beta: the role of T regulatory cells. *Immunology*, 117, 4, (Apr, 2006) pp. 433-442

Therasse, P., *et al.* (2000). New guidelines to evaluate the response to treatment in solid tumors. European Organization for Research and Treatment of Cancer, National Cancer Institute of the United States, National Cancer Institute of Canada. *J Natl Cancer Inst*, 92, 3, (Feb 2, 2000) pp. 205-216

Thompson, R. H., *et al.* (2005). Costimulatory molecule B7-H1 in primary and metastatic clear cell renal cell carcinoma. *Cancer*, 104, 10, (Nov 15, 2005) pp. 2084-2091

Thornton, A. M. & E. M. Shevach (2000). Suppressor effector function of CD4+CD25+ immunoregulatory T cells is antigen nonspecific. *J Immunol*, 164, 1, (Jan 1, 2000) pp. 183-190

Topalian, S. L., *et al.* (1988). Immunotherapy of patients with advanced cancer using tumor-infiltrating lymphocytes and recombinant interleukin-2: a pilot study. *J Clin Oncol*, 6, 5, (May, 1988) pp. 839-853

Toussaint, N. C. & O. Kohlbacher (2009). OptiTope--a web server for the selection of an optimal set of peptides for epitope-based vaccines. *Nucleic Acids Res*, 37, Web Server issue, (Jul, 2009) pp. W617--W622

Tureci, O., *et al.* (2005). Identification of tumor-associated autoantigens with SEREX. *Methods Mol Med*, 109, pp. 137-154

Tykodi, S. S., *et al.* (2004). Allogeneic hematopoietic cell transplantation for metastatic renal cell carcinoma after nonmyeloablative conditioning: toxicity, clinical response, and immunological response to minor histocompatibility antigens. *Clin Cancer Res*, 10, 23, (Dec 1, 2004) pp. 7799-7811

Uemura, H., *et al.* (2006). A phase I trial of vaccination of CA9-derived peptides for HLA-A24-positive patients with cytokine-refractory metastatic renal cell carcinoma. *Clin Cancer Res*, 12, 6, (Mar 15, 2006) pp. 1768-1775

Uyttenhove, C., *et al.* (2003). Evidence for a tumoral immune resistance mechanism based on tryptophan degradation by indoleamine 2,3-dioxygenase. *Nat Med*, 9, 10, (Oct, 2003) pp. 1269-1274

Van den Hove, L. E., *et al.* (1997). Phenotype, cytokine production and cytolytic capacity of fresh (uncultured) tumour-infiltrating T lymphocytes in human renal cell carcinoma. *Clin Exp Immunol*, 109, 3, (Sep, 1997) pp. 501-509

Visvader, J. E. & G. J. Lindeman (2008). Cancer stem cells in solid tumours: accumulating evidence and unresolved questions. *Nat Rev Cancer*, 8, 10, (Oct, 2008) pp. 755-768

von Boehmer, H. (2005). Mechanisms of suppression by suppressor T cells. *Nat Immunol*, 6, 4, (Apr, 2005) pp. 338-344

Wang, H. Y., *et al.* (2004). Tumor-specific human CD4+ regulatory T cells and their ligands: implications for immunotherapy. *Immunity*, 20, 1, (Jan, 2004) pp. 107-118

Wang, J. C. & J. E. Dick (2005). Cancer stem cells: lessons from leukemia. *Trends Cell Biol*, 15, 9, (Sep, 2005) pp. 494-501

Wang, K., *et al.* (2009). Identification of tumor-associated antigens by using SEREX in hepatocellular carcinoma. *Cancer Lett*, 281, 2, (Aug 28, 2009) pp. 144-150

Weber, F., *et al.* (2005). Variability in organ-specific EGFR mutational spectra in tumour epithelium and stroma may be the biological basis for differential responses to tyrosine kinase inhibitors. *Br J Cancer*, 92, 10, (May 23, 2005) pp. 1922-1926

Wei, Y. C., *et al.* (2007). Combined treatment of dendritoma vaccine and low-dose interleukin-2 in stage IV renal cell carcinoma patients induced clinical response: A pilot study. *Oncol Rep*, 18, 3, (Sep, 2007) pp. 665-671

Weinzierl, A. O., *et al.* (2007). Distorted relation between mRNA copy number and corresponding major histocompatibility complex ligand density on the cell surface. *Mol Cell Proteomics*, 6, 1, (Jan, 2007) pp. 102-113

Welters, M. J., *et al.* (2009). Report on the sixth annual meeting of the Association for Immunotherapy of Cancer (CIMT), May 15 and 16, 2008 in Mainz, Germany. *Cancer Immunol Immunother*, 58, 5, (May, 2009) pp. 777-787

Wierecky, J., *et al.* (2006). Immunologic and clinical responses after vaccinations with peptide-pulsed dendritic cells in metastatic renal cancer patients. *Cancer Res*, 66, 11, (Jun 1, 2006) pp. 5910-5918

Wolchok, J. D., *et al.* (2009). Guidelines for the evaluation of immune therapy activity in solid tumors: immune-related response criteria. *Clin Cancer Res*, 15, 23, (Dec 1, 2009) pp. 7412-7420

Wong, K. M., *et al.* (2011). Unraveling the Genetics of Cancer: Genome Sequencing and Beyond. *Annu Rev Genomics Hum Genet*, (Jun 2, 2011)

Woo, E. Y., *et al.* (2001). Regulatory CD4(+)CD25(+) T cells in tumors from patients with early-stage non-small cell lung cancer and late-stage ovarian cancer. *Cancer Res*, 61, 12, (Jun 15, 2001) pp. 4766-4772

Wood, C., *et al.* (2008). An adjuvant autologous therapeutic vaccine (HSPPC-96; vitespen) versus observation alone for patients at high risk of recurrence after nephrectomy for renal cell carcinoma: a multicentre, open-label, randomised phase III trial. *Lancet*, 372, 9633, (Jul 12, 2008) pp. 145-154

World Health Organization., (1979). *WHO handbook for reporting results of cancer treatment*, World Health Organization, ISBN: 9241700483, Geneva, Albany, N.Y.

Yates, J. R., *et al.* (2009). Proteomics by mass spectrometry: approaches, advances, and applications. *Annu Rev Biomed Eng*, 11, 2009) pp. 49-79

Young, M. R., *et al.* (1997). Increased recurrence and metastasis in patients whose primary head and neck squamous cell carcinomas secreted granulocyte-macrophage colony-stimulating factor and contained CD34+ natural suppressor cells. *Int J Cancer*, 74, 1, (Feb 20, 1997) pp. 69-74

Zea, A. H., *et al.* (2005). Arginase-producing myeloid suppressor cells in renal cell carcinoma patients: a mechanism of tumor evasion. *Cancer Res*, 65, 8, (Apr 15, 2005) pp. 3044-3048

Zou, W. (2006). Regulatory T cells, tumour immunity and immunotherapy. *Nat Rev Immunol*, 6, 4, (Apr, 2006) pp. 295-307

9

Oxidative Stress and Redox-Signaling in Renal Cell Cancer

Karen Block

The Veterans Health Care System, ALMD and
The University of Texas Health Science Center at San Antonio
USA

1. Introduction

Worldwide, approximately 150,000 people are diagnosed with Renal Cell Carcinoma (RCC) and 78,000 deaths are reported each year with the incidence on the rise (Jemel et al, 2010). Renal tumors are classified according to the "Heidelberg classification" where the tumors are separated based on their location within the nephron and linked to morphologic and genetic abnormalities (Schullerus et al, 1997). While most cases of RCC occur sporadically, inherited predisposition to renal cancer accounts for ~5% of cases. Hereditary and sporadic gene mutations associated with renal carcinoma include, von Hippel-Lindau *(VHL)* (Maher & Kaelin, 1997; Tory et al, 1989; Latif et al, 1993), tuberous sclerosis 2 *(TSC2)*, (Washecka & Hanna, 1991), fumarate hydratase *(FH)* (Pfaffenroth & Linehan, 2008), succinate dehydrogenase *(SDH)* (Vanharanta et al, 2004; Henderson et al, 2009; Ricketts et al, 2008), MET (Schmidt et al, 1997; Lubensky et al, 1999), and Birt-Hogg-Dube' *(BHD)* (Pavlovich et al, 2002; Khoo et al, 2001, Schmidt et al, 2001). The diverse nature of these genes and the histologically distinct tumors they give rise to implicates various mechanisms and biological pathways in renal tumorigenesis. On the cellular level, inactivation of common pathogenic pathways and mechanisms involve oxidative stress. Oxidative stress is caused by an imbalance between the production of reactive oxygen species and the cells ability to neutralize the reactive intermediates. Adverse effects occur when the excess reactive oxygen species damage a cell's lipids, protein or DNA; together contributing to genomic instability and tumorigenesis. Additionally, reactive oxygen species can serve as important upstream regulators as well as downstream mediators of action through redox-signaling. Two major sources of oxidative stress in the kidney include the Mitochondria and NAD(P)H oxidases of the Nox family. Unlike natural byproducts of mitochondrial metabolism or mitochondrial dysfunction, reactive oxygen species generated by Nox oxidases function as signaling molecules that initiate and/or modulate different regulatory pathways involved in tumorigenesis and metastasis. Clinically, efforts to target specific enzymatic sources of reactive oxygen species production, that result in alterations of signaling and metabolism, represents novel therapeutic approaches to treat renal cancer. This chapter will review the links between genes inactivated in RCC that lead to enhanced oxidative stress, mediated by different enzymatic sources, and the biological pathways activated by redox-sensitive signaling molecules involved in cell growth, cell survival, and metastasis in RCC.

2. Sources of oxidative stress in renal cancer

Renal cell carcinoma, as is the case in many cancers, demonstrate oxidative stress (Szatrowski et al, 1991). Oxidative stress is defined as an imbalance between the production of reactive oxygen species and a biological system's ability to readily detoxify the reactive intermediates (Fridovich, 1978). Oxidative stress not only causes direct and irreversible oxidative damage to macromolecules but also disrupts key redox-dependent signaling processes. Reactive oxygen species include hydrogen peroxide (H_2O_2), hydroxyl radical ($OH·$), peroxynitrite ($ONOO·$), and superoxide ($O_2−$), many of which have been detected in renal cell carcinoma (Wickramasinghe, 1975; Block et al, 2007, 2010). Intracellular generation of the superoxide anion $O_2·^-$ occurs, in part, by the semi-ubiquinone compound of the mitochondrial electron transport chain (Cadenas & Davies, 2000; Evans & Halliwell, 1999) and through NADPH-oxidases of the Nox family (Nox) (Babior, 1999; Vignais, 2002). Superoxide can interact with nitric oxide (NO) to produce peroxynitrite ($OONO·$), a very reactive intermediate. Superoxide is converted into hydrogen peroxide enzymatically by the cytosolic antioxidant, superoxide-dismutase-1 (SOD1) or the mitochondrial superoxide-dismutase-2 (SOD2) and is then converted to water by glutathione peroxidase (GPX); however, this conversion is not 100% efficient and expression and activity of SOD1 is reduced in conventional renal cell carcinoma (Sarto et al, 1999; Fukai & Ushio-Fukai, 2011). Superoxide poorly crosses biological membranes (Evans & Halliwell, 1999); however, hydrogen peroxide can easily diffuse across biological membranes and is then removed by the antioxidant, catalase. Superoxide (O_2^-) and hydrogen peroxide (H_2O_2) can react to form a highly reactive and damaging hydroxyl ($•OH$) radical, which can not diffuse from the site of generation and quickly damages surrounding macromolecules such as amino acids, carbohydrates, lipids, and nucleic acids. Oxidative damage on nuclei acids form adducts such as deoxyguanidine (8-OH-dG), which if not cleared can potentially generate mutations (Novo & Parola, 2008). 8-OH-dG is often used an intracellular marker of oxidative stress. Together, overproduction of reactive oxygen species and/or alterations of the antioxidant system are key pathological triggers of cancer. Major sources of reactive oxygen species in renal cell carcinoma are NADPH oxidases of the Nox family and mitochondria. Unlike the mitochondria, which generate reactive oxygen species as a byproduct of cellular metabolism, NADPH oxidases of the Nox family generate reactive oxygen species that modulate redox-sensitive cellular responses and are essential mediators of normal cell physiology. However, as discussed below, excessive reactive oxygen species production by an overactive NADPH oxidase system, likely mediates constitutive activation of signaling pathways involved in the initiation and progression of renal carcinogenesis. This occurs through the selective oxidation of specific signaling enzymes/proteins that are linked to processes such as activation of transcription factors, secretion of cytokines or altering signaling proteins such as protein kinases and phosphatases. Redox research is providing evidence that increased and/or sustained levels of oxidative stress play a large role in the genesis of human cancers, including renal cancer.

2.1 NAD(P)H Oxidases of the Nox family as a source of oxidative stress in renal cell carcinoma

Figure 1. NAD(P)H oxidases of the Nox family are major sources of reactive oxygen species in renal cancer. Nox oxidases have six N-terminal transmembrane regions which contain four heme-binding histidines and in the C-terminal cytosolic region, they have an FAD and a NADPH-binding domain which together catalyse the reduction of molecular oxygen, using NADPH as an electron donor, to generate superoxide, (O_2^-) which is dismutated to hydrogen peroxide (H_2O_2) by superoxide dismutase (SOD). Although these oxidases are proposed to play a role in a variety of signaling events, such as cell growth, cell survival, oxygen sensing and inflammatory processes, their *bona fide* functions and regulation, as well as molecular composition, are largely unknown. Early studies on NAD(P)H oxidases were performed in neutrophils and phagocytic cells, investigating the respiratory burst NAD(P)H oxidase system. The molecular composition of the phagocyte respiratory burst oxidase or phagocyte NAD(P)H oxidase consists of two plasma membrane-associated proteins, gp91phox (the catalytic Nox subunit, now called Nox2) and the small regulatory subunit, p22phox, which comprise flavocytochrome b558. In addition to the membrane bound components, cytosolic factors, p47phox p67phox p40phox, and the small GTPase Rac are also necessary to activate the phagocyte NAD(P)H oxidase. Upon activation, the pg91phox phagocyte Nox oxidase generates a "burst" of reactive oxygen species, which functions in immunity. Homologs of Nox2, termed Nox (for NAD(P)H oxidase) proteins have been identified in somatic cells and generate reactive oxygen species at a much lower concentration than the phagocyte Nox oxidase. To date, the Nox family comprises seven members: Nox1-5 and the dual oxidases Duox-1 and -2 (Suh et al, 1999; Royer-Pokora et al, 1986; Cheng et al, 2001; Geiszt et al, 2000; Banfi et al, 2001; Dupuy et al, 1999; Deken et al, 2000). For the purpose of this chapter, Nox isoforms will only be considered. Nox1, Nox2, and Nox4, are the NAD(P)H oxidase isoforms that are predominantly expressed in the various renal cells (Bondi et al, 2010; Gorin et al, 2003, 2005; Block et al, 2007, 2009; Eid et al, 2009). The isoform Nox4/Renox was cloned from the kidney (Geiszt et al, 2000; Shiose et al, 2001). It is a 578-amino-acid protein that exhibits 39% identity to the phagocyte Nox2 with special conservation in the six membrane-spanning regions and binding sites for NAD(P)H, flavin adenine dinucleotide (FAD), and heme, the electron transfer centers that are required to pass electrons from NAD(P)H to oxygen to form superoxide and hydrogen peroxide (Lassegue & Griendling, 2010; Bedard & Krause, 2007; Brown & Griendling 2009; Geiszt, 2006; Selemidis et al, 2008; Geiszt et al, 2000; Shiose et al, 2001). The dehydrogenase domain of Nox4 exists in a conformation that allows spontaneous transfer of electrons from NAD(P)H to FAD, suggesting the enzyme has constitutive activity that is regulated primarily at the level of its expression in response to various stimuli (Nisimoto et al, 2010). Additional evidence suggests that in the presence of certain stimuli, Nox4 activity is enhanced when bound to p22phox, but does not require cytosolic subunits that are essential to activate other Nox isoforms (Bedard et al, 2007; Geiszt, 2006; Selemidis et al, 2008; Ambasta et al, 2004; Martyn et al, 2006). The localization of Nox4 may be cell type specific and has been documented to localize to intracellular membranes of the endoplasmic reticulum, focal adhesions and nucleus (Lassegue & Griendling, 2010; Bedard et al, 2007; Brown et al, 2009; Martyn et al, 2006; Pedruzzi et al, 2004; Hilenski et al, 2004). Nox4 harbors internal sequences that are predictive of a mitochondrial targeting sequence. Indeed, in the kidney, Nox4, unlike other Nox isoforms Nox4 localizes to the mitochondria (Block et al, 2009; Kuroda et al, 2010). This finding may suggest novel cross talk of the Nox oxidases and mitochondria in renal cancer. Nox1 is expressed in renal proximal tubular cells, glomerular mesangial cells, and podocytes. Activation mechanisms for Nox1 are similar to those of Nox2 and involve complex formation with regulatory cytosolic subunits upon agonist stimulation. However, in contrast to Nox2, Nox1 primarily interacts with the p47phox homolog, NoxO1 (Nox organizer 1), the p67phox homolog, NoxA1 (Nox activator 1), and

Rac upon activation (Lassegue & Griendling, 2010; Lambeth, 2007; Bedard & Krause, 2007; Brandes & Schroder, 2008; Geiszt, 2006; Selemidis et al, 2008). The expression of Nox regulatory subunits, p22phox, p47phox and p67phox are also expressed in renal cells (Jones et al, 1995). While Nox4 and p22phox over-expression seems to be a feature of renal cancer cells, ongoing studies are addressing the mechanisms by which Nox enzymes play a causal role in the renal cancer phenotype. Nox-dependent effects on cell division, angiogenesis, cell survival, mitogen, and cytokine signaling in a subset of human cancers provide putative mechanisms by which Nox enzymes may be linked to cancer development. For example, Nox1 over-expression transforms normal fibroblasts and creates a cell that is tumorigenic in athymic mice (Suh et al, 1999). Furthermore, Nox1 triggers an angiogenic switch and converts tumors from dormant to aggressive growth (Arbiser et al, 2002). Nox4 was found to regulate growth of malignant melanoma cells and to inhibit apoptosis of pancreatic cancer cells (Mochizuki et al, 2006; Vaquero et al, 2004). Nox5 mediates growth of prostate cancer cells (Brar et al, 2003). Overexpression of p22phox in normal proximal tubular epithelial cells can activate signaling pathways known to be constitutively active in the majority of renal cancers (Block et al, 2010). Nox activity is higher in renal cell carcinoma

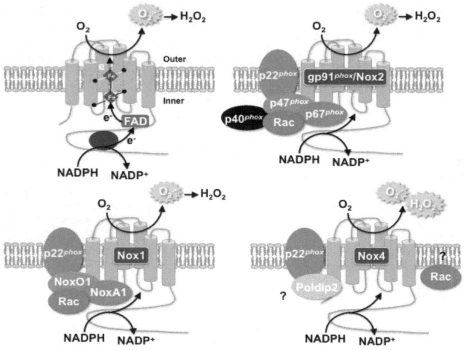

Fig. 1. Structure and molecular organization of the nicotinamide adenine dinucleotide phosphate, NAD(P)H oxidases of the Nox family. The top left panel illustrates the topology and the enzymatic reaction catalyzed by the Nox enzymes. The other panels represent the molecular structure of the different isoforms of Nox oxidases predominantly expressed in renal carcinoma cells, gp91phox/Nox2, Nox1, and Nox4. All Nox proteins can form a complex with p22phox, but the cytosolic subunits differ from the Nox oxidase isoforms. FAD, flavin adenine dinucleotide; H2O2, hydrogen peroxide; O_2^-, superoxide.

compared to normal proximal tubular epithelial cells and the expression of cytosolic SOD1 is reduced (Block et al, 2010). It has been demonstrated that superoxide is the main reactive oxygen species necessary for maintaining the expression of a critical protein involved in renal carcinogenesis, HIF-2alpha (Block et al, 2010).

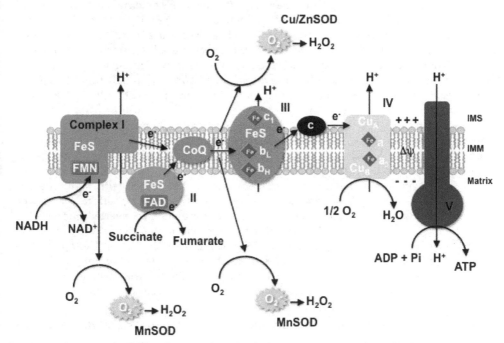

Fig. 2. Production of ROS by the mitochondrial electron-transport chain. IMS, intermembrane space; IMM, inner mitochondrial membrane; $\Delta\psi m$, mitochondrial membrane potential.

2.2 Mitochondria as a source of oxidative stress in renal cell carcinoma

Mitochondria play a central role in the generation of reactive oxygen species in cells and tissues. Aerobic energy metabolism relies on oxidative phosphorylation, a crucial process by which the oxidoreduction energy of mitochondrial electron transport is converted to the high-energy phosphate bond of ATP. During mitochondrial oxidative phosphorylation, superoxide anion and hydrogen peroxide can be formed. In normal respiratory cells, approximately 5% of electrons flowing through the electron transport chain can be diverted to form $O_2^{\cdot-}$ at the levels of complex I (NADH/ubiquinone oxidoreductase) and complex III (ubiquinol/cytochrome c oxidoreductase) (Cadenas & Davies, 2000; Halliwell et al, 1999) (**Figure 2**). $O_2^{\cdot-}$ is then converted by mitochondrial SOD (SOD2) into hydrogen peroxide (H_2O_2). Mitochondrial dysfunction, enhanced metabolism, or genetic alterations in mitochondrial DNA are potential mechanisms by which mitochondria-dependent reactive oxygen species generation is enhanced in cancer cells. Within the mitochondria, elements that are particularly vulnerable to free radicals include lipids, proteins, and mitochondrial DNA (mtDNA). Mitochondrial DNA is highly susceptible to damage because it is not protected by histones and is directly exposed to reactive oxygen species generated by the respiratory chain and DNA repair capacity is less efficient in the mitochondria. Free radical damage to mitochondrial proteins decrease their affinity for substrates or coenzymes resulting in reduced function and thus the production of more free radicals, which cause additional mitochondrial damage. Mitochondrial dysfunction is determined by a decrease in mitochondrial membrane potential and reduction of mitochondrial respiration with decreased ETC complex I and III activity while increasing mitochondrial-produced hydrogen peroxide. Tumor cells shown to exhibit mitochondrial dysfunction are those that have mutations in the tricarboxylic acid (TCA) cycle enzymes succinate dehydrogenase (SDH) or fumarate hydratase (FH). Electron microscopy of renal tumors has also demonstrated changes in the number, shape and function of mitochondria (Tickoo et al, 2000). Mitochondrial dysfunction in renal oncocytomas (BHD) are linked to mutations in subunits of complex I (Mayr et al, 2008). Additionally, chromophobe renal carcinoma exhibit abnormal mitochondria with altered cristae suggesting compromised mitochondrial function (Moreno et al, 2005). Alternatively, the production of reactive oxygen species may be altered by changes in mitochondrial metabolism. Cancer cells have enhanced expression of glucose transporters allowing increased consumption of glucose with high detectable levels of secreted lactate. This phenomenon, known as the "Warburg" effect, occurs when glucose is processed to pyruvate (via glycolysis) and pyruvate is converted into lactate in lieu of acetyl CoA (the primary intermediate of citric acid cycle) giving rise to glycolytic ATP production in the presence of oxygen (Warburg et al, 1924; Bui & Thompson, 2006; Brahimi-Horn et al, 2007). Overall, this altered metabolism, known as "tumor metabolism", mediates mitochondrial dysfunction and enhanced mitochondrial-dependent reactive oxygen species generation leading to enhanced cell growth and cell survival.

3. Gene inactivation and cellular factors that give rise to oxidative stress in RCC

Gene inactivation associated with oxidative stress

3.1 Loss of VHL

The von Hippel-Lindau gene (*VHL*) is inactivated in ~80% of renal cell carcinomas due to inherited or sporadic point mutations, deletions or promoter hypermethylation (Gnarra et al, 1994; Pfaffenroth & Linehan, 2008). Histologically, VHL-deficient tumors present as clear cell as the cytoplasm of these tumors are rich in lipids and glycogen, which provide the characteristic clear cytoplasm. Clear cell renal carcinoma is histologically the most common form of renal cancer and is likely derived from the renal tubular epithelium. The importance of VHL inactivation in renal carcinogenesis is underscored by the finding that restoration of VHL function in VHL-defective renal carcinoma cells suppresses tumor formation in nude mice (Gnarra et al, 1996; Iliopoulos et al, 1995). VHL is the substrate recognition module of an E3 ubiquitin ligase complex that contains elongin B, elongin C, Cul2, and Rbx1 (Kibel et al, 1995; Kamura et al, 1999). This complex targets the alpha subunits of the heterodimeric transcription factor HIF (hypoxia-inducible factor) for polyubiquitination and proteasomal degradation. Cells lacking wild-type VHL fail to degrade HIF-alpha subunits, thus hypoxia-inducible gene products are constitutively overproduced. Loss of VHL, and clear cell renal carcinoma in general, are associated with enhanced oxidative stress, mediated in large part by Nox oxidases. Nox-dependent superoxide generation is higher in cultured VHL-deficient

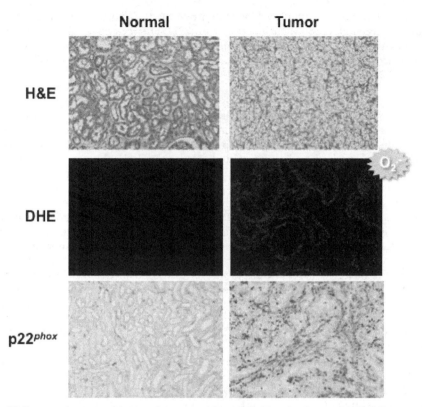

Fig. 3. p22*phox* protein expression and superoxide production is elevated in RCC tumors compared to normal adjacent renal tissue. Adapted from Block et al, 2010. *Top panel*, H&E staining. *Middle panel*, Detection of superoxide (O_2^-) in frozen 30-um–thick RCC sections, with dihydroethidium (DHE). *Bottom panel*, p22phox was detected by immunoperoxidase staining.

RCC cells compared to normal epithelial cells, mediated through p22phox-based Nox oxidases, **Figure 3**, (Block et al, 2007, 2010). p22phox protein expression, the Nox regulatory subunit necessary for Nox4 and Nox1 activation, is higher in VHL-deficient cultured renal cancer cells and in human renal tumors compared to normal controls (Block et al, 2007, 2010). Although the mechanism has not been fully defined, p22phox is an ubiquitinated protein and can associate with the von Hippel-Lindau protein *in vivo*, suggesting that p22phox-based Nox oxidase complexes may be stabilized upon the loss of the tumor suppressor protein, von Hippel-Lindau (pVHL). The Nox catalytic subunit, Nox4 is also overexpressed in VHL-deficient cells and in a subset of human RCCs at the mRNA and protein level (Maranchie & Zhan, 2005; Block et al, 2007, 2010). Although the mechanisms remain unclear, the Nox4 promoter harbors hypoxia responsive elements (HRE) known to be transcriptionally activated by HIFs (Diebold et al, 2010). Nox1 is expressed in renal tubular epithelial cells and is overexpressed in a subset of human RCC tumors compared to normal adjacent tissue (Block, 2010). Nox1 play a role in Nox-dependent reactive oxygen species and the genesis of RCC. Finally, it is clear in other cell types that Nox subunits and

Nox-derived ROS can be upregulated/activated by growth factors (Gorin et al, 2005; Bondi et al, 2010; Meng et al, 2008; Michaeloudes et al, 2011; Sturrock et al, 2006). Although the role of growth factor-induced Nox expression has not been explored, it is likely an alternative mechanism for enhanced Nox-derived reactive oxygen species in RCC.

3.2 TSC2

Tuberous sclerosis complex (TSC) is a multi-system genetic disease that causes tumors to form in several different organs, primarily in the kidney, brain, eyes, heart, skin and lungs. Tuberous sclerosis complex, like von Hippel–Lindau disease, are autosomal dominant tumor suppressor syndromes that can exhibit similar renal phenotypes and seem to share some signaling pathway components. TSC is caused by mutations in either the *TSC1* gene, located on chromosome 9 (Slegtenhorst et al, 1997) or the *TSC2* gene, located on chromosome 16 (European Chromosome 16 Tuberous Sclerosis Consortium, 1993). The TSC complex integrates cellular signaling inputs such as growth factors and cellular energy supply and regulates cell growth, proliferation, and survival. *TSC1* encodes hamartin and *TSC2* encodes tuberin, which form a heterodimer that inhibit mammalian target of rapamycin (mTOR) activity. mTOR is a key upstream regulator of protein synthesis activated in the majority of renal cancers and is discussed in detail below. Mutations in *TSC1* or *TSC2* genes give rise to tumors exhibiting increased phosphorylation of mTOR substrates and readouts of active mRNA translation, p70S6 kinase and 4E-BP1. Inactivation of TSC1/2 results in HIF accumulation through increased HIF mRNA translation by activated mTOR signaling. Rodent models harboring heterozygous mutations in the TSC2 gene develop spontaneous RCC, due to loss of heterozygosity (LOH). Kidneys of TSC2-/- rats demonstrate higher levels of the oxidative stress marker, 8-oxo-dG. In humans, between 60 and 80% of TSC patients have benign renal tumors called angiomyolipomas (AML) (Crino et al, 2006). These tumors are composed of vascular tissue (angio-), smooth muscle (– myo–), and fat (–lipoma). The discrepancy of benign and malignant TSC2-deficient tumors in the human and rodent disease respectively is unclear. In human AMLs, upregulation of the tumor suppressor phosphatase and tensin homolog (PTEN) by HIF-1 alpha was demonstrated to reduce Akt activation suggesting that PTEN may safeguard against developing malignant tumors in patients with TSC deficiency (Mahimainathan et al, 2009). A minority of TSC patients progress to renal cell carcinoma. Although the mechanisms remain unclear, oxidative stress may play a role. The DNA lesion caused by oxidative stress, 8-oxoguanine (8-oxy-dG), is normally excised and repaired by 8-oxoguanine DNA glycosylase 1 (hOGG1), which localizes in the nucleus and the mitochondria. Down regulation of OGG1 has also been linked to TSC-deficiency (Habib et al, 2008, 2009). Alternatively, *OGG1* is located on a chromosome region often demonstrating LOH, 3p25-26 in renal cell carcinoma (Gokden et al, 2008). Although genetic mutations in *TSC2* have not been detected in conventional clear cell renal carcinoma, Nox-dependent reactive oxygen species generation has been identified to post-translationally inactivate tuberin (Block et al, 2010). Taken together, reactive oxygen species may play a role in TSC inactivation, downregulation of OGG and DNA and lipid damage.

3.3 Tricarboxylic acid (Krebs) cycle genes, fumarate hydratase (FH)/succinate dehyrdogenase (SDH)

The tricarboxylic acid (TCA)/Krebs cycle is part of a metabolic pathway coupled to mitochondrial oxidative phosphorylation that converts nutrients to energy in aerobic cells.

The fumarate hydratase (*FH*) and succinate dehydrogenase (*SDH*) genes encode mitochondrial TCA cycle enzymes that play an essential role in energy production by catalyzing the conversion of fumarate to malate and succinate to fumarate respectively. Individuals who harbor germline mutations in either of these TCA cycle enzymes have an increased risk for developing renal tumors. Mutations in fumarate hydratase *(FH)* gene give rise to a rare form of hereditary leiomyomatosis and renal cell carcinoma (HLRCC). Renal tumors arising from genetic loss of FH range from type 2 papillary to tubulo-papillary to collecting-duct carcinomas. These tumors have significantly impaired oxidative phosphorylation and thus demonstrate aerobic glycolysis (Warburg effect) and are aggressive (Warburg et al, 1924). Positron emission tomography (PET) imaging demonstrates high glucose uptake in FH-deficient renal tumors lead to enhanced reactive oxygen species, mediated by a p47phox-based Nox oxidase, suggesting a role for the Nox oxidase isoform, Nox1 or Nox2 (Sudarshan, 2009). There is no evidence of genetic mutations in *FH* in sporadic conventional renal cell carcinoma; however, it has been demonstrated that mRNA and protein levels of FH are reduced in clear cell renal carcinoma (Sudarshan et al, 2011). Reduced levels of fumarate hydratase in clear cell renal carcinoma is associated with stabilized HIF-2alpha levels, likely mediated through an Akt-dependent mRNA translational pathway (Sudarshan et al, 2011). Additionally, overexpression of FH in VHL-deficient cells reduced cell invasion, suggesting that reduced levels of FH play a role in metastasis in clear cell renal carcinoma. Succinate dehydrogenase, SDH (complex II) is a functional member of both the Krebs cycle and the aerobic respiratory chain. Complex II couples the oxidation of succinate to fumarate in the mitochondrial matrix with the reduction of ubiquinone in the membrane (Cecchini et al, 2002). Mutations of the nuclear encoded genes of the mitochondrial oxidative phosphorylation complex, succinate dehyrdogenase B gene (SDHB) are associated with renal cell carcinoma (Vanharanta et al, 2004; Henderson et al, 2009; Ricketts et al, 2008). There is no detectable enhanced reactive oxygen species production in SDH mutated cells (Pollard & Tomlinson, 2005; King et al, 2006).

Cellular factors associated with oxidative stress

3.4 Hypoxia

Solid tumors exhibit intratumor hypoxic states, where regions of low oxygen (hypoxia) and necrosis is common Semenza, 2002; Maxwell et al, 1997). Hypoxia sensing and related signaling events, including activation of hypoxia-inducible factor 1 (HIF-1) now suggest that NAD(P)H oxidases, Nox1 and Nox4 serve as oxygen sensors. The human Nox4 promoter harbors putative hypoxia responsive element (HRE), which binds hypoxia-inducible factor-1 alpha (HIF-1a) (Diebold et al, 2010). Similarly, Nox1 mRNA and protein expression is enhanced in lung cells exposed to hypoxia (Goyal et al, 2004). Hypoxia-induced activation of Nox1-dependent reactive oxygen species generation was necessary for activation of HIF-1-dependent gene expression, which was blocked by the anti-oxidant, catalase (Goyal et al, 2004). In support of these conclusions, Nox1 and Nox4 are increased by chronic exposure of mice to hypoxia (Mittal et al, 2007). In RCC, the biological significance of hypoxia-induced Nox4 and Nox1 is unclear but may mediate HIF- and NF-kB-dependent signaling. In endothelial cells exposed to hypoxic conditions, superoxide is formed at the ubisemiquinone site of complex III in the mitochondria (Chandel et al, 2000). However, it is unclear if mitochondria participate in hypoxia-induced reactive oxygen species generation in renal cell carcinoma.

3.5 Growth factors

Stabilization of HIF-alpha binds to the HIF-beta subunit (ARNT) and the dimer translocates to the nucleus and binds to HIF-responsive elements, HREs (core sequence of 5'-RCGTG-3' in the enhancer elements of target genes) which drives the transcriptional activation of over a hundred genes that support renal carcinogenesis including, but limited to, vascular endothelial growth factor (VEGF) and platelet-derived growth factor-beta (PDGF-b), implicated in angiogenesis and transforming growth factor alpha (TGF-a), which can establish a mitogenic autocrine loop with the epidermal growth factor (EGF) receptor (EGFR) (Knebelmann et al, 1998; Maxwell & van den Berg, 1999; de Paulsen et al, 2001) in renal epithelial cells. The growth factors bind to their respective receptors (VEGF-R, PDGF-R and EGF-R), which are each tyrosine kinase receptors. Growth factor-induced redox signaling by Nox oxidases is well established and involves several redox-sensitive steps. Activation of signaling pathways, mediated by the aforementioned tyrosine kinases, requires inactivation of a large family of enzymes that dephosphorylate tyrosine residues, protein tyrosine phosphatases (PTPs). All PTPs contain an essential cysteine residue, which is highly susceptible to oxidation by reactive oxygen species, especially by hydrogen peroxide, leading to reversible inhibition (Rhee et al, 2003; Chiarugi & Cirri, 2003; Lee et al, 1998). By inhibiting the activity of PTPs, NADPH oxidase derived reactive oxygen species can affect the activity of tyrosine kinase signaling pathways. For example, Nox4 has been implicated in modulating PDGF-induced cell growth, VEGF-induced angiogenic responses, insulin induced glucose uptake, and insulin-like growth factor-1-induced antiapoptotic effects, although in different types of cells (Mahadev et al, 2004; Datla et al, 2007; Wagner et al, 2007). Another kinase activated in the majority of RCCs is the phosphatidylinositol 3-kinase (PI3K). PI3K signaling is regulated by the tumor suppressor phosphatase and tensin

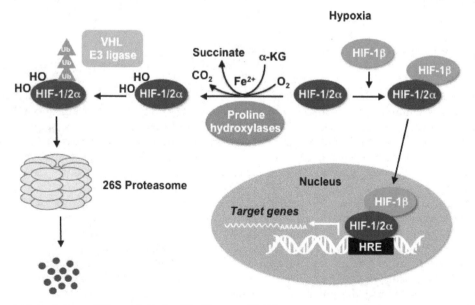

Fig. 4. Regulation of Hypoxia Inducible Factors (HIFs).

homolog (PTEN). PTEN dephosphorylates phosphatidylinositol 3,4,5-triphosphate, a product of the PI3 kinase (PI3K) reaction. In various cell types, overexpression of the Nox catalytic subunit, Nox1, potentiates PIP3 generation and activation of the protein kinase Akt induced by EGF, PDGF, and insulin as a result of hydrogen peroxide-dependent oxidation of essential cysteine residue of PTEN (Cho et al, 2004; Mahadev et al, 2004). Mutations in PTEN, although common in a number of cancers, are not commonly detected in RCC. However, reactive oxygen species -induced inactivation of PTEN has not been examined in RCC.

4. Redox-signaling in renal cancer

4.1 Redox regulation of hypoxia inducible factors (HIFs)

A common endpoint in the majority of RCC, independent of histological type, is the stabilization of HIF-alpha subunits through multi-step processes regulated at several levels by redox-sensitive pathways. HIF-alpha contains two highly conserved proline residues, located at the NH2-terminus in the oxygen-dependent degradation domains (ODDs), which are modified by a family of 4-prolyl hydroxylases (Epstein et al, 2001; Bruick & McKnight, 2001). Proline hydroxylases (PHDs) catalyze the hydroxylation reaction, which requires oxygen and 2-oxoglutarate (2-OG) as substrates and iron and ascorbate as cofactors. Proline hydroxylation promotes HIF-alpha binding to the multimeric VHL E3 ubiquitin ligase complex (Kamura et al, 1999). When hydroxylated and bound to VHL, HIF-alpha is polyubiquitinated and targeted for regulated protein degradation through the 26S proteasome (Jaakkola et al, 2001; Maxwell et al, 1999). HIF-alpha can also be hydroxylated at the COOH-terminus by asparaginyl hydroxylases which are Fe(II)- and 2-oxoglutarate (2-OG)–dependent family of dioxygenases (Masson & Ratcliffe 2003; Lando et al, 2002). Asparagine hydroxylation silences the COOH-terminal transactivation domains of HIF-alpha by preventing their interaction with the p300/CBP coactivator (Mahon et al, 2001). Reactive oxygen species inhibit PHD activity by oxidizing the PHD cofactors ferrous iron (Fe2+) to Fe3+ (Gerald et al, 2004). In solid VHL-competent tumors (hypoxic conditions), where mTOR is inactivated, reactive oxygen species are enhanced, likely stabilizing HIF-alpha subunits by inactivation of PHDs. Inactivation or loss of Fumarate Hydratase (FH) or Succinate dehydrogenase (SDH) can also lead to the inactivation of PHDs through different mechanisms. In FH-deficient cells, fumarate can competitively inhibit 2-OG-dependent HIF-hydroxylation resulting in the escape of VHL-dependent degradation (O'Flaherty et al, 2010), providing a VHL independent mechanism for dysregulation of HIF expression. Mutations in the Succinate dehydrogenase (SDH) gene promote the accumulation of succinate. Succinate is one of the end products of prolyl hydroxylase activity. Thus, succinate accumulation can block proly hydroxylase function and cause an accumulation of HIF-alpha (Pollard et al, 2005). In summary, loss of FH or SDH plays a role in HIF-alpha stabilization through inhibition of PHDs through metabolites and likely not through reactive oxygen species. Whereas, when VHL is mutated, expression of HIF-alpha subunits is maintained through Nox-dependent redox-sensitive pathways that mediate ongoing mRNA translation, discussed below (Block et al, 2007).

4.2 Redox regulation of PI3K-Akt signaling

The PI3K/Akt/mTOR signaling pathway is activated in the majority of renal cell carcinomas and mediates biological outputs such as cell growth, cell proliferation, metabolism, and cell survival (Manning & Cantley, 2007; Porta & Figlin, 2009). The PtdIns(3,4,5)P3 phosphatase PTEN that blocks PI3-kinase signaling is mutated in ~30% of renal cell carcinomas. Reactive oxygen species -dependent inactivation of PTEN in renal cell carcinoma has not been studied, but likely to occur. When PI3-kinase is activated, protein kinase B (Akt) and phosphoinositide-dependent protein kinase 1 (PDK1) translocate to the membrane and binds to PtdIns(3,4,5)P3 and PtdIns(3,4)P2 through the pleckstrin domain (Franke et al, 1997). The colocalization of activated PDK1 and Akt allows Akt to be phosphorylated by PDK1 on threonine 308, leading to partial activation of Akt. Full activation of Akt occurs upon phosphorylation of serine 473 by a Rictor-associated mTORC2 complex (see below). There are three isoforms of serine/threonine Akt in humans; Akt1, Akt2, and Akt3. In renal cell carcinoma, the Akt2 isoform maintains HIF-alpha expression in the absence of VHL (Toschi et al, 2008). The PI3K/Akt signaling pathway is regulated by reactive oxygen species produced by p22phox-based Nox oxidases (Block et al, 2007). Furthermore, the catalytic subunit implicated in reactive oxygen species-dependent Akt activation appears to be Nox1 and Nox4 (Block et al, 2007). Treatment of renal carcinoma cells with the PI3K inhibitor, LY29002 or wortmannin has no effect on Nox activity, suggesting Nox-derived reactive oxygen species act as an upstream regulator of PI3K/Akt signaling cascade (Block et al, 2007).

4.3 Redox regulation of mTOR signaling

Translational control of existing mRNAs allows for quick changes in cellular concentrations of encoded proteins. Regulation of the rate of translation is complex and occurs at several steps. One major step of translational regulation occurs at the cap-recognition stage. This is controlled by the formation of the eIF4F complex, which include the cap-binding factor eukaryotic translation initiation factor 4E, eIF4E, and its binding partners, eIF4G and the RNA helicase, eIF4A. Binding of eIF4F complex to the mRNA cap structure is inhibited by eIF4E- binding protein 1, 4E-BP1 (Gingras et al, 2004). 4E-BP1 competes with eIF4G for a common binding site within eIF4E (Marcotrigiano et al, 1999). Therefore, when eIF4E is bound to 4E-BP1, cap-dependent translation is inhibited. Release of 4E-BP1 from heterdimerization with eIF4E is regulated by mammalian target of rapamycin (mTOR)-dependent phosphorylation of 4E-BP1. Activation of mTOR is controlled by upstream kinases known to be constitutively active in most renal cancers, the PI3K/Akt- and the RAS/MAPK-signaling pathways. The regulation of the PI3K/Akt/mTOR signaling is redox-sensitive and is regulated by p22phox-based Nox oxidases (Block et al, 2007, 2009). The Nox catalytic isoforms, Nox1 and Nox4 play an important role in stabilizing/maintaining HIF-alpha protein expression in the absence of VHL through an Akt-mTOR signaling mRNA translational pathway. As previously discussed, activation of Akt signaling is likely mediated, in part, through inactivation of the PI3K-dependent phosphatase, PTEN. The hamartin/tuberin (TSC1/TSC2) complex is an upstream negative regulator of mammalian target of rapamycin complex 1 (mTORC1). Activation of Akt leads to Akt-mediated phosphorylation of TSC2 at amino acid, T1462, which leads to TSC2 dissociation from TSC1 and is targeted for regulated protein degradation through the 26S proteasome (Plas & Thompson, 2003). Post-translational inactivation of tuberin/TCS2 has been identified in conventional clear cell renal carcinoma, which exhibits hyperactive Akt signaling (Block et al, 2010). In cultured and human RCC where p22phox and Nox-derived reactive oxygen species are high, protein expression of TSC2 is significantly reduced due to

Akt-dependent phosphorylation and degradation. Activation of mTOR, in turn, phosphorylates, several substrates necessary to activate mRNA translation. Phosphorylation of 4E-BP1 results in its dissociation from eIF4E. mTOR-dependent phosphorylation of S6K leads to its activation and downstream phosphorylation of other proteins, which collectively affect translation initiation and elongation (Holz et al, 2005; Yang et al, 2003). The RAS/MAPK pathway mediates translation by phosphorylation of translational elongation factors, including eIF4E. eIF4E is a bonafide oncogene, that when activated, through phosphorylation, inhibits its binding to the translational repressor 4E-BP1 leading to aberrant and unregulated ongoing mRNA translation of oncogenes (Mamane et al, 2004). Therefore, eIF4E is considered an oncogene involved in cell cycle progression, cell transformation, and cell survival. Misregulation of mRNA translation and constitutive activation of mTOR contributes to renal cancer. mTOR is the catalytic subunit of two distinct complexes, mTOR complex 1 (mTORC1) and mTORC2. mTORC1 and mTORC2 are part of a multimeric complex commonly referred to as the Raptor-associated mTORC1 (Rapamycin sensitive), and Rictor-associated mTORC2 (rapamycin-insensitive). Raptor and Rictor are scaffolding proteins within each complex allowing the assembly of other proteins. mTORC1 complex consists of mTOR, Raptor, mammalian LST8/G-protein β-subunit like protein (mLST8/GβL), PRAS40 and Deptor (Kim et al, 2002, 2003; Harris & Lawrence, 2003). mTORC2 complex consists of mTOR, Rictor, GβL, and mammalian stress-activated protein kinase interacting protein 1 (mSIN1) (Sarbassov et al, 2004, 2005; Frias et al, 2006), Protor and Deptor. Unlike mTORC1, the regulation and downstream substrates of mTORC2 are less understood. mTORC2 phosphorylates AGC kinases such as the serine/threonine protein kinase Akt, at the hydrophobic motif (HM) site, Ser473 in the presence of growth factors, which is enhanced by PI3K activity. Rapamycin, a natural inhibitor of mTOR signaling, binds the FK506-binding protein (FKBP12) and, in turn, rapamycin–FKBP12 binds mTOR inhibiting phosphorylation of raptor-associated mTOR (mTORC1) substrates, but not rictor-associated mTOR (mTORC2) substrates. Prolonged treatment and higher dosage of rapamycin has been reported to inhibit mTORC2 in a subset of cell lines. Rapamycin analogues (mTORC1 inhibitors) have been utilized for the treatment for RCC. Despite initial excitement, objective response rates to these drugs remain low. One reason for rapamycin resistance of RCC may be due to absent and/or incomplete mTORC2 inhibition. In support of these clinical findings, *in vitro* studies have demonstrated that shRNA-mediated knockdown of Rictor (TORC2 complex) but not Raptor (TORC1 complex) reduces HIF-2alpha protein expression, suggesting TORC2 signals through yet unidentified pathways involved in mRNA translation to maintain HIF-2alpha protein expression (Toschi et al, 2008). A role for mTORC2 in mRNA translation is now becoming evident. mTORC2 complex has been found to associate with ribosomes in a PI3K-dependent manner and phosphorylates nascent Akt at the turn motif (TM; Thr450) site, which is not inducible by growth factors (Oh et al, 2010). In cancer cells, including renal cancer, where PI3K is constitutively active, mTORC2 binding to the ribosomes is enhanced. Additionally, it has been demonstrated that treatment of some cancer cell lines with rapamycin and rapalogs increase Akt and eIF4E phosphorylation involving PI3K and Mnk kinases (Wang et al, 2007, 2008). Importantly, cultured VHL-deficient cell lines and RCC cell lines cultured from patient tumors exhibit this phenomenon. Together, this provides an alternative mechanism for rapamycin resistance of RCC and may explain why so few patients respond to rapalog therapy.

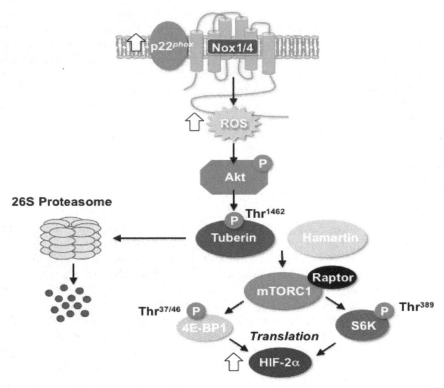

Fig. 5. Proposed mechanism of reactive oxygen species derived from p22phox-dependent Nox oxidases in the regulation of HIF-2alpha mRNA translation in RCC.

4.4 Redox regulation of nuclear factor kappa B (NF-kB) signaling

Nuclear factor kappa B (NF-κB) is a family of redox-sensitive dimeric transcription factors that regulate hundreds of genes involved in inflammation, proliferation, angiogenesis, and cell survival (Pande & Ramos, 2005). NFkB is constitutively expressed in a number of cancers, including renal cancer. It has been proposed that the resistance of RCC to chemotherapy and radiotherapy is due to increased levels of the nuclear factor kB activity and resistance to apoptosis (Oya et al, 2001; Qi & Ohh, 2003). In an unstimulated state, NF-kB binds a member of the inhibitory (IkB) family in the cytoplasm. Activation of NF-kB occurs in response to a wide variety of extracellular stimuli resulting in IkB phosphorylation and subsequent regulated protein degradation. The dissociation of IkB unmasks the NF-kB nuclear localization sequence allowing NF-kB to localize to into the nucleus where it heterodimerizes with a member of the NF-kB/Rel/Dorsal (NRD) family of proteins (Pande & Ramos, 2005). Although there are five known NRD members, RelA, cRel, RelB, p50 and p65, the classical dimer is composed of p50 and RelA. Reactive oxygen species have been implicated as second messengers involved in the activation of NF-kB as several studies have demonstrated that activation of NF-kB by nearly all stimuli can be blocked by antioxidants (Schulze-Osthoff et al, 1997, 1998; Giri & Aggarwal, 1998). Reactive oxygen species on NF-kB activation is further supported by studies demonstrating that hydrogen peroxide induces

NF-κB-dependent interleukin-8 expression in endothelial cells, which contributes to the angiogenic phenotype (Shono et al, 1996). Nox oxidase catalytic subunits, Nox1 and Nox4 have been implicated in the activation of NF-kB. Although the mechanisms remain to be determined, it is likely through regulation of IkK phosphorylation and degradation (Dröge, 2002). More recent studies suggest that NF-kB upregulates Nox oxidase expression and production of Nox-dependent reactive oxygen species. Here, overexpression of p65/RelA or IKKβ up-regulated Nox1, Nox4, and p22phox, mRNA, and protein expression through direct binding of the respective promoters (Manea, et al 2007, 2010). In contrast, NADPH-dependent superoxide production (Nox activity) was reduced in the presence of NF-kB inhibitors. Together, this suggests that NF-kB acts upstream to mediate Nox-dependent reactive oxygen species production and downstream NF-kB activity is positively regulated by Nox-generated reactive oxygen species.

5. Cell growth, survival and metastatic pathways regulated by redox-signaling in renal cancer

5.1 Mitochondrial-derived reactive oxygen species as a mediator of cell proliferation

Cancer cells utilize aerobic glycolysis and glutamine metabolism to generate the necessary resources for rapid cell proliferation and anchorage-independent cell growth. Altered glucose metabolism in cancer cells is termed the Warburg effect, which describes the propensity for most cancer cells to take up glucose avidly and convert it primarily to lactate, despite available oxygen (aerobic glycolysis) (Warburg et al, 1924). In addition to enhanced glucose metabolism, cancer cells also depend on continued mitochondrial function for metabolism, specifically glutaminolysis or glutamine metabolism. Glutamine's importance in tumor cell metabolism derives from characteristics it shares with glucose. The glutamine-fueled TCA cycle leads to the generation of reactive oxygen species by mitochondrial complexes of the electron transport chain and results in generation of ATP, NADPH, amino acids, nucleotides, and lipids (Wise et al, 2008; DeBerardinis, 2008). Mitochondrial metabolism of glutamine is elevated in cancer cells and the type of oncogenes activated in the tumor cells influences glutamine metabolism. For example, tumor cells that exhibit K-ras activation results in enhanced glutamine metabolism, fueling mitochondrial metabolism and mitochondrial derived reactive oxygen species-generation through complex III, independent of OXPHOS, which is necessary for cellular proliferation and anchorage-independent cell growth (Chandel et al, 2000). Additionally, c-Myc enhances glutamine metabolism in cancer cells by enhancing glutaminase (GLS), an amidohydrolase enzyme, which generates glutamate from glutamine. In prostate cancer cells, GLS is important for Myc-induced cell proliferation. K-ras and c-Myc amplification has been detected in RCC. Deciphering the pathways that fuel the TCA cycle differentially in renal cancer cells of various histologies will be important to elucidate the role of mitochondria in RCC cell proliferation and anchorage-independent growth.

5.2 Nox oxidase-derived reactive oxygen species as a mediator of cell proliferation

In renal cell carcinoma, inhibition of Nox oxidases using the NAD(P)H oxidase flavoprotein inhibitor diphenylene iodonium, DPI, reduces cell number and tumor growth in a xenograft nude mouse model; however, the mechanisms by which Nox-derived reactive oxygen species mediate cell proliferation remain unclear (Block et al, 2007). Kidney cancers demonstrate enhanced activation of redox-sensitive signaling pathways involved in cell proliferation. Notably, HIF-2alpha, rather than HIF-1alpha, has been shown to play a critical role in renal tumorigenesis due to HIF-2alpha driven TGF-alpha expression, the mitogen for proximal tubular epithelial cells. Up-regulation of TGF-alpha leads to its binding to the epidermal growth factor receptor (EGFR) with subsequent activation of the PI3K/Akt signaling pathway. As discussed earlier, growing evidence suggest that Nox-derived reactive oxygen species can stimulate signal transduction cascades through the EGFR likely through protein tyrosine phosphatase (PTP) inhibition. A role for Nox oxidases in agonist-induced cell proliferation has been demonstrated in a variety of other cell types; for example, proliferating keratinocytes showed higher reactive oxygen species generation and Nox1 expression than quiescent cells (Chamulitrat et al, 2003). Over-expression of Nox1 in several cell types is associated with increased cell division (Suh et al, 1999; Ranjan et al, 2006; Kamata et al, 2005). In addition, Nox overexpression has been seen in human renal, colon, prostate cancers and melanomas. In the case of Nox4 in melanoma cells and Nox5 in prostate cancer cells, inhibition of reactive oxygen species resulted in inhibition of cell proliferation, supporting a role for reactive oxygen species in mitogenic signaling (Lassegue & Clempus, 2003).

5.3 Reactive oxygen species as a mediator of cell survival

Increased reactive oxygen species is normally linked to cell death. However, in a subset of cancers, Nox-dependent reactive oxygen species has been associated with cell survival. For example, Nox4- and Nox1-derived reactive oxygen species inhibits apoptosis in pancreatic cancer cells and colon cancer cells respectively in a NF kappa-B- (Fukuyama et al, 2005) and Akt-dependent manner (Mochizuki et al, 2006). It is still unknown what role Nox oxidases and/or mitochondrial-derived reactive oxygen species play in RCC cell survival.

5.4 Reactive oxygen species as a mediator of angiogenesis

Renal tumors are known to be a highly vascular due to enhanced angiogenesis. Angiogenesis is the process in which tissue recruits blood vessels to form a neovasculature to vascularize the tissue. In most cases, the intratumor tissue experiences physiologic hypoxia and generates the angiogenic growth factor vascular endothelial growth factor (VEGF). VEGF induces angiogenesis by stimulating endothelial cell proliferation and migration primarily through the receptor tyrosine kinase VEGF receptor-2. VEGF binding initiates tyrosine phosphorylation of KDR, which results in activation of downstream signaling enzymes including ERK, Akt and eNOS, which contribute to angiogenic-related responses in endothelial cells (Colavitti et al, 2002; Matsumoto & Claesson-Welsh, 2001). Although NADPH oxidases are important for maintaining HIF-alpha expression in RCC, it is likely that Nox oxidases play a broader role in angiogenesis. Nox-derived reactive oxygen species function as signaling molecules to mediate various angiogenic-related responses such as cell proliferation, migration and angiogenic gene expression in endothelial cells (Ushio-Fukai et al, 2002, 2004, 2006). In endothelial cells, NADPH oxidase is activated by numerous stimuli including VEGF, EGF, cytokines, and hypoxia. Downregulation of Nox4 inhibits VEGF-induced endothelial cell migration and proliferation (Datla et al, 2007). Nox4 expression is upregulated in new capillaries in brain ischemia-induced angiogenesis of mice (Vallet et al, 2005). In animals of prostate cancer, Nox1 over-expression markedly increased angiogenesis by inducing the angiogenic factor VEGF correlating with an aggressive tumor phenotype (Lim et al, 2005). Nox1-induced hydrogen peroxide increases VEGF and VEGF receptor expression and MMP activity, markers of the angiogenic switch, thereby promoting vascularization and rapid expansion of melanoma tumors (Arbiser et al, 2002). Nox2 generates reactive oxygen species in endothelial cells by a number of agonists including VEGF and Ang 1, which are involved in angiogenesis (Ushio-Fukai et al, 2002; Gorlach et al, 2000; Li & Shah, 2002; Frey et al, 2002; Fürst et al., 2005; Harfouche et al, 2005). Neovascularization in response to ischemia or VEGF is inhibited in Nox2−/− mice and in wild-type mice treated with a NADPH oxidase inhibitor (Ushio-Fukai et al, 2002; Tojo et al, 2005; Al-Shabrawey et al, 2005). Taken together, accumulating evidence suggest that reactive oxygen species derived from NADPH oxidases play an important role in physiological and pathological angiogenesis; however, the enzymatic sources and role of reactive oxygen species involved in renal cancer angiogenesis remain undetermined.

6. Oxidative stress as potential novel biomarkers or therapeutic treatments in renal cancer

6.1 Novel biomarkers

Metabolites are the intermediates and products of metabolism. Whether its mitochondrial dysfunction, mutation in TCA cycle genes, or abnormal oxygen consumption, metabolic profiling can provide a metabolite fingerprint of intracellular physiology within a tumor. As the kidney is an organ, which secretes the water and waste drain from each kidney to the bladder and are eliminated from the body as urine, small-molecule metabolites are likely to be found in the urine. Metabolic profiling may be used for the establishment of non-invasive urinary biomarkers for the prediction of renal cancer, prognostic indicator, or responsiveness to therapy. A comprehensive metabolomics-driven approach is needed for the identification of biomarkers in various histologies of RCC. The most representative product that may reflect oxidative damage induced by reactive oxygen species detectable in the urine is 8-hydroxy-2'-deoxyguanosine (8-OHdG) (Sakano et al, 2009). F2-Isoprostanes and malondialdehyde (MDA) are considered reliable markers of lipid peroxidation *in vivo* and can also be detected in the urine. However, the use of oxidative stress markers as biomarkers for RCC may be challenging as many co-morbidities such as diabetes and hypertension induce oxidative stress that may be detected in the urine.

6.2 Antioxidants

The use of antioxidants to prevent disease is controversial. Antioxidants are manufactured within the body and are naturally found in fruits and vegetable food sources. As this chapter has just revealed a broad role for reactive oxygen species in renal tumorigenesis, it would be rational to think that antioxidants will slow or prevent activation of oncogene signaling in tumor cells. Indeed, *in vitro* studies demonstrate some beneficial effects of antioxidants on tumor cells and observational studies suggested a diet high in fruits and vegetables, both of which are rich with antioxidants, may prevent cancer development. However, many randomized trials have indicated that there is no benefit in preventing cancer or affecting mortality with antioxidant supplementation using vitamin C, vitamin E, or beta carotene in human patients (Lin et al, 2009). Supplementation with vitamin C, along with vitamins A, E, and beta-carotene did not prevent gastrointestinal cancer (Bjelakovic et al, 2004) did not lower the risk of prostate cancer (Kirsh et al, 2006) however, one study did find an association between the intake of vitamins A, C, or E and a reduced risk for cervical cancer (Kim et al, 2010). Are the successes or failure of antioxidants organ or genetic specific? All cells have intracellular antioxidant defense systems. However, as discussed, neutralization of free radicals are not 100% efficient and some proteins that function to neutralize the antioxidants are significantly reduced or inactivated in cancers, including renal cancer. Moreover, the enzymatic sources that generate reactive oxygen species are overactive and are not "turned off" by antioxidants. Here, it is likely that co-morbidities such as diabetes and hypertension play a systemic biological role in antioxidant failures, as diabetes and hypertension are known to induce oxidative stress alone, without the compounding issues of a tumor and tumor environment. Taken together, it is evident that a successful approach for antioxidant therapy will be to target the enzymatic sources that produce the reactive oxygen species such as NADPH oxidases or the mitochondria. Targeting Nox enzymes in an isoform-selective manner is likely to offer therapeutic advantages.

6.3 Novel therapeutic targets

Hypoxia inducible factors are master transcriptional regulators that activate over 100 genes involved in renal tumorigenesis. Therefore, targeting HIF-alpha subunits is an attractive therapeutic clinical goal. To date, agents with anti-angiogenic activity that inhibit VEGFR and PDGFR signaling (e.g. sorafenib, sunitinib), the VEGF ligand (bevacizumab), and the EGF ligand (cetuximab) have demonstrated some effectiveness in the management of renal cell cancer to different degrees (Patel et al, 2006; Sosman et al, 2007). However, these agents target only a small portion of the downstream genes regulated by HIF. As outlined here, the majority of renal cancer exhibits stabilization of HIF-alpha through the loss of VHL function or inhibition of proline hydroxylation activity together resulting in HIF-alpha overexpression. In the absence of VHL, maintaining HIF-alpha expression is dependent on ongoing mRNA translation, regulated by mTOR signaling. However, clinical trials using approved mTOR inhibitors such as temsirolimus (CCI-779) and everolimus (RAD001) do not exhibit beneficial outcomes long term. Importantly, renal carcinoma cells express HIF-2alpha or HIF-1alpha/HIF-2alpha and knockout and molecular studies have revealed that HIF-1alpha translation is dependent on mTORC1 signaling, whereas HIF-2alpha is downstream of the mTORC2 pathway; therefore, rapalogs have little to no effect on reducing HIF-2alpha expression in renal cell carcinoma (Toschi et al, 2008). Because Nox-dependent reactive oxygen species production maintain HIF-2alpha in the absence of proteasomal degradation by VHL and the broader role Nox oxidases play in other signaling pathways that mediate the genesis of RCC, suggest that novel development of specific inhibitors of NADPH oxidases may provide a novel approach for therapeutic targeting. For now, based on the literature and molecular mechanisms of mTOR signaling, new agents that target both the mTORC1 and mTORC2 pathways have the potential to downregulate both HIF-1alpha and HIF-2alpha in clear cell kidney cancers and could provide more antitumor activity than temsirolimus and everolimus, which again primarily target the mTORC1 pathway. Agents, which inhibit mTORC1, mTORC2 and PI3K pathways, such as AZD8055, demonstrates potent anti-tumor activity in *in vitro* and *in vivo* model systems (Chresta et al, 2010). It is unclear, if these inhibitors have indirect antioxidant effects.

7. Acknowledgement

I would like to thank my colleague, Dr. Yves Gorin for the creative design of the figures and critical reading of this chapter. KB is supported by Veterans Career Development Award & NIH/NCI CΛ131272.

8. References

Al-Shabrawey, M; Bartoli, M; El-Remessy, AB; Platt, DH; Matragoon, S; Behzadian, MA; Caldwell, RW; & Caldwell, RB. Inhibition of NAD(P)H oxidase activity blocks vascular endothelial growth factor overexpression and neovascularization during ischemic retinopathy. *Am J Pathol.* 167, (2005), 599-607.

Ambasta, RK; Kumar, P; Griendling, KK; Schmidt, HH; Busse, R; & Brandes, RP. Direct interaction of the novel Nox proteins with p22phox is required for the formation of a functionally active NADPH oxidase. *J Biol Chem* 279, (2004), 45935–45941.

Arbiser, JL; Petros, J; Klafter, R; Govindajaran, B; McLaughlin, ER; Brown, LF; Cohen, C; Moses, M; Kilroy, S; Arnold, RS; & Lambeth, JD. Reactive oxygen generated by Nox1 triggers the angiogenic switch. *Proc Natl Acad Sci U S A.* 99, (2002), 715-720.

Babior, BM. NADPH oxidase: an update. *Blood.* 93, (1999) 464-476.

Bánfi, B; Malgrange, B; Knisz, J; Steger, K; Dubois-Dauphin, M; & Krause, KH. NOX3, a superoxide-generating NADPH oxidase of the inner ear. *J Biol Chem.* 279, (2004), 46065-46072.

Bedard, K; & Krause, KH. The NOX family of ROS-generating NADPH oxidases: physiology and pathophysiology. *Physiol Rev* 87, (2007), 245–313.

Bjelakovic, G; Nikolova, D; Simonetti, RG; & Gluud, C. Antioxidant supplements for prevention of gastrointestinal cancers: a systematic review and meta-analysis. *Lancet.* 364, (2004), 1219-1228.

Block, K; Gorin; Hoover, P, Williams, P; Chelmicki, T; Clark, RA; Yoneda, T; & Abboud, HE. NAD(P)H oxidases regulate HIF-2alpha protein expression. *J Biol Chem.* 282, (2007), 8019-8026.

Block, K; Gorin, Y; & Abboud, HE. Subcellular localization of Nox4 and regulation in diabetes. *Proc Natl Acad Sci USA* 106, (2009), 14385–14390.

Block, K; Gorin, Y; New, DD; Eid, A; Chelmicki; T, Reed, A; Choudhury, GG; Parekh, DJ; & Abboud HE. The NADPH oxidase subunit p22phox inhibits the function of the tumor suppressor protein tuberin. *Am J Pathol.* 176, (2010), 2447-5245.

Bondi, CD; Manickam, N; Lee, DY; Block, K; Gorin, Y; Abboud, HE; & Barnes JL. NAD(P)H oxidase mediates TGF-beta1-induced activation of kidney myofibroblasts. *J Am Soc Nephrol.* 21, (2010), 93-102.

Brahimi-Horn, MC; Chiche, J; & Pouysségur, J. Hypoxia signalling controls metabolic demand. *Curr Opin Cell Biol.* 19, (2007), 223-239.

Brandes, RP; & Schroder, K. Composition and functions of vascular nicotinamide adenine dinucleotide phosphate oxidases. *Trends Cardiovasc Med.* 18, (2008), 15–19.

Brar, SS; Corbin, Z; Kennedy, TP; Hemendinger, R; Thornton, L; Bommarius, B; Arnold, RS; Whorton, AR; Sturrock, AB; Huecksteadt, TP; Quinn, MT; Krenitsky, K; Ardie, KG; Lambeth, JD; & Hoidal, JR. NOX5 NAD(P)H oxidase regulates growth and apoptosis in DU 145 prostate cancer cells. *Am J Physiol Cell Physiol.* 285, (2003) C353-C369.

Bruick, RK; & McKnight, SL. *Science.* 294, (2001), 1337-1340. A conserved family of prolyl-4-hydroxylases that modify HIF.

Brown, DI; & Griendling, KK. Nox proteins in signal transduction. *Free Radic Biol Med* 47, (2009), 1239–1253.

Bui, T; & Thompson, CB. Cancer's sweet tooth. *Cancer Cell.* 9 (2006) 419-420.

Cadenas, E; & Davies, KJ. Mitochondrial free radical generation, oxidative stress, and aging. *Free Radic Biol Med.* 29, (2000), 222-230.

Cecchini, G; Schröder, I; Gunsalus, RP; & Maklashina, E. Succinate dehydrogenase and fumarate reductase from Escherichia coli. *Biochim Biophys Acta.* 1553, (2002), 140-157.

Chamulitrat, W; Schmidt, R; Tomakidi, P; Stremmel, W; Chunglok, W; Kawahara, T; & Rokutan, K. Association of gp91phox homolog Nox1 with anchorage-independent growth and MAP kinase-activation of transformed human keratinocytes. *Oncogene.* 22, (2003), 6045-6053.

Chandel, NS; McClintock, DS; Feliciano, CE; Wood, TM; Melendez, JA; Rodriguez, AM; & Schumacker, PT. Reactive oxygen species generated at mitochondrial complex III stabilize hypoxia-inducible factor-1alpha during hypoxia: a mechanism of O2 sensing. *J Biol Chem.* 275, (2000) 25130-15138.

Cheng, G; Cao, Z; Xu, X; van Meir, EG; & Lambeth, JD. Homologs of gp91phox: cloning and tissue expression of Nox3, Nox4, and Nox5. *Gene.* 269, (2001) 131-140.

Chiarugi, P; & Cirri, P. Redox regulation of protein tyrosine phosphatases during receptor tyrosine kinase signal transduction. *Trends Biochem Sci.* 28, (2003), 509-514

Cho, SH; Lee, CH; Ahn, Y; Kim, H; Kim, H; Ahn, CY; Yang, KS; & Lee, SR. Redox regulation of PTEN and protein tyrosine phosphatases in H(2)O(2) mediated cell signaling. *FEBS Lett.* 560, (2004), 7-13.

Chresta, CM; Davies, BR; Hickson, I; Harding, T; Cosulich, S; Critchlow, SE; Vincent, JP; Ellston, R; Jones, D; Sini, P; James, D; Howard, Z; Dudley, P; Hughes, G; Smith, L; Maguire, S; Hummersone, M; Malagu, K; Menear, K; Jenkins, R; Jacobsen, M; Smith, GC; Guichard, S; & Pass, M. AZD8055 is a potent, selective, and orally bioavailable ATP-competitive mammalian target of rapamycin kinase inhibitor with in vitro and in vivo antitumor activity. *Cancer Res.* 70, (2010), 288-298.

Colavitti, R; Pani, G; Bedogni, B; Anzevino, R; Borrello, S; Waltenberger, J; & Galeotti, T. Reactive oxygen species as downstream mediators of angiogenic signaling by vascular endothelial growth factor receptor-2/KDR. *J Biol Chem.* 277, (2002), 3101-3108.

Crino, PB; Nathanson, KL; & Henske, EP. The tuberous sclerosis complex. *N Engl J Med.* 355, (2006), 1345-1356.

Dang, CV; Resar, LM,; Emison, E; Kim, S; Li, Q; Prescott, JE; Wonsey, D; & Zeller, K. Function of the c-Myc oncogenic transcription factor. *Exp Cell Res.* 253, (1999), 63-77.

Datla, SR; Peshavariya, H; Dusting, GJ; Mahadev, K; Goldstein, BJ; & Jiang, F. Important role of Nox4 type NADPH oxidase in angiogenic responses in human microvascular endothelial cells in vitro. *Arterioscler Thromb Vasc Biol.* 27, (2007), 2319-2324.

DeBerardinis, RJ. Is cancer a disease of abnormal cellular metabolism? New angles on an old idea. *Genet Med.* 10, (2008), 767-777.

Deken, X; Wang, D; Many, MC; Costagliola, S; Libert, F; Vassart, G; Dumont, JE; & Miot, F. Cloning of two human thyroid cDNAs encoding new members of the NADPH oxidase family. *J Biol Chem.* 275, (2000), 23227-23233. de Paulsen, N; Brychzy, A; Fournier, MC; Klausner, RD; Gnarra, JR; Pause, A; & Lee, S. Role of transforming growth factor-alpha in von Hippel--Lindau (VHL)(-/-) clear cell renal carcinoma cell proliferation: a possible mechanism coupling VHL tumor suppressor inactivation and tumorigenesis. *Proc. Natl. Acad. Sci. U. S. A.* 98, (2001), 1387-1392.

Diebold, I, Petry, A, Hess, J, & Görlach, A. The NADPH oxidase subunit NOX4 is a new target gene of the hypoxia-inducible factor-1. *Mol Biol Cell.* 21, (2010), 2087-2096.

Dröge, W. Free radicals in the physiological control of cell function. *Physiol Rev.* 82, (2002) 47-95.

Dupuy, C, Ohayon, R, Valent, A, Noël-Hudson, MS, Dème, D, & Virion, A. Purification of a novel flavoprotein involved in the thyroid NADPH oxidase. Cloning of the porcine and human cdnas. *J Biol Chem.* 274, (1999), 37265-37269.

Eid, AA; Gorin, Y; Fagg, BM; Kasinath, BS; Gorin, Y; Ghosh-Choudhury, G; Barnes, JL; & Abboud, HE. Mechanisms of podocyte injury in diabetes: role of cytochrome P450 and NADPH oxidases. *Diabetes* 58, (2009), 1201–1211.

Epstein, AC; Gleadle, JM; McNeill, LA; Hewitson, KS; O'Rourke, J; Mole, DR; Mukherji, M; Metzen, E; Wilson, MI; Dhanda, A; Tian, YM; Masson, N; Hamilton, DL; Jaakkola, P; Barstead, R; Hodgkin, J; Maxwell, PH; Pugh, CW; Schofield, CJ; & Ratcliffe, PJ; C. elegans EGL-9 and mammalian homologs define a family of dioxygenases that regulate HIF by prolyl hydroxylation. *Cell.* 107, (2001), 43-54.

European Chromosome 16 Tuberous Sclerosis Consortium. Identification and characterization of the tuberous sclerosis gene on chromosome 16. *Cell.* 75, (1993), 1305-1315.

Evans, P; & Halliwell, B. Free radicals and hearing. Cause, consequence, and criteria. *Ann N Y Acad Sci.* 884, (1999), 19-40.

Franke, TF; Kaplan, DR; Cantley, LC; & Toker, A. Direct regulation of the Akt proto-oncogene product by phosphatidylinositol-3,4-bisphosphate. *Science.* 275, (1997), 665-668.

Frey, RS; Rahman, A; Kefer, JC; Minshall, RD; & Malik, AB. PKCzeta regulates TNF-alpha-induced activation of NADPH oxidase in endothelial cells. *Circ Res.* 90, (2002), 1012-1019.

Frias, MA; Thoreen, CC; Jaffe, JD; Schroder, W; Sculley, T; Carr, SA; & Sabatini, DM. mSin1 is necessary for Akt/PKB phosphorylation, and its isoforms define three distinct mTORC2s. *Curr Biol.* 16, (2006), 1865-1870.

Fridovich I. The biology of oxygen radicals. *Science.* 201,(1978), 875-880.

Fürst, R; Brueckl, C; Kuebler, WM; Zahler, S; Krötz, F; Görlach, A; Vollmar, AM; & Kiemer, AK. Atrial natriuretic peptide induces mitogen-activated protein kinase phosphatase-1 in human endothelial cells via Rac1 and NAD(P)H oxidase/Nox2-activation. *Circ Res.* 96, (2005), 43-53.

Fukai, T, & Ushio-Fukai, M. Superoxide Dismutases: Role in Redox Signaling, Vascular Function, and Diseases. *Antioxid Redox Signal.* (2011).

Fukuyama, M; Rokutan, K; Sano, T; Miyake, H; Shimada, M; & Tashiro, S. Overexpression of a novel superoxide-producing enzyme, NADPH oxidase 1, in adenoma and well differentiated adenocarcinoma of the human colon. *Cancer Lett.* 221, (2005), 97-104.

Geiszt, M; Kopp, JB; Várnai, P; & Leto, TL. Identification of renox, an NAD(P)H oxidase in kidney. *Proc Natl Acad Sci U S A.* 97, (2000), 8010-8014.

Geiszt, M. NADPH oxidases: new kids on the block. *Cardiovasc Res* 71, (2006), 289–299.

Gerald, D; Berra, E; Frapart, YM; Chan, DA; Giaccia, AJ; Mansuy, D; Pouysségur, J; Yaniv, M; & Mechta-Grigoriou, F. JunD reduces tumor angiogenesis by protecting cells from oxidative stress. *Cell.* 118, (2004), 781-794.

Gingras, AC, Raught, B, & Sonenberg, N. mTOR signaling to translation. *Curr Top Microbiol Immunol.* 279, (2004), 169-97.

Giri, DK; & Aggarwal, BB. Constitutive activation of NF-kappaB causes resistance to apoptosis in human cutaneous T cell lymphoma HuT-78 cells. Autocrine role of tumor necrosis factor and reactive oxygen intermediates. J Biol Chem. 273, (1998), 14008-14014.

Gnarra, JR; Tory, K; Weng ,Y; Schmidt, L; Wei, MH; Li, H; Latif, F; Liu, S; Chen, F; Duh, FM; et al. Mutations of the VHL tumour suppressor gene in renal carcinoma. *Nat Genet.* 7, (1994), 85-90.

Gnarra, JR; Duan, DR; Weng, Y; Humphrey, JS; Chen, DY; Lee, S; Pause, A; Dudley, CF; Latif, F; Kuzmin, I; Schmidt, L; Duh, FM; Stackhouse, T; Chen, F; Kishida, T; Wei, MH; Lerman, MI; Zbar, B; Klausner, RD; & Linehan, WM. Molecular cloning of the von Hippel-Lindau tumor suppressor gene and its role in renal carcinoma. *Biochim Biophys Acta.* 1242, (1996), 201-210.

Gokden, N; Li, L; Zhang, H; Schafer, RF; Schichman, S; Scott, MA; Smoller, BR; & Fan, CY. Loss of heterozygosity of DNA repair gene, hOGG1, in renal cell carcinoma but not in renal papillary adenoma. *Pathol Int.* 58, (2008), 339-343.

Gorin, Y; Ricono, JM; Kim, NH; Bhandari, B, Choudhury, GG; & Abboud, HE. Nox4 mediates angiotensin II-induced activation of Akt/protein kinase B in mesangial cells. *Am J Physiol Renal Physiol.* 285, (2003), F219–F229.

Gorin, Y; Block, K; Hernandez, J; Bhandari, B; Wagner, B; Barnes, JL; & Abboud, HE. Nox4 NAD(P)H oxidase mediates hypertrophy and fibronectin expression in the diabetic kidney. *J Biol Chem* 280, (2005), 39616–39626.

Goyal, P; Weissmann, N; Grimminger, F; Hegel, C; Bader, L; Rose, F; Fink, L; Ghofrani, HA;, Schermuly, RT; Schmidt, HH; Seeger, W; & Hänze, J. Upregulation of NAD(P)H oxidase 1 in hypoxia activates hypoxia-inducible factor 1 via increase in reactive oxygen species. *Free Radic Biol Med.* 36, (2004), 1279-1288.

Habib SL. Molecular mechanism of regulation of OGG1: tuberin deficiency results in cytoplasmic redistribution of transcriptional factor NF-YA. *J Mol Signal.* 4, (2009), 8.

Habib, SL, Simone, S, Barnes, JJ, & Abboud, HE. Tuberin haploinsufficiency is associated with the loss of OGG1 in rat kidney tumors. *Mol Cancer.* 24, 7, (2008), 10.

Harfouche, R; Malak, NA; Brandes, RP; Karsan, A; Irani, K; & Hussain, SN. Roles of reactive oxygen species in angiopoietin-1/tie-2 receptor signaling. FASEB J. 12, (2005), 1728-1730.

Harris ,TE; & Lawrence, JC Jr. TOR signaling. Sci STKE. 212, (2003), 15.

Henderson, A; Douglas, F; Perros, P; Morgan, C; & Maher, ER. SDHB-associated renal oncocytoma suggests a broadening of the renal phenotype in hereditary paragangliomatosis. Fam Cancer. 8, (2009), 257-260.

Hilenski, LL; Clempus, RE; Quinn, MT; Lambeth, JD; Griendling, KK. Distinct subcellular localizations of Nox1 and Nox4 in vascular smooth muscle cells. Arterioscler Thromb Vasc Biol 24, (2004), 677–683.

Holz, MK; Ballif, BA; Gygi, SP; & Blenis, J. mTOR and S6K1 mediate assembly of the translation preinitiation complex through dynamic protein interchange and ordered phosphorylation events. Cell. 123, (2005), 569-580.

Iliopoulos, O; Kibel, A; Gray, S; & Kaelin, WG Jr. Tumour suppression by the human von Hippel-Lindau gene product. Nat Med. 1, (1995), 822-826.

Jaakkola, P; Mole, DR; Tian, YM; Wilson, MI; Gielbert, J; Gaskell, SJ; Kriegsheim, Av; Hebestreit, HF; Mukherji, M; Schofield, CJ; Maxwell, PH; Pugh, CW; & Ratcliffe, PJ. Targeting of HIF-alpha to the von Hippel-Lindau ubiquitylation complex by O2-regulated prolyl hydroxylation. Science. 292, (2001), 468-472.

Jemal, A; Murray, T; Ward, E; Samuels, A; Tiwari, RC; Ghafoor, A; Feuer, EJ; & Thun, MJ. Cancer statistics. CA. Cancer J. Clin. 55, (2005), 10-30.

Jones, SA, Hancock, JT, Jones, OT, Neubauer, A, & Topley, N. The expression of NADPH oxidase components in human glomerular mesangial cells: detection of protein and mRNA for p47phox, p67phox, and p22phox. J Am Soc Nephrol. 5, (1995), 1483-1491.

Kamata, H; Honda, S; Maeda, S; Chang, L; Hirata, H; & Karin, M. Reactive oxygen species promote TNFalpha-induced death and sustained JNK activation by inhibiting MAP kinase phosphatases. Cell. 120, (2005), 649-661.

Kamura, T; Koepp, DM; Conrad, MN; Skowyra, D; Moreland, RJ; Iliopoulos, O; Lane, WS; Kaelin, WG Jr; Elledge, SJ; Conaway, RC; Harper, JW; & Conaway, JW. Rbx1, a component of the VHL tumor suppressor complex and SCF ubiquitin ligase. Science. 284, (1999), 657-661.

Khoo, SK; Bradley, M; Wong, FK; Hedblad, MA; Nordenskjöld, M; & Teh, BT. Birt-Hogg-Dubé syndrome: mapping of a novel hereditary neoplasia gene to chromosome 17p12-q11.2. Oncogene. 20, (2001), 5239-5242.

Kibel, A; Iliopoulos, O; DeCaprio, JA; & Kaelin, WG Jr. Binding of the von Hippel-Lindau tumor suppressor protein to Elongin B and C. Science. 269, (1995), 1444-1446.

Kim, DH; Sarbassov, DD; Ali, SM; King, JE; Latek, RR, Erdjument-Bromage, H; Tempst, P; & Sabatini, DM. mTOR interacts with raptor to form a nutrient-sensitive complex that signals to the cell growth machinery. Cell. 110, (2002), 163-175.

Kim, J; Kim, MK; Lee, JK; Kim, JH; Son, SK; Song, ES; Lee, KB; Lee, JP, Lee, JM; & Yun, YM. Intakes of vitamin A, C, and E, and beta-carotene are associated with risk of cervical cancer: a case-control study in Korea. Nutr Cancer. 62, (2010), 181-189.

King, A; Selak, MA; & Gottlieb, E. Succinate dehydrogenase and fumarate hydratase: linking mitochondrial dysfunction and cancer. Oncogene. 25, (2006), 4675-4682.

Kirsh, VA; Hayes, RB; Mayne, ST; Chatterjee, N; Subar, AF; Dixon, LB; Albanes, D; Andriole, GL; Urban, DA; & Peters U. PLCO Trial. Supplemental and dietary vitamin E, beta-carotene, and vitamin C intakes and prostate cancer risk. *J Natl Cancer Inst.* 98, (2006), 245-254.

Knebelmann, B; Ananth, S; Cohen, HT; & Sukhatme, VP. Transforming growth factor alpha is a target for the von Hippel-Lindau tumor suppressor. *Cancer Res.* 58, (1998), 226-231.

Kuroda, J; Ago, T; Matsushima, S; Zhai, P; Schneider, MD; & Sadoshima, J. NADPH oxidase 4 (Nox4) is a major source of oxidative stress in the failing heart. *Proc Natl Acad Sci U S A.* 107, (2010), 15565-15570.

Lambeth, JD. Nox enzymes, ROS, and chronic disease: an example of antagonistic pleiotropy. *Free Radic Biol Med* 43, (2007), 332–347.

Lassegue, B; & Clempus, RE. Vascular NAD(P)H oxidases: specific features, expression, and regulation. *Am J Physiol Reg Integr Compar Physiol* 285, (2003), R277–R297.

Lassègue, B; & Griendling, KK. NADPH oxidases: functions and pathologies in the vasculature. *Arterioscler Thromb Vasc Biol.* 30, (2010), 653-661.

Latif, F; Tory, K; Gnarra, J; Yao, M; Duh, FM; Orcutt, ML; Stackhouse, T; Kuzmin, I; Modi, W; Geil, L, et al. Identification of the von Hippel-Lindau disease tumor suppressor gene. *Science.* 260, (1993), 1317-1320.

Lee, SR; Kwon, KS; Kim, SR; & Rhee, SG. Reversible inactivation of protein-tyrosine phosphatase 1B in A431 cells stimulated with epidermal growth factor. *J Biol Chem.* 273, (1998), 15366-15372.

Li, JM; & Shah, AM. Intracellular localization and preassembly of the NADPH oxidase complex in cultured endothelial cells. *J Biol Chem.* 277, (2002), 19952-19960.

Lim, SD; Sun, C; Lambeth, JD; Marshall, F; Amin, M; Chung, L; Petros, JA; Arnold, RS. Increased Nox1 and hydrogen peroxide in prostate cancer. *Prostate.* 62, (2005), 200-207.

Lin, J; Cook, NR; Albert, C; Zaharris, E; Gaziano, JM; Van Denburgh, M; Buring, JE; & Manson, JE. Vitamins C and E and beta carotene supplementation and cancer risk: a randomized controlled trial. *J Natl Cancer Inst.* 101, (2009), 14-23.

Lubensky, IA; Schmidt, L; Zhuang, Z; Weirich, G; Pack, S, Zambrano, N; Walther, MM; Choyke, P; Linehan, WM; & Zbar, B. Hereditary and sporadic papillary renal carcinomas with c-met mutations share a distinct morphological phenotype. *Am J Pathol.* 155, (1999), 517-526.

Mahadev, K; Motoshima, H; Wu, X; Ruddy, JM; Arnold, RS; Cheng, G; Lambeth, JD; & Goldstein, BJ. The NAD(P)H oxidase homolog Nox4 modulates insulin-stimulated generation of H2O2 and plays an integral role in insulin signal transduction. *Mol Cell Biol.* 24, (2004), 1844-1854.

Maher, ER; & Kaelin, WG Jr. von Hippel-Lindau disease. *Medicine (Baltimore).* 76, (1997), 381-391.

Mahimainathan, L; Ghosh-Choudhury, N; Venkatesan, B; Das, F; Mandal, CC; Dey, N; Habib, SL; Kasinath, BS; Abboud, HE; & Ghosh Choudhury, G. TSC2 deficiency increases PTEN via HIF1alpha. *J Biol Chem.* 284, (2009), 27790-27798.

Mahon, PC; Hirota, K; & Semenza, GL. FIH-1: a novel protein that interacts with HIF-1alpha and VHL to mediate repression of HIF-1 transcriptional activity. *Genes Dev.* 15, (2001), 2675-2686.

Mamane, Y; Petroulakis, E; Rong, L; Yoshida, K; Ler, LW; Sonenberg, N. eIF4E--from translation to transformation. *Oncogene.* 23, (2004), 3172-3179.

Manea, A; Manea, SA; Gafencu, AV; & Raicu, M. Regulation of NADPH oxidase subunit p22(phox) by NF-kB in human aortic smooth muscle cells. *Arch Physiol Biochem.* 113, (2007), 163-172.

Manea, A; Tanase, LI; Raicu, M; & Simionescu, M. Transcriptional regulation of NADPH oxidase isoforms, Nox1 and Nox4, by nuclear factor-kappaB in human aortic smooth muscle cells. *Biochem Biophys Res Commun.* 396, (2010), 901-907.

Manning, BD; & Cantley, LC. AKT/PKB signaling: navigating downstream. *Cell.* 129, (2007), 1261-1274.

Maranchie, JK; & Zhan, Y. Nox4 is critical for hypoxia-inducible factor 2-alpha transcriptional activity in von Hippel-Lindau-deficient renal cell carcinoma. *Cancer Res.* 65, (2005), 9190-9193.

Marcotrigiano, J, Gingras, AC, Sonenberg, N, & Burley, SK. Cap-dependent translation initiation in eukaryotes is regulated by a molecular mimic of eIF4G. *Mol Cell.* 3, (1999), 707-716.

Martyn, KD; Frederick, LM; von Loehneysen, K; Dinauer, MC; & Knaus, UG. Functional analysis of Nox4 reveals unique characteristics compared to other NADPH oxidases. *Cell Signal* 18, (2006), 69–82.

Masson, N; & Ratcliffe, PJ. HIF prolyl and asparaginyl hydroxylases in the biological response to intracellular O(2) levels. *J Cell Sci.* 116, (2003), 3041-3049.

Matsumoto, T; & Claesson-Welsh, L. VEGF receptor signal transduction. *Sci STKE.* 112, (2001), re21.

Maxwell, PH, Dachs, GU; Gleadle, JM; Nicholls, LG; Harris, AL; Stratford, IJ; Hankinson, O; Pugh, CW; & Ratcliffe, PJ. Hypoxia-inducible factor-1 modulates gene expression in solid tumors and influences both angiogenesis and tumor growth. *Proc Natl Acad Sci U S A.* 94, (1997), 8104-8109.

Maxwell, PH; Wiesener, MS; Chang, GW; Clifford, SC; Vaux, EC; Cockman, ME; Wykoff, CC; Pugh, CW; Maher, ER; & Ratcliffe, PJ. The tumour suppressor protein VHL targets hypoxia-inducible factors for oxygen-dependent proteolysis. *Nature.* 399, (1999), 271-275.

Maxwell, P; & van den Berg, HW. Changes in the secretion of insulin-like growth factor binding proteins -2 and -4 associated with the development of tamoxifen resistance and estrogen independence in human breast cancer cell lines. *Cancer Lett.* 139, (1999), 121-127.

Mayr, JA; Meierhofer, D; Zimmermann, F; Feichtinger, R; Kögler, C; Ratschek, M; Schmeller, N; Sperl, W; & Kofler, B. Loss of complex I due to mitochondrial DNA mutations in renal oncocytoma. *Clin Cancer Res.* 14, (2008), 2270-2275.

Meng, D; Lv, DD; & Fang, J. Insulin-like growth factor-I induces reactive oxygen species production and cell migration through Nox4 and Rac1 in vascular smooth muscle cells. *Cardiovasc Res.* 80, (2008), 299-308.

Michaeloudes, C; Sukkar, MB; Khorasani, NM; Bhavsar, PK; & Chung, KF. TGF-β regulates Nox4, MnSOD and catalase expression, and IL-6 release in airway smooth muscle cells. *Am J Physiol Lung Cell Mol Physiol.* (2011).

Mochizuki, T; Furuta, S; Mitsushita J; Shang, WH; Ito, M; Yokoo, Y; Yamaura, M; Ishizone, S, Nakayama, J; Konagai, A; Hirose, K; Kiyosawa, K; & Kamata, T. Inhibition of NADPH oxidase 4 activates apoptosis via the AKT/apoptosis signal-regulating kinase 1 pathway in pancreatic cancer PANC-1 cells. *Oncogene.* 25, (2006), 3699-36707.

Moreno, SM; Benítez, IA; & Martínez González, MA. Ultrastructural studies in a series of 18 cases of chromophobe renal cell carcinoma. *Ultrastruct Pathol.* 29, (2005), 377-387.

Nisimoto, Y; Jackson, HM; Ogawa, H; Kawahara, T; & Lambeth, JD. Constitutive NADPH-dependent electron transferase activity of the Nox4 dehydrogenase domain. *Biochemistry.* 49, (2010), 2433-2442.

Novo, E; & Parola, M. Redox mechanisms in hepatic chronic wound healing and fibrogenesis. *Fibrogenesis Tissue Repair.* (2008).

O'Flaherty, L; Adam, J; Heather, LC; Zhdanov, AV; Chung, YL; Miranda, MX; Croft, J; Olpin, S; Clarke, K; Pugh, CW,; Griffiths, J; Papkovsky, D; Ashrafian, H; Ratcliffe, PJ; & Pollard, PJ. Dysregulation of hypoxia pathways in fumarate hydratase-deficient cells is independent of defective mitochondrial metabolism. *Hum Mol Genet.* 19, (2010), 3844-3851.

Oya, M; Ohtsubo, M; Takayanagi, A; Tachibana, M;Shimizu, N; & Murai, M. Constitutive activation of nuclear factor-kappaB prevents TRAIL-induced apoptosis in renal cancer cells. *Oncogene.* 20, (2001), 3888-3896.

Pande, V; & Ramos, MJ. NF-kappaB in human disease: current inhibitors and prospects for de novo structure based design of inhibitors. *Curr Med Chem.* 12, (2005), 357-374.

Patel, PH, Chaganti, RS, & Motzer, RJ. Targeted therapy for metastatic renal cell carcinoma. *Br J Cancer.* 94, (2006), 614-619.

Plas, DR, & Thompson, CB. Akt activation promotes degradation of tuberin and FOXO3a via the proteasome. *J Biol Chem.* 278, (2003), 12361-12366.

Pavlovich, CP; Walther, MM; Eyler, RA; Hewitt, SM; Zbar, B; Linehan, WM; & Merino, MJ. Renal tumors in the Birt-Hogg-Dubé syndrome. *Am J Surg Pathol.* 26, (2002), 1542-1552.

Pedruzzi, E; Guichard, C; Ollivier, V; Driss, F; Fay, M; Prunet, C; Marie. JC; Pouzet, C; Samadi, M; Elbim, C; O'dowd, Y; Bens, M; Vandewalle, A; Gougerot-Pocidalo, MA; Lizard, G; & Ogier-Denis, E. NAD(P)H oxidase Nox-4 mediates 7-ketocholesterol-induced endoplasmic reticulum stress and apoptosis in human aortic smooth muscle cells. *Mol Cell Biol* 24, (2004), 10703-10717.

Pfaffenroth, EC: & Linehan, WM. Genetic basis for kidney cancer: opportunity for disease-specific approaches to therapy. *Expert Opin Biol Ther.* 8, (2008), 779-790.

Pollard, PJ; Brière, JJ; Alam, NA; Barwell, J; Barclay, E; Wortham, NC; Hunt, T; Mitchell, M; Olpin, S; Moat, SJ; Hargreaves, IP; Heales, SJ; Chung, YL; Griffiths, JR; Dalgleish, A; McGrath, JA; Gleeson, MJ; Hodgson, SV; Poulsom, R; Rustin, P; Tomlinson, IP. Accumulation of Krebs cycle intermediates and over-expression of HIF1alpha in tumours which result from germline FH and SDH mutations. *Hum Mol Genet.* 14, (2005), 2231-2239.

Porta, C; & Figlin, RA. Phosphatidylinositol-3-kinase/Akt signaling pathway and kidney cancer, and the therapeutic potential of phosphatidylinositol-3-kinase/Akt inhibitors. *J Urol.* 182, (2009), 2569-2577.

Oh, WJ; Wu, CC; Kim, SJ; Facchinetti, V; Julien, LA; Finlan, M; Roux, PP; Su, B; & Jacinto, E. mTORC2 can associate with ribosomes to promote cotranslational phosphorylation and stability of nascent Akt polypeptide. *EMBO J.* 29, (2010), 3939-3951.

Qi, H; & Ohh, M. The von Hippel-Lindau tumor suppressor protein sensitizes renal cell carcinoma cells to tumor necrosis factor-induced cytotoxicity by suppressing the nuclear factor-kappaB-dependent antiapoptotic pathway. *Cancer Res.* 63, (2003), 7076-7080.

Ranjan, P; Anathy, V; Burch, PM; Weirather, K; Lambeth, JD; Heintz, NH. Redox-dependent expression of cyclin D1 and cell proliferation by Nox1 in mouse lung epithelial cells. *Antioxid Redox Signal.* 8, (2006), 1447-1459.

Rhee, SG; Chang, TS; Bae, YS; Lee, SR; Kang, SW. Cellular regulation by hydrogen peroxide. *J Am Soc Nephrol.* 14, (2003), S211-S215.

Ricketts, C; Woodward, ER; Killick, P; Morris, MR; Astuti, D; Latif, F; & Maher, ER. Germline SDHB mutations and familial renal cell carcinoma. *J Natl Cancer Inst.* 100, (2008), 1260-1262.

Royer-Pokora, B; Kunkel, LM; Monaco, AP; Goff, SC; Newburger, PE; Baehner, RL; Cole, FS; Curnutte, JT; & Orkin, SH. Cloning the gene for an inherited human disorder--chronic granulomatous disease--on the basis of its chromosomal location. Nature. 322, (1986), 32-38.

Sakano, N; Wang, DH; Takahashi, N; Wang, B; Sauriasari, R; Kanbara, S; Sato, Y; Takigawa, T; Takaki, J; & Ogino, K. Oxidative stress biomarkers and lifestyles in Japanese healthy people. *J Clin Biochem Nutr.* 44, (2009), 185-195.

Sarbassov DD, Guertin DA, Ali SM, Sabatini DM. Phosphorylation and regulation of Akt/PKB by the rictor-mTOR complex. Science. 2005 Feb 18;307(5712):1098-101.

Sarbassov, DD; Ali, SM; Kim, DH; Guertin, DA; Latek, RR; Erdjument-Bromage, H; Tempst, P; & Sabatini, DM. Rictor, a novel binding partner of mTOR, defines a rapamycin-insensitive and raptor-independent pathway that regulates the cytoskeleton. *Curr Biol.* 14, (2004), 1296-1302.

Sarto, C; Frutiger, S; Cappellano, F; Sanchez, JC; Doro, G; Catanzaro, F; Hughes, GJ; Hochstrasser, DF; & Mocarelli, P. Modified expression of plasma glutathione peroxidase and manganese superoxide dismutase in human renal cell carcinoma. *Electrophoresis.* 20, (1999), 3458-3466.

Schmidt, L; Duh, FM; Chen, F; Kishida, T; Glenn, G; Choyke, P; Scherer, SW; Zhuang, Z; Lubensky, I; Dean, M; Allikmets, R; Chidambaram, A; Bergerheim, UR; Feltis, JT; Casadevall, C; Zamarron, A; Bernues, M; Richard, S; Lips, CJ; Walther, MM; Tsui, LC; Geil, L; Orcutt, ML; Stackhouse, T; Lipan, J; Slife, L; Brauch, H; Decker, J; Niehans, G; Hughson, MD; Moch, H; Storkel S; Lerman, MI; Linehan, WM; Zbar, B. Germline and somatic mutations in the tyrosine kinase domain of the MET proto-oncogene in papillary renal carcinomas. *Nat Genet.* 16, (1997), 68-73.

Schmidt, LS; Warren, MB; Nickerson, ML; Weirich, G; Matrosova, V; Toro, JR; Turner, ML; Duray, P; Merino, M; Hewitt, S; Pavlovich, CP; Glenn, G; Greenberg, CR; Linehan, WM; & Zbar B. Birt-Hogg-Dubé syndrome, a genodermatosis associated with spontaneous pneumothorax and kidney neoplasia, maps to chromosome 17p11.2. Am J Hum Genet. 69, (2001), 876-882.

Schullerus, D; Herbers, J; Chudek, J; Kanamaru, H; & Kovacs, G. Loss of heterozygosity at chromosomes 8p, 9p, and 14q is associated with stage and grade of non-papillary renal cell carcinomas. *J Pathol.* 183, (1997), 151-155.

Schulze-Osthoff, K; Ferrari, D; Riehemann, K; & Wesselborg, S. Regulation of NF-kappa B activation by MAP kinase cascades. Immunobiology. 198, (1997), 35-49.

Schulze-Osthoff, K; Ferrari, D; Los, M; Wesselborg, S; & Peter, ME. Apoptosis signaling by death receptors. *Eur J Biochem.* 254, (1998), 439-459.

Selemidis, S; Sobey, CG; Wingler, K; Schmidt, HH; Drummond, GR. NADPH oxidases in the vasculature: molecular features, roles in disease and pharmacological inhibition. *Pharmacol Ther.* 120, (2008), 254-291.

Semenza, GL. HIF-1 and tumor progression: pathophysiology and therapeutics. *Trends Mol Med.* 8, (2002), S62-S67.

Shiose, A; Kuroda, J; Tsuruya, K; Hirai, M; Hirakata, H; Naito, S; Hattori, M; Sakaki, Y; & Sumimoto, H. A novel superoxide-producing NAD(P)H oxidase in kidney. *J Biol Chem* 276, (2001), 1417-1423.

Shono, T; Ono, M; Izumi, H; Jimi, SI; Matsushima, K; Okamoto, T; Kohno, K; & Kuwano, M. Involvement of the transcription factor NF-kappaB in tubular morphogenesis of human microvascular endothelial cells by oxidative stress. *Mol Cell Biol.* 16, (1996), 4231-4239.

Sturrock, A; Cahill, B; Norman, K; Huecksteadt, TP; Hill, K; Sanders, K; Karwande, SV; Stringham, JC; Bull, DA; Gleich, M; Kennedy, TP; & Hoidal, JR. Transforming growth factor-beta1 induces Nox4 NAD(P)H oxidase and reactive oxygen species-dependent proliferation in human pulmonary artery smooth muscle cells. *Am J Physiol Lung Cell Mol Physiol.* 290, (2006), L661-L673.

Sudarshan, S; Sourbier, C; Kong, HS; Block, K; Valera, Romero, VA; Yang, Y; Galindo, C; Mollapour, M; Scroggins, B; Goode, N; Lee, MJ; Gourlay, CW; Trepel, J; Linehan, WM; & Neckers, L. Fumarate hydratase deficiency in renal cancer induces glycolytic addiction and hypoxia-inducible transcription factor 1alpha stabilization by glucose-dependent generation of reactive oxygen species. *Mol Cell Biol.* 29, (2009), 4080-4090.

Sudarshan, S; Shanmugasundaram, K; Naylor, SL; Lin, S; Livi, CB; O'Neill, CF; Parekh, DJ; Yeh, IT;Sun, LZ; & Block, K. Reduced Expression of Fumarate Hydratase in Clear Cell Renal Cancer Mediates HIF-2α Accumulation and Promotes Migration and Invasion. *PLoS One.* 6, (2011), e21037.

Suh, YA; Arnold, RS; Lassegue, B; Shi, J; Xu, X; Sorescu, D; Chung, AB; Griendling, KK; & Lambeth, JD. Cell transformation by the superoxide-generating oxidase Mox1. *Nature.* 401, (1999), 79-82.

Sosman, JA; Puzanov, I; & Atkins, MB. Opportunities and obstacles to combination targeted therapy in renal cell cancer. *Clin Cancer Res.* 13, (2007), 764s-769s.

Szatrowski, TP; & Nathan, CF. Production of large amounts of hydrogen peroxide by human tumor cells. *Cancer Res.* 51, (1991), 794-798.

Tickoo, SK; Lee, MW; Eble, JN; Amin, M; Christopherson, T; Zarbo, RJ; & Amin, MB. Ultrastructural observations on mitochondria and microvesicles in renal oncocytoma, chromophobe renal cell carcinoma, and eosinophilic variant of conventional (clear cell) renal cell carcinoma. *Am J Surg Pathol.* 24, (2000), 1247-1256.

Tojo, T; Ushio-Fukai, M; Yamaoka-Tojo, M; Ikeda, S; Patrushev, N; & Alexander, RW. Role of gp91phox (Nox2)-containing NAD(P)H oxidase in angiogenesis in response to hindlimb ischemia. *Circulation.* 111, (2005), 2347-2355.

Tory, K; Brauch, H; Linehan, M; Barba, D; Oldfield, E; Filling-Katz; M, Seizinger, B; Nakamura, Y; White, R; Marshall, FF, et al. Specific genetic change in tumors associated with von Hippel-Lindau disease. *J Natl Cancer Inst*. 81, (1989), 1097-1101.

Toschi, A; Lee, E; Gadir, N; Ohh, M; & Foster, DA. Differential dependence of hypoxia-inducible factors 1 alpha and 2 alpha on mTORC1 and mTORC2. *J Biol Chem*. 283, (2008), 34495-34499.

Ushio-Fukai, M; Tang, Y; Fukai, T; Dikalov, SI; Ma, Y; Fujimoto, M; Quinn, MT; Pagano, PJ; Johnson, C; & Alexander, RW. Novel role of gp91(phox)-containing NAD(P)H oxidase in vascular endothelial growth factor-induced signaling and angiogenesis. *Circ Res*. 91, (2002), 1160-1167.

Ushio-Fukai, M, & Alexander, RW. Reactive oxygen species as mediators of angiogenesis signaling: role of NAD(P)H oxidase. *Mol Cell Biochem*. 264, (2004), 85-97.

Ushio-Fukai M. Redox signaling in angiogenesis: role of NADPH oxidase. *Cardiovasc Res*. 71, (2006), 226-235.

Vallet, P; Charnay, Y; Steger, K; Ogier-Denis, E; Kovari, E; Herrmann, F; Michel, JP; & Szanto, I. Neuronal expression of the NADPH oxidase NOX4, and its regulation in mouse experimental brain ischemia. *Neuroscience*. 132, (2005), 233-238.

van Slegtenhorst, M; de Hoogt, R; Hermans, C; Nellist, M; Janssen, B; Verhoef, S; Lindhout, D; van den Ouweland, A; Halley, D; Young, J; Burley, M; Jeremiah, S; Woodward, K; Nahmias, J; Fox, M; Ekong, R; Osborne, J; Wolfe, J; Povey, S; Snell, RG; Cheadle, JP; Jones, AC; Tachataki, M; Ravine, D; Sampson, JR; Reeve, MP; Richardson, P; Wilmer, F; Munro, C; Hawkins, TL; Sepp, T; Ali, JB; Ward, S; Green, AJ; Yates, JR; Kwiatkowska, J; Henske, EP; Short, MP; Haines, JH; Jozwiak, S; & Kwiatkowski, DJ. Identification of the tuberous sclerosis gene TSC1 on chromosome 9q34. *Science*. 277, (1997), 805-808.

Vaquero, EC; Edderkaoui, M; Pandol, SJ; Gukovsky, I; & Gukovskaya, AS. Reactive oxygen species produced by NAD(P)H oxidase inhibit apoptosis in pancreatic cancer cells. *J Biol Chem*. 279, (2004), 34643-34654.

Vanharanta, S; Buchta, M; McWhinney, SR; Virta, SK; Peçzkowska, M; Morrison, CD; Lehtonen, R; Januszewicz, A; Järvinen, H; Juhola, M; Mecklin, JP; Pukkala, E; Herva, R; Kiuru, M; Nupponen, NN; Aaltonen, LA; Neumann, HP; & Eng, C. Early-onset renal cell carcinoma as a novel extraparaganglial component of SDHB-associated heritable paraganglioma. *Am J Hum Genet*. 74, (2004), 153-159.

Vignais, PV. The superoxide-generating NADPH oxidase: structural aspects and activation mechanism. *Cell Mol Life Sci*. 59, (2002), 1428-1459.

Wagner, B; Ricono, JM; Gorin, Y; Block, K; Arar, M; Riley, D; Choudhury, GG; & Abboud, HE. Mitogenic signaling via platelet-derived growth factor beta in metanephric mesenchymal cells. *J Am Soc Nephrol*. 18, (2007), 2903-2911.

Wang, X; Hawk, N; Yue, P; Kauh, J; Ramalingam, SS; Fu, H; Khuri, FR; & Sun, SY. Overcoming mTOR inhibition-induced paradoxical activation of survival signaling pathways enhances mTOR inhibitors' anticancer efficacy. *Cancer Biol Ther*. 7, (2008), 1952-1958.

Wang, X; Yue, P; Chan, CB; Ye, K; Ueda, T; Watanabe-Fukunaga, R; Fukunaga, R; Fu, H, Khuri; FR, & Sun, SY. Inhibition of mammalian target of rapamycin induces phosphatidylinositol 3-kinase-dependent and Mnk-mediated eukaryotic translation initiation factor 4E phosphorylation. *Mol Cell Biol*. 27, (2007), 7405-7413.

Warburg, O; Posener, K; & Negelein, E. Úber den Stoffwechsel der Tumoren. *Biochem. Z.* 152,319-344, (1924).

Washecka, R; & Hanna, M. Malignant renal tumors in tuberous sclerosis. *Urology.* 37, (1991), 340-343.

Wickramasinghe, RH. Biological aspects of cytochrome P450 and associated hydroxylation reactions. *Enzyme.* 19, (1975), 348-376.

Wise, DR; DeBerardinis, RJ; Mancuso, A; Sayed, N; Zhang, XY; Pfeiffer, HK; Nissim, I; Daikhin, E; Yudkoff, M; McMahon, SB, & Thompson, CB. Myc regulates a transcriptional program that stimulates mitochondrial glutaminolysis and leads to glutamine addiction. *Proc Natl Acad Sci U S A.* 105, (2008), 18782-18787.

Yang, HS; Jansen, AP; Komar, AA; Zheng, X; Merrick, WC; Costes, S; Lockett, SJ; Sonenberg, N; & Colburn, NH. The transformation suppressor Pdcd4 is a novel eukaryotic translation initiation factor 4A binding protein that inhibits translation. *Mol Cell Biol.* 23, (2003), 26-37.

Permissions

The contributors of this book come from diverse backgrounds, making this book a truly international effort. This book will bring forth new frontiers with its revolutionizing research information and detailed analysis of the nascent developments around the world.

We would like to thank Robert J. Amato, D.O., for lending his expertise to make the book truly unique. He has played a crucial role in the development of this book. Without his invaluable contribution this book wouldn't have been possible. He has made vital efforts to compile up to date information on the varied aspects of this subject to make this book a valuable addition to the collection of many professionals and students.

This book was conceptualized with the vision of imparting up-to-date information and advanced data in this field. To ensure the same, a matchless editorial board was set up. Every individual on the board went through rigorous rounds of assessment to prove their worth. After which they invested a large part of their time researching and compiling the most relevant data for our readers. Conferences and sessions were held from time to time between the editorial board and the contributing authors to present the data in the most comprehensible form. The editorial team has worked tirelessly to provide valuable and valid information to help people across the globe.

Every chapter published in this book has been scrutinized by our experts. Their significance has been extensively debated. The topics covered herein carry significant findings which will fuel the growth of the discipline. They may even be implemented as practical applications or may be referred to as a beginning point for another development. Chapters in this book were first published by InTech; hereby published with permission under the Creative Commons Attribution License or equivalent.

The editorial board has been involved in producing this book since its inception. They have spent rigorous hours researching and exploring the diverse topics which have resulted in the successful publishing of this book. They have passed on their knowledge of decades through this book. To expedite this challenging task, the publisher supported the team at every step. A small team of assistant editors was also appointed to further simplify the editing procedure and attain best results for the readers.

Our editorial team has been hand-picked from every corner of the world. Their multi-ethnicity adds dynamic inputs to the discussions which result in innovative outcomes. These outcomes are then further discussed with the researchers and contributors who give their valuable feedback and opinion regarding the same. The feedback is then collaborated with the researches and they are edited in a comprehensive manner to aid the understanding of the subject.

Apart from the editorial board, the designing team has also invested a significant amount of their time in understanding the subject and creating the most relevant covers. They scrutinized every image to scout for the most suitable representation of the subject and create an appropriate cover for the book.

The publishing team has been involved in this book since its early stages. They were actively engaged in every process, be it collecting the data, connecting with the contributors or procuring relevant information. The team has been an ardent support to the editorial, designing and production team. Their endless efforts to recruit the best for this project, has resulted in the accomplishment of this book. They are a veteran in the field of academics and their pool of knowledge is as vast as their experience in printing. Their expertise and guidance has proved useful at every step. Their uncompromising quality standards have made this book an exceptional effort. Their encouragement from time to time has been an inspiration for everyone.

The publisher and the editorial board hope that this book will prove to be a valuable piece of knowledge for researchers, students, practitioners and scholars across the globe.

List of Contributors

Israel Gomy and Wilson Araújo Silva Jr.
University of São Paulo, Medical School of Ribeirão Preto, Genetics Department, Ribeirão Preto, Brazil

Cristina Battaglia
Dept. of Biomedical Sciences and Technologies, University of Milano, Milano, Italy
Doctoral School of Molecular Medicine, University of Milano, Milano, Italy

Valentina Tinaglia
Dept. of Biomedical Sciences and Technologies, University of Milano, Milano, Italy
Doctoral School of Molecular Medicine, University of Milano, Milano, Italy

Eleonora Mangano, Ingrid Cifola and Fabio Frascati
Institute for Biomedical Technologies, National Research Council, Segrate, Italy

Silvio Bicciato and Simona Nuzzo
Center for Genome Research, University of Modena and Reggio Emilia, Modena, Italy

Cristina Bianchi and Roberto A. Perego
Dept. of Experimental Medicine, University of Milano-Bicocca, Milano, Italy

Michele Guida and Giuseppe Colucci
Department of Medical Oncology National Cancer Institute Viale Orazio Flacco Bari, Italy

Evgeny Yakirevich, Andres Matoso, David J. Morris and Murray B. Resnick
Department of Pathology and Laboratory Medicine, Rhode Island Hospital and Alpert Medical School of Brown University, USA

Christudas Morais, David W. Johnson and Glenda C. Gobe
Centre for Kidney Disease Research, School of Medicine, The University of Queensland, Australia

David W. Johnson
Department of Renal Medicine, The University of Queensland at Princess Alexandra Hospital, Brisbane, Australia

Tomoaki Tanaka and Tatsuya Nakatani
Osaka City University Graduate School of Medicine, Department of Urology, Japan

Vanessa Medina Villaamil and Guadalupe Aparicio Gallego
INIBIC, A Coruña University Hospital, A Coruña, Spain

Luis Miguel Antón Aparicio
Medical Oncology Service, A Coruña University Hospital, A Coruña, Spain
Medicine Department, University of A Coruña, A Coruña, Spain

Heiko Schuster, Mathias Walzer and Stefan Stevanović
Department of Immunology, Institute for Cell Biology, University of Tübingen, Germany

Mathias Walzer
Applied Bioinformatics Group, Center for Bioinformatics, University of Tübingen, Germany

Karen Block
The Veterans Health Care System, ALMD and The University of Texas Health Science Center at San Antonio, USA

Printed in the USA
CPSIA information can be obtained
at www.ICGtesting.com
JSHW011423221024
72173JS00004B/657

9 781632 423566